The
Bethesda Review
of Clinical Oncology

The Bethesda Review of Clinical Oncology

EDITORS

JAME ABRAHAM, MD, FACP

Director, Breast Oncology Program Taussig Cancer Institute,
Professor of Medicine, Lerner College of Medicine,
Cleveland Clinic, Cleveland, Ohio

JAMES L. GULLEY, MD, PHD, FACP

Director, Medical Oncology Service
Center for Cancer Research
National Cancer Institute
National Institutes of Health
Bethesda, Maryland
Formerly of Emory University School of Medicine
And Loma Linda University School of Medicine

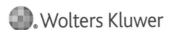 Wolters Kluwer

Philadelphia • Baltimore • New York • London
Buenos Aires • Hong Kong • Sydney • Tokyo

Senior Acquisitions Editor: Ryan Shaw
Editorial Coordinator: John Larkin
Marketing Manager: Rachel Mante Leung
Production Project Manager: Kim Cox
Design Coordinator: Joan Wendt
Manufacturing Coordinator: Beth Welsh
Prepress Vendor: Newgen Knowledge Works Pvt. Ltd., Chennai, India

First Edition
Copyright © 2019 Wolters Kluwer.

Printed in China

Library of Congress Cataloging-in-Publication Data
Names: Abraham, Jame, editor. | Gulley, James L. (James Leonard), 1964– editor.
Title: The Bethesda review of clinical oncology / editors, Jame Abraham, James L. Gulley.
Other titles: Review of clinical oncology
Description: Philadelphia : Wolters Kluwer, [2019]
Identifiers: LCCN 2017057996 | ISBN 9781496354884 (Hardback)
Subjects: | MESH: Neoplasms–therapy | Examination Questions
Classification: LCC RC266.5 | NLM QZ 18.2 | DDC 616.99/40076–dc23
LC record available at https://lccn.loc.gov/2017057996

LWW.com

We dedicate this book to those lives that are touched by cancer and to their caregivers who spend endless hours taking care of them.

"May I never forget that the patient is a fellow creature in pain. May I never consider him merely a vessel of disease."
—Maimonides *(Twelfth-century philosopher and physician)*

Contributors

Jame Abraham, MD, FACP Director, Breast Oncology Program, Taussig Cancer Institute, Professor of Medicine, Lerner College of Medicine, Cleveland Clinic, Cleveland, Ohio

David J. Adelstein, MD Professor, Department of Medicine, Cleveland Clinic, Lerner College of Medicine of Case Western Reserve University, Cleveland, Ohio; Staff, Department of Hematology and Medical Oncology, Cleveland Clinic, Taussig Cancer Institute, Cleveland, Ohio

Piyush K. Agarwal, MD Head, Bladder Cancer Section, Urologic Oncology Branch, Center for Cancer Research, National Cancer Institute, National Institutes of Health, Bethesda, Maryland; Tenure-Track Investigator, Urologic Oncology Branch, Center for Cancer Research, National Cancer Institute, National Institutes of Health, Bethesda, Maryland

Sanjiv S. Agarwala, MD Professor, Temple University School of Medicine, Philadelphia, Pennsylvania; Chief of Medical Oncology and Hematology; Director, Melanoma and Immunology Program, St. Luke's Cancer Center, Easton, Pennsylvania

Christina M. Annunziata, MD, PhD Investigator, Women's Malignancies Branch, National Cancer Institute, Bethesda, Maryland

Andrea B. Apolo, MD Chief, Bladder Cancer Section, Investigator and Lasker Scholar, Center for Cancer Research, Genitourinary Malignancies Branch, National Cancer Institute, National Institutes of Health, Bethesda, Maryland

Ananth K. Arjunan, MD Fellow, Division of Hematology and Oncology, University of Pittsburgh, Pittsburgh, Pennsylvania

Philip M. Arlen, MD Attending Physician, National Cancer Institute, National Institutes of Health, Bethesda, Maryland

Ann Berger MSN MD Chief of Pain and Palliative Care, National Institutes of Health, Clinical Center, Bethesda, Maryland

Christina Brzezniak, DO Chief of Thoracic Oncology, John P. Murtha Cancer Center, Walter Reed National Military Medical Center, Bethesda, Maryland

Brian Burkey, MD Professor, Otolaryngology—Head and Neck Surgery, Vice-Chairman, Head and Neck Institute, Cleveland Clinic and Foundation, Cleveland, Ohio

George Carter, MMS PA-C National Institutes of Health, NCL, Medical Oncology Branch, Bethesda, Maryland

Julia Cheringal, MD Medical Oncology Fellow, John P. Murtha Cancer Center, Walter Reed National Military Medical Center, Bethesda, Maryland

Michael Craig, MD Professor, Department of Medicine, Section Chief, West Virginia University Cancer Institute, Morgantown, West Virginia

William L. Dahut, MD Senior Investigator, Genitourinary Malignancies Branch, National Institutes of Health, Bethesda, Maryland

Erin F. Damery, PharmD, BCOP Clinical Oncology Pharmacist, Pharmacy Department, University of Kansas Health System, Kansas City, Kansas

Robert Dean, MD Department of Hematology/Oncology, Taussig Cancer Institute, Cleveland Clinic, Cleveland, Ohio

Jaydira Del Rivero, MD Staff Clinician, Medical Oncology Service, Center for Cancer Research, National Cancer Institutes, National Institutes of Health, North Bethesda, Maryland

Marnie Grant Dobbin, MS, RDN, CNSC Clinical Research Dietitian, Nutrition Department, National Institutes of Health, Bethesda, Maryland

Daniel E. Elswick, MD, FAPM Clinical Associate Professor, Behavioral Medicine and Psychiatry, West Virginia University School of Medicine, Morgantown, West Virginia

Bassam Estfan, MD Assistant Professor of Medicine, Taussig Cancer Institute, Cleveland Clinic, Lerner College of Medicine, Case Western Reserve University, Cleveland, Ohio; Staff, Hematology/Oncology, Cleveland Clinic, Cleveland, Ohio

Sheryl B. Fleisch, MD Assistant Professor, Psychiatry and Behavioral Sciences, Vanderbilt University Medical Center, Nashville, Tennessee

Juan C. Gea-Banacloche, MD Senior Clinician, Experimental Transplantation and Immunology Branch, National Cancer Institute, National Institutes of Health, Bethesda, Maryland; Chief, Infectious Diseases Consultation Service, NIAID/NCI, NIH Clinical Center, Bethesda, Maryland

Thomas J. George, Jr., MD, FACP Associate Professor, Department of Medicine, University of Florida, Gainesville, Florida; Director, GI Oncology Program, Department of Medicine, University of Florida Health Cancer Center, Gainesville, Florida

Aaron T. Gerds, MD, MS Assistant Professor of Medicine, Hematology and Medical Oncology, Cleveland Clinic, Cleveland, Ohio; Staff, Leukemia Program, Cleveland Clinic, Cleveland, Ohio

Azam Ghafoor, MD Oncology Fellow, Medical Oncology Branch, National Cancer Institute, Bethesda, Maryland

Mark R. Gilbert, MD Senior Investigator and Chief, Neuro-Oncology Branch, National Institutes of Health/National Institute of Neurologic Disorders and Stroke, National Institutes of Health, Bethesda, Maryland

Ann W. Gramza, MD Medical Oncologist, Division of Hematology and Oncology, Lombardi Comprehensive Cancer Center, Georgetown University, Washington, DC

Megan Greally MB, BCh, BAO Advanced Oncology Fellow, Gastrointestinal Oncology, Memorial Sloan Kettering Cancer Center, New York

F. Anthony Greco, MD Director Sarah Cannon Cancer Center, Centennial Medical Center Sarah Cannon Cancer Center, Nashville, Tennessee

James L. Gulley, MD, PhD, FACP Director, Medical Oncology Service, Center for Cancer Research, National Cancer Institute, National Institutes of Health, Bethesda, Maryland; Formerly of Emory University School of Medicine, and Loma Linda University School of Medicine

Mehdi Hamadani, MD Associate Professor of Medicine, Hematology/Oncology, CIBMTR & Medical College of Wisconsin, Milwaukee, Wisconsin; Director, Blood and Marrow Transplant Program, Hematology/Oncology, Froedtert Hosptial, Milwaukee, Wisconsin

Hannah W. Hazard-Jenkins, MD, FACS Associate Professor, Department of Surgery, Director of Clinical Services, WVU Cancer Institute, West Virginia University Hospital, Morgantown, West Virginia

Brandie Heald, MS, LGC Licensed Genetic Counselor, Genomic Medicine Institute, Cleveland Clinic, Cleveland, Ohio

Upendra P. Hegde, MD Associate Professor, Department of Medicine, University of Connecticut, Farmington, Connecticut; Associate Director, Melanoma and Cutaneous Oncology Program, Neag Comprehensive Cancer Center, John Dempsey Hospital, Farmington, Connecticut

Thomas E. Hughes, PharmD, BCOP Clinical Pharmacy Specialist, Pharmacy Department, National Institutes of Health, Clinical Research Center, Bethesda, Maryland

Nikhil P. Joshi, MD Assistant Professor of Medicine, Cleveland Clinic, Lerner College of Medicine, Cleveland, Ohio; Staff Physician, College of Medicine, California; Staff Physician, Department of Radiation Oncology, Cleveland Clinic Foundation, California

Matt Kalaycio, MD Department of Hematology/Oncology, Taussig Cancer Institute, Cleveland Clinic, Cleveland, Ohio

Abraham S. Kanate, MD Assistant Professor of Internal Medicine, Osborn Hematopoietic Malignancy and Transplantation Program, West Virginia University, Morgantown, West Virginia

Alok A. Khorana, MD, FACP Professor of Medicine, Taussig Cancer Institute, Cleveland Clinic Lerner College of Medicine, Case Western Reserve University, Cleveland, Ohio; Staff, Hematology/Oncology, Cleveland Clinic, Cleveland, Ohio

David R. Kohler, PharmD Oncology Clinical Pharmacy Specialist, Pharmacy Department, National Institutes of Health Clinical Center, Bethesda, Maryland

Elise C. Kohn, MD, CAPT (ret), USPHS Head, Gynecologic Cancer Therapeutics, Clinical Investigations Branch, Cancer Therapy Evaluation Program, National Cancer Institute, Bethesda, Maryland

Megan Kruse, MD Department of Hematology-Oncology, Cleveland Clinic, Cleveland, Ohio

Chaoyuan Kuang, MD, PhD Fellow, Division of Hematology and Oncology, University of Pittsburgh, Pittsburgh, Pennsylvania; Fellow, Division of Hematology and Oncology, University of Pittsburgh Medical Center, Pittsburgh, Pennsylvania

Shaji K. Kumar, MD. Professor of Medicine, Consultant, Division of Hematology, Chair, Dysproteinemia Group; Medical Director, Cancer Clinical Research Office, Rochester, Minnesota

Charles A. Kunos, MD, PhD Medical Officer and Coordinator, Investigational Therapeutics & Radiation, Investigational Drug Branch, Cancer Therapy Evaluation Program, Division of Cancer Treatment and Diagnosis, National Cancer Institute, National Institutes of Health, Rockville, Maryland

Arjun Lakshman, MD, MRCP Post-doctoral Research Fellow, Division of Hematology, Mayo Clinic, Rochester, Minnesota; Post-doctoral Research Fellow, Division of Hematology, Mayo Clinic, Rochester, Minnesota

Paulette Lebda, MD Department of Radiology, Cleveland Clinic, Cleveland, Ohio

James J. Lee, MD, PhD Associate Professor of Medicine, Division of Hematology-Oncology, Department of Medicine, University of Pittsburgh School of Medicine, Pittsburgh, Pennsylvania

Jung-min Lee, MD Investigator and Lasker Clinical Research Scholar, Women's Malignancies Branch, Center for Cancer Research, National Cancer Institute, Bethesda, Maryland

Gregory D. Leonard University Hospital Galway, Galway, Ireland

Ravi A. Madan, MD Clinical Director of the Genitourinary Malignancies Branch at the National Cancer Institute, National Institutes of Health, Bethesda, Maryland

Bindu Manyam, MD Department of Radiation Oncology, Cleveland Clinic, Cleveland, Ohio

Christopher Melani, MD Staff Clinician, Lymphoid Malignancies Branch, National Cancer Institute, National Institutes of Health, Bethesda, Maryland; Staff Clinician, Lymphoid Malignancies Branch, National Cancer Institute, National Institutes of Health, Bethesda, Maryland

Lekha Mikkilineni, MD, MA Fellow in Hematology/Oncology, National Cancer Institute, National Institutes of Health, Bethesda, Maryland; Clinical Fellow, National Cancer Institute, Clinical Center - NIH, Bethesda, Maryland

Emanuela Molinari Neurology Department, Neuroscience Division, The Queen Elizabeth University Hospital, Glasgow, United Kingdom; Consultant Neurologist, Neurology, The Queen Elizabeth University Hospital, Glasgow, United Kingom

Andreas Niethammer, MD, PhD Associate Professor of Experimental Oncology, Department of Radiation Oncology, Ruprecht-Karls-Universitaet Heidelberg, Heidelberg, Germany

Michelle A. Ojemuyiwa, MD Assistant Professor, Department of Medicine, Hematology Oncology Uniformed Services, University of Health Sciences Walter Reed National Military Medical Center, Bethesda, Maryland

Maryland Pao, MD Clinical Professor, Department of Psychiatry, Georgetown University School of Medicine, Washington, DC; Clinical & Deputy Scientific Director, National Institute of Mental Health, National Institutes of Health, Bethesda, Maryland

Hiral Parekh, MD, MPH Assistant Professor, Department of Medicine, University of Florida, Gainesville, Florida; Oncologist, Department of Medicine, University of Florida Health Cancer Center, Gainesville, Florida

Holly Jane Pederson, MD Associate Professor, Medicine, Cleveland Clinic, Lerner College of Medicine, Cleveland, Ohio; Director, Medical Breast Services, Breast Services, Department of General Surgery, Cleveland Clinic, Cleveland, Ohio

Jean-Paul Pinzon, DO Medical Director, Palliative Care, Inova Schar Cancer Institute, Fairfax, Virginia

Muzaffar H. Qazilbash, MD Professor of Medicine, Stem Cell Transplantation and Cellular Therapy, University of Texas, MD Anderson Cancer Center, Houston, Texas

Jason M. Redman, MD Medical Oncology Fellow, Medical Oncology Service, National Cancer Institute, National Institutes of Health, Bethesda, Maryland

Kevin R. Rice, MD Associate Professor of Surgery, Urology Service Uniformed Services, University of Health Sciences, Walter Reed National Military Medical Center, Bethesda, Maryland

Mark Roschewski, MD Staff Clinician, Lymphoid Malignancies Branch, National Cancer Institute, National Institutes of Health, Bethesda, Maryland; Staff Clinician, Lymphoid Malignancies Branch, National Cancer Institute, National Institutes of Health, Bethesda, Maryland

Donald L. Rosenstein, MD Professor and Vice Chair for Hospital Psychiatry, Psychiatry and Medicine, University of North Carolina at Chapel Hill, Chapel Hill, North Carolina; Director, Comprehensive Cancer Support Program, North Carolina Cancer Hospital, Chapel Hill, North Carolina

Inger L. Rosner, MD Associate Professor, Department of Surgery, Uniformed Services University, Bethesda, Maryland; Director, Urologic Oncology, Department of Surgery, Walter Reed National Military Medical Center, Bethesda, Maryland

Kerry Ryan, MPH, MS PA-C National Institutes of Health, NHLBI, Pulmonary Branch, Bethesda, Maryland

Meena Sadaps, MD Medical Resident, Department of Internal Medicine, Cleveland Clinic Foundation, Cleveland, Ohio

Yogen Saunthararajah, MD Professor of Medicine, Hematology and Oncology, Case Western Reserve University, Cleveland, Ohio; Staff, Hematology and Oncology, Cleveland Clinic, Cleveland, Ohio

Mikkael A. Sekeres, MD, MS Professor of Medicine, Director, Leukemia Program, Cleveland Clinic, Cleveland, Ohio; Director, Leukemia Program, Cleveland Clinic, Cleveland, Ohio

Chirag Shah, MD Associate Professor, Department of Radiation Oncology, Cleveland Clinic Lerner College of Medicine, Cleveland, Ohio; Staff Physician, Director of Clinical Research, Department of Radiation Oncology, Cleveland Clinic, Cleveland, Ohio

Dale R. Shepard, MD, PhD Director, Taussig Cancer Institute Phase I and Sarcoma Programs; Staff, Hematology and Medical Oncology and Center for Geriatric Medicine, Cleveland Clinic, Cleveland, Ohio; Assistant Professor of Medicine, Internal Medicine, Cleveland Clinic, Lerner College of Medicine, Cleveland, Ohio; Director, Taussig Institute Phase I and Sarcoma Programs, Hematology and Medical Oncology, Cleveland Clinic, Cleveland, Ohio

Davendra P. S. Sohal, MD, MPH Assistant Professor of Medicine, Taussig Cancer Institute, Cleveland Clinic, Lerner College of Medicine, Case Western Reserve University, Cleveland, Ohio; Staff, Hematology/Oncology, Cleveland Clinic, Cleveland, Ohio

Ramaprasad Srinivasan, MD, PhD Investigator and Head, Molecular Cancer Section, Urologic Oncology Branch, Center for Cancer Research, National Cancer Institute, Bethesda, Maryland

Samer A. Srour, MB ChB, MS Assistant Professor of Medicine, Department of Medicine, Dan L. Duncan Comprehensive Cancer Center, Hematology and Oncology Section, Baylor College of Medicine, Houston, Texas

Jason S. Starr, DO Assistant Professor, Department of Medicine, University of Florida, Gainesville, Florida; Oncologist, Department of Medicine, University of Florida Health Cancer Center, Gainesville, Florida

James P. Stevenson, MD Vice-Chairman, Department of Hematology and Medical Oncology, Cleveland Clinic, Taussig Cancer Institute, Cleveland, Ohio

Julius Strauss, MD Staff Clinician, Laboratory of Tumor Immunology and Biology, Center for Cancer Research, National Cancer Institute, National Institutes of Health, Bethesda, Maryland

Christina Tafe, MSN, ACNP-BC, ACHPN Nurse Practitioner, Advanced Disease Management, Heartland Care Partners, Fairfax, Virginia

Sarah M. Temkin, MD Professor, Massey Cancer Center, Virginia Commonwealth University, Richmond, Virginia; Division Director, Gynecologic Oncology, Virginia Commonwealth University, Richmond, Virginia

Anish Thomas, MBBS, MD Investigator, Developmental Therapeutics Branch, National Cancer Institute, Bethesda, Maryland

Neel Trivedi, MD Hematology/Oncology Fellow, Division of Hematology/Oncology, Lombardi Comprehensive Cancer Center, Washington, DC

Chaitra Ujjani, MD Associate Professor, Division of Hematology/Oncology, Lombardi Comprehensive Cancer Center, Washington, DC

Stephanie Valente, DO Department of Surgery, Cleveland Clinic, Cleveland, Ohio

Leticia Varella, MD Assistant Professor, Department of Medicine, Division of Hematology & Oncology, Weill Cornell Medicine, Cornell University, New York, New York

Andrew Vassil, MD Department of Radiation Oncology, Cleveland Clinic, Cleveland, Ohio

Christopher E. Wee, MD Chief Medical Resident, Department of Internal Medicine, Cleveland Clinic Foundation, Cleveland, Ohio

Kristen P. Zeligs, MD Gynecologic Oncologist, Department of Obstetrics and Gynecology, Walter Reed National Military Medical Center, Bethesda, Maryland

Peter A. Zmijewski, MD Chief Resident, West Virginia University General Surgery Residency, West Virginia University School of Medicine, Morgantown, West Virginia

Preface

The Bethesda Handbook of Clinical Oncology is a clear, concise, and comprehensive reference book for the busy clinician to use in his or her daily patient encounters. The book has been compiled by clinicians who are working at the National Cancer Institute, National Institutes of Health, Cleveland Clinic, M.D. Anderson, Mayo Clinic as well as scholars from other academic institutions. To limit the size of the book, less space is dedicated to etiology, pathophysiology, and epidemiology and greater emphasis is placed on practical clinical information. For easy accessibility to the pertinent information, long descriptions are avoided, and more tables, pictures, algorithms, and phrases are included.

The Bethesda Handbook of Clinical Oncology is not intended as a substitute for the many excellent oncology reference textbooks available that are essential for a more complete understanding of the pathophysiology and management of complicated oncology patients. We hope that the reader-friendly format with its comprehensive review of the management of each disease with treatment regimens, including dosing and schedule, makes this book unique and useful for oncologists, oncology fellows, residents, students, oncology nurses, and allied health professionals.

The landscape of oncology has changed substantially since we published the first edition of this book more than 16 years ago. For the fifth edition, we have updated all chapters and added two new chapters, "Clinical Genetics" and "Diagnosis-Driven Individualization of Cancer Care." Since we are publishing a companion Board Review Book *The Bethesda Review of Clinical Oncology*, in this edition we have eliminated the questions at the end of each chapters.

As always, we have attempted to capture the advances in the field and listened to the feedback from readers to improve this edition. We hope that anyone needing a comprehensive review of oncology will find *The Bethesda Handbook of Clinical Oncology* to be an indispensable resource.

Jame Abraham and James L. Gulley

Acknowledgments

Our sincere thanks to all our esteemed colleagues and friends who contributed to this book.

We thank our publisher, Wolters Kluwer, and dedicated staff members at the company who have been supporting this book for more than 13 years. We would like to thank Ms. Grace Caputo for carefully editing many chapters and offering suggestions.

We thank our wives, Shyla, and Trenise, for their encouragement and support in this endeavor.

Above all, we thank you for your support and feedback.

Contents

Contributors v
Preface xi
Acknowledgments xiii

Chapter 1   **Head and Neck** 1
Nikhil P. Joshi, David J. Adelstein, and Brian Burkey

Chapter 2   **Non–Small Cell Lung Cancer** 9
Christina Brzezniak, Julia Cheringal, and Anish Thomas

Chapter 3   **Small Cell Lung Cancer** 29
Christopher E. Wee and James P. Stevenson

Chapter 4   **Esophageal Cancer** 35
Megan Greally and Gregory D. Leonard

Chapter 5   **Gastric Cancers** 41
Hiral Parekh and Thomas J. George, Jr.

Chapter 6   **Biliary Tract Cancer** 51
Davendra P. S. Sohal and Alok A. Khorana

Chapter 7   **Primary Cancers of the Liver** 55
Bassam Estfan and Alok A. Khorana

Chapter 8   **Gastrointestinal Stromal Tumors (GIST)** 61
Dale R. Shepard and Alok A. Khorana

Chapter 9   **Colorectal Cancer** 65
Jason S. Starr and Thomas J. George, Jr.

Chapter 10   **Pancreatic Cancer** 85
Ananth K. Arjunan and James J. Lee

Chapter 11   **Anal Cancer** 89
Chaoyuan Kuang and James J. Lee

Chapter 12   **Breast Cancer** 93
Megan Kruse, Leticia Varella, Stephanie Valente, Paulette Lebda,
Andrew Vassil, and Jame Abraham

Chapter 13   **Renal Cell Cancer** 129
Ramaprasad Srinivasan, Azam Ghafoor, and Inger L. Rosner

Chapter 14   **Prostate Cancer** 139
Ravi A. Madan and William L. Dahut

Chapter 15   **Bladder Cancer** 153
Andrea B. Apolo, Piyush K. Agarwal, and William L. Dahut

Chapter 16   **Testicular Carcinoma** 161
Kevin R. Rice, Michelle A. Ojemuyiwa, and Ravi A. Madan

Chapter 17   **Ovarian Cancer** 167
Jung-min Lee and Elise C. Kohn

Chapter 18   **Endometrial Cancer** 181
Kristen P. Zeligs and Christina M. Annunziata

Chapter 19   **Cervical Cancer** 187
Sarah M. Temkin and Charles A. Kunos

Chapter 20   **Vulvar Cancer** 193
Kristen P. Zeligs and Christina M. Annunziata

Chapter 21   **Sarcomas and Malignancies of the Bone** 197
Dale R. Shepard

Chapter 22   **Skin Cancers and Melanoma** 205
Upendra P. Hegde and Sanjiv S. Agarwala

Chapter 23   **Acute Leukemia** 221
Aaron T. Gerds and Mikkael A. Sekeres

Chapter 24   **Chronic Lymphoid Leukemias** 233
Neel Trivedi and Chaitra Ujjani

Chapter 25   **Chronic Myeloid Leukemias** 237
Samer A. Srour and Muzaffar H. Qazilbash

Chapter 26   **Chronic Myeloproliferative Neoplasms** 241
Yogen Saunthararajah

Chapter 27   **Multiple Myeloma** 247
Arjun Lakshman and Shaji K. Kumar

Chapter 28   **Non-Hodgkin's Lymphoma** 251
Christopher Melani and Mark Roschewski

Chapter 29   **Hodgkin Lymphoma** 267
Robert Dean and Matt Kalaycio

Chapter 30   **Hematopoietic Cell Transplantation** 271
Abraham S. Kanate, Michael Craig, and Mehdi Hamadani

Chapter 31   **Carcinoma of Unknown Primary** 279
F. Anthony Greco

Chapter 32   **Central Nervous System Tumors** 285
Emanuela Molinari and Mark R. Gilbert

Chapter 33   **Endocrine Tumors** 297
Jaydira Del Rivero and Ann W. Gramza

Chapter 34   **Hematopoietic Growth Factors** 307
Philip M. Arlen and Andreas Niethammer

Chapter 35   **Infectious Complications in Oncology** 313
Lekha Mikkilineni and Juan C. Gea-Banacloche

Chapter 36   **Oncologic Emergencies and Paraneoplastic Syndromes** 323
Meena Sadaps and James P. Stevenson

Chapter 37   **Psychopharmacologic Management in Oncology**   329
Donald L. Rosenstein, Maryland Pao, Sheryl B. Fleisch, and Daniel E. Elswick

Chapter 38   **Management of Emesis**   333
David R. Kohler

Chapter 39   **Nutrition**   355
Marnie Grant Dobbin

Chapter 40   **Pain and Palliative Care**   361
Christina Tafe, Jean-Paul Pinzon, and Ann Berger

Chapter 41   **Central Venous Access Device**   391
Peter A. Zmijewski and Hannah W. Hazard-Jenkins

Chapter 42   **Procedures in Medical Oncology**   395
Kerry Ryan and George Carter

Chapter 43   **Basic Principles of Radiation Oncology**   399
Chirag Shah, Nikhil P. Joshi, and Bindu Manyam

Chapter 44   **Clinical Genetics**   405
Holly Jane Pederson and Brandie Heald

Chapter 45   **Basic Principles of Immuno-Oncology**   413
Jason M. Redman, Julius Strauss, and Ravi A. Madan

Chapter 46   **Anticancer Agents**   423
Erin F. Damery and Thomas E. Hughes

Head and Neck 1

Nikhil P. Joshi, David J. Adelstein, and Brian Burkey

REVIEW QUESTIONS

1. A 57-year-old man presents with a neck mass and sore throat. He has a 15-year history of smoking 1 pack per day, but has not smoked since the last 10 years, and drinks one to two glasses of wine per week. He has been married for 15 years. He works as a financial consultant. Examination shows two 2 cm level II nodes in the left neck, and fiberoptic examination shows a mass in the left tonsil well away from midline and not involving the soft palate or tongue base. Biopsy shows squamous carcinoma and staining for p16 is positive. PET/CT shows a 2.2 cm mass in the left tonsil, as well as two 2 cm nodes in the left neck at level II. He is staged as $T_2 N_{2b} M_0$ stage IVA.

    Recommendations for treatment could include the following:

    A. Induction chemotherapy with docetaxel, cisplatin, and 5-FU

    B. Definitive concurrent cisplatin and radiation to both necks

    C. Treatment on a clinical trial for HPV+ head and neck cancer

    D. Definitive chemoradiation to left tonsil and left neck

    E. Stereotactic body radiotherapy

2. A 31-year-old man presents with a sore tongue. Examination shows a 4.0 cm raised tender mass in the left floor of mouth. He is a nonsmoker but has chewed tobacco for 10 years. He is married. Biopsy of the tongue lesion showed squamous cell carcinoma. PET/CT shows a 4 cm floor of

mouth tumor with a 1 cm submental node with no metastatic disease elsewhere.

   Which of the following is TRUE?

   A. Definitive chemoradiation is the standard of care.

   B. Surgery followed by adjuvant radiation/chemoradiation per pathology is indicated.

   C. Adjuvant chemotherapy has a proven role in this case.

   D. Surgery alone will be enough in this case.

   E. None of the above.

3. A 58-year-old man who emigrated from southern China 10 years ago is evaluated for a 3-month history of an enlarging neck mass. Neck examination reveals two firm lymph nodes: a 4 cm left level III node and a 2 cm left supraclavicular lymph node. Fiberoptic endoscopy reveals a mass in the left nasopharynx. Biopsy revealed WHO type III nasopharyngeal carcinoma. Contrast-enhanced CT shows a 4.5 cm left level III lymph node, a 2.4 cm left supraclavicular node, as well as a mass localized to the nasopharynx with parapharyngeal extension. These were the only regions to show FDG uptake on PET/CT.

   Which of the following is TRUE?

   A. Surgical resection of the primary tumor with left neck dissection followed as needed by chemoradiation is the treatment of choice.

   B. This represents one of a minority of head and neck cancers in which a strong association with EBV has not been established.

   C. The recommended treatment is concurrent cisplatin chemotherapy and radiation followed by adjuvant cisplatin and 5-FU chemotherapy.

   D. This is a uniformly fatal disease.

   E. Induction chemotherapy with paclitaxel and carboplatin is indicated.

4. A 62-year-old woman presented with a 2 cm oropharyngeal SCC (base of tongue) with spread to a 6 cm lymph node spanning left levels II and III. She began treatment with concurrent cisplatin and radiation. She developed oral candidiasis in her fourth week of treatment. She also experienced mucositis and throat pain with attendant anorexia and weight

loss that required percutaneous feeding tube placement and narcotic pain medications. She is being seen for her end-of-treatment visit today and her weight has stabilized. She continues to use narcotics regularly for throat pain and mucositis.

Which of the following is TRUE?

A. Prophylactic anticandida treatment should be initiated for all such patients beginning concurrent chemoradiation.

B. Her percutaneous feeding tube should be scheduled for removal within 1 month following treatment completion.

C. Any necessary dental extractions should be carried out before treatment starts.

D. Xerostomia is unlikely to occur in this patient.

E. After definitive chemoradiation, salvage neck dissection for this patient is ill advised.

5. A 68-year-old man with an 80-pack-year smoking history and a history of alcohol intake consisting of 12 beers on most weekends presents with a stage IVA squamous carcinoma of the glottic larynx (T_3 N_{2c} M_0). His weight is 68 kg and height is 66″. His performance status is good, and he has no other medical problems except mild emphysema. He lives with his wife of 42 years and is retired from a machining company where he worked for 35 years. His past history includes military service in Vietnam, with exposure to Agent Orange. Which is the best treatment choice for this patient?

A. Cisplatin with concurrent radiation.

B. Radiation as definitive treatment.

C. Surgery followed by postoperative concurrent cisplatin and radiation if nodal extracapsular extension of disease or positive margins on pathological examination.

D. Cetuximab and concurrent cisplatin-based chemotherapy and radiation.

E. A or C.

6. An otherwise healthy 53-year-old wood worker presents with a large right maxillary sinus mass with involvement of the skin of his cheek. Systemic staging scans are negative for distant disease. He has a 25-pack-year

smoking history with moderate alcohol intake. The best treatment option for treatment is

    A. Definitive radiation therapy

    B. Definitive chemoradiation therapy

    C. Surgery followed adjuvant radiation with chemotherapy as indicated by pathology

    D. Surgery alone

    E. Palliative chemotherapy or radiation based on patient preference

7. A 65-year-old otherwise healthy gentleman presents with a right preauricular mass with deviation of his face and failure to close the right eye. CT scan shows a large right parotid mass. Biopsy is positive for adenoid cystic carcinoma. The best treatment option for treatment is

    A. Total parotidectomy with facial nerve sacrifice followed by adjuvant chemotherapy

    B. Total parotidectomy with facial nerve sacrifice followed by adjuvant radiation

    C. Total parotidectomy with facial nerve preservation followed by adjuvant radiation

    D. Subtotal parotidectomy with facial nerve preservation followed by adjuvant chemotherapy

    E. Total parotidectomy with facial nerve sacrifice followed by adjuvant radiation to the skull base

8. A 60-year-old lady presents with a 4 cm right piriform sinus SCC involving the larynx causing airway obstruction necessitating a tracheostomy. She also needed a feeding tube for nutrition due to near total dysphagia. She has a 35-pack-year smoking history and is a chronic alcohol abuser. Imaging shows the disease penetrating through the right ala of the thyroid cartilage. The best treatment option for her is

    A. Total laryngopharyngectomy followed by adjuvant chemotherapy

    B. High-dose chemotherapy with stem cell rescue

    C. Total laryngopharyngectomy followed by adjuvant radiation and chemotherapy per pathology

D. Total laryngopharyngectomy alone

E. Definitive chemoradiation for laryngeal salvage

9. A 55-year-old gentleman with a 25-pack-year history of smoking presents with hoarseness. An in-office endoscopy shows disease limited to the right true vocal cord with good cord mobility. Biopsy is positive for SCC. He is staged as T1aN0M0 SCC of the glottis. Acceptable treatment options include all except

   A. Definitive radiation to 70 Gy at 2 Gy fractions given daily

   B. Definitive radiation to 63 Gy at 2.25 Gy per day

   C. Laryngeal microsurgery

   D. Definitive chemotherapy with docetaxel, cisplatin, and 5-FU

   E. Both A and D

10. A 52-year-old man with an 8-pack-year history of smoking and no alcohol intake presents with a 2.7 cm left level II node with a 1 cm left tongue base mass. Biopsy from the tongue base mass is positive for SCC and stains positive for p16. He had an MI 3 months ago. Staging is negative for distant metastatic disease. He is staged as T1N1M0, stage III left tongue base SCC, p16+. The best treatment option in this case is

    A. Definitive radiation alone

    B. Definitive chemoradiation

    C. Induction docetaxel, cisplatin, and 5-FU

    D. Definitive radiation and cetuximab

    E. Ipilimumab combined with nivolumab

ANSWERS TO REVIEW QUESTIONS

1. ANSWER: D. This patient likely has HPV-associated oropharynx cancer, which tends to occur at a slightly younger age than smoking- and alcohol-related cancers. He is expected to have a 30% to 50% better prognosis compared to patients with the same site and stage of cancer who have a history of smoking and alcohol abuse. Because of the stage of disease, considerations for cure include definitive chemoradiation. This gentleman is a candidate for left-sided radiation to the tonsil and involved neck. Distance from the midline and noninvolvement of midline structures like tongue base and soft palate makes him eligible for this treatment. Alternatively, surgery followed by adjuvant radiation/chemoradiation is also an option.

2. ANSWER: B. This is a young patient with no smoking history but a positive history of tobacco chewing and an oral cancer. The limited stage of disease and the risk of more primaries in the oral cavity make surgery (in this case, wide local excision or partial glossectomy) the best choice of treatment. Due to the size of the primary tumor and presence of neck node on imaging, he should have neck dissection. This should be followed by adjuvant radiation/chemoradiation as indicated (chemotherapy is added for extracapsular spread or positive margins).

3. ANSWER: C. This is a patient who emigrated from a region where nasopharyngeal carcinoma is endemic. Supraclavicular lymph node-positive nasopharyngeal carcinoma qualifies as locally advanced disease (stage IVB in this case). Nasopharyngeal carcinoma does have a strong association with EBV, unlike other head and neck malignancies, some of which are associated with HPV infection. The recommended treatment for locally advanced nasopharyngeal carcinoma is concurrent cisplatin chemotherapy and radiation with adjuvant chemotherapy with cisplatin and 5-FU. Surgery is rarely indicated for nasopharyngeal carcinoma.

4. ANSWER: C. This is a relatively typical course for a patient receiving concurrent chemoradiation for an oropharyngeal squamous cell carcinoma. Oral candidiasis is not uncommon in this setting and is treated with antifungal medications at the time it is discovered; prophylactic treatment is not generally indicated. Percutaneous feeding tube removal is not scheduled for a specific time frame, but is only done once the patient can demonstrate a sustained ability to take adequate nutrition orally. A thorough dental evaluation and any procedures, particularly extractions, should be done before initiating chemoradiation. Healing ability will be impaired after chemoradiation, and extractions pose a risk for the development of osteoradionecrosis. Cholinergic agonists can be considered for xerostomia that persists for 1 to 2 years after chemoradiation and is troublesome. For large (>6 cm, N_3) adenopathy, a salvage neck dissection might be needed for residual disease.

5. ANSWER: E. In locally advanced carcinoma of the larynx, cisplatin and concurrent radiation results in improved larynx preservation and similar survival compared to surgery followed by radiation and compared with chemotherapy followed by radiation or radiation alone. However, adding cetuximab to the combination of cisplatin and radiation has not been shown to improve outcomes over those achieved with just concurrent cisplatin and radiation. Postoperative cisplatin and radiation do improve local control and PFS in patients with nodal extracapsular extension and positive margins. The choice of treatment will depend on the patient's overall condition, the likelihood that voice can be preserved with nonoperative primary treatment, and the patient's preference. Radiation alone could be considered for a patient that cannot tolerate combined chemoradiation or surgery followed by combined chemoradiation, but this patient has a good performance status and medical condition, as well as family support.

6. ANSWER: C. Locally advanced maxillary sinus cancer is best managed with a total maxillectomy followed by adjuvant radiation with chemotherapy added for positive margins or extracapsular extension of involved lymph nodes. This approach is associated with the best locoregional control. Medically inoperable or unresectable lesions might be treated with Options A or B but are generally associated with a poor outcome—likely reflecting the extent of disease.

7. ANSWER: E. Locally advanced parotid cancer causing facial nerve dysfunction mandates a total parotid resection with sacrifice of the facial nerve. Adenoid cystic carcinoma has a predilection for cranial nerve involvement and spread to the skull base. Adjuvant radiation including the skull base improves local control for these cancers. The role of chemotherapy for salivary gland cancers is controversial and its role in the adjuvant setting is being studied (RTOG 1008).

8. ANSWER: C. Laryngopharyngeal dysfunction at baseline due to locally advanced hypopharynx cancer is best treated with surgery followed by adjuvant radiation and chemotherapy. Such patients should not be considered for laryngeal preservation strategies.

9. ANSWER: E. Early-stage glottic cancer can be treated with either definitive radiation or laryngeal microsurgery with equally good oncologic outcomes. 2.25 Gy is better than 2 Gy fractions for local control and should be considered standard. Chemotherapy has no role in the management of early-stage larynx cancer.

10. ANSWER: A. This gentleman is best treated with definitive radiation alone and is associated with excellent locoregional control and survival. Chemotherapy is not recommended. While transoral surgery and neck dissection might be appropriate, adjuvant radiation will be needed if both necks are not addressed. His MI 3 months ago makes him a less than ideal candidate for this approach. Immunotherapy has no role in the management of early oropharynx cancer.

Non–Small Cell Lung Cancer 2

Christina Brzezniak, Julia Cheringal, and Anish Thomas

REVIEW QUESTIONS

1. A 70-year-old otherwise healthy former smoker presents with persistent cough and hemoptysis of 2 months' duration. Further workup reveals a 3 cm cavitating hilar mass, multiple bilateral parenchymal lung nodules and a 2 cm hypodense lesion in the right hepatic lobe. Biopsies of the lung and liver masses are consistent with squamous cell lung carcinoma. Tumor molecular analysis shows absence of EGFR, KRAS mutations, and ALK fusion. MRI brain shows no evidence of metastatic disease. Which of the following combinations would be the best choice for first-line chemotherapy?

   A. Cisplatin and gemcitabine

   B. Cisplatin and pemetrexed

   C. Carboplatin, paclitaxel, and bevacizumab

   D. Carboplatin, pemetrexed, and bevacizumab

2. Based on available data, which of the following is true regarding screening for lung cancer in a 54-year-old man with 20-pack-year history of smoking who quit smoking 3 years ago?

   A. Annual low dose CT screening is expected to result in a reduction in lung cancer–related mortality

   B. Annual low dose CT screening is expected to result in a reduction in all cause mortality

C. Chest X-ray and sputum cytology is expected to result in a reduction in lung cancer–related mortality

D. Chest X-ray and sputum cytology is expected to result in a reduction in all cause mortality

E. None of the above

---

3. A 70-year-old otherwise healthy woman came to medical attention with long standing cough. CT scan showed a 4 cm left hilar mass and right hilar lymphadenopathy. Patient underwent bronchoscopy, right video-assisted thoracic surgery, wedge biopsy, and cervical mediastinoscopy with biopsy. Pathology showed lung adenocarcinoma with involvement of right hilar lymph nodes. Tissue is inadequate for molecular analyses. Which of the following is the best treatment option?

A. Surgical resection of the primary mass and lymph nodes followed by adjuvant chemoradiation

B. Concurrent chemotherapy and radiation

C. Neoadjuvant chemotherapy followed by surgery

D. Sequential chemotherapy and radiation

---

4. A 50-year-old Korean woman was evaluated by her primary care doctor for a 2 month history of cough. CXR revealed a large mediastinal mass and blunting of the costophrenic angles consistent with a pleural effusion. A follow-up CT scan revealed bulky mediastinal lymph nodes and a 2.4 cm RML mass as well as a right-sided pleural effusion. Thoracentesis revealed abnormal cells that were TTF-1 and napsin positive. Mutational testing revealed a point mutation of EGFR exon 21 L858R. What is the most appropriate first-line therapy for this patient?

A. Check point inhibition with pembrolizumab

B. Definitive concurrent chemotherapy plus radiation therapy

C. Oral erlotinib

D. Single-agent chemotherapy with pemetrexed

---

5. A patient with newly diagnosed EGFR mutated lung adenocarcinoma has been on treatment with erlotinib for 14 months. She has had minimal side effects of rash, which is well managed with topical therapy and minimal

diarrhea managed with imodium as needed. She now has worsening cough and restaging images reveal two new pulmonary masses and reaccumlation of her pleural effusion. What is the next step in management?

A. Switch to platinum-based doublet chemotherapy

B. Single agent pemetrexed

C. Check point inhibitor with nivolumab

D. Rebiopsy and send for molecular testing

6. A 73-year-old male with greater than 100-pack-year smoking history presents to his doctor because he is short of breath when having to walk up the steps in his three story home. His primary care provider enrolled him in a lung cancer screening event hosted at the local hospital and he underwent low dose CT scan imaging. This revealed a 4 × 6 cm mass of the LUL with surrounding bronchiectasis and a small left pleural effusion. Staging imaging revealed a liver lesion that was biopsied and consistent with pulmonary adenocarcinoma. Mutational testing revealed a KRAS mutation and he was started on platinum doublet therapy with carboplatin plus paclitaxel. He completed 4 cycles of chemotherapy which he tolerated well and continued to work full time as a banker. Re-staging imaging revealed progressive disease to his liver with numerous new lesions, he has a PS of 1 and would like to be aggressive. What is the next best step in treatment?

A. Immune check point inhibitor

B. Single agent docetaxel

C. Radiation to the liver

D. Hospice referral and transition to comfort care

7. A 45-year-old female never smoker presents with shortness of breath on exertion, cough, and fatigue of 3 months' duration. Her past medical history is unremarkable. CT scan reveals a peripheral right lung nodule which is biopsy-proven to be adenocarcinoma. Molecular analysis reveals ALK translocation. Staging evaluation shows extensive metastatic involvement of bilateral adrenals, bones, and a 2 cm left parietofrontal lesion with no evidence of edema or mass effect. What is the next best step in treatment?

A. Refer to hospice

B. Whole brain radiation followed by platinum-based chemotherapy

   C. SBRT followed by platinum based chemotherapy

   D. Crizotinib

   E. Ceritinib

8. A 65-year-old male smoker with 10-pack-year history of smoking presents with newly diagnosed metastatic lung adenocarcinoma. What is the best way to proceed with molecular analysis of this patient's tumor?

   A. Sequencing of EGFR, KRAS, BRAF

   B. Sequencing of EGFR, KRAS, BRAF and FISH for ALK, ROS

   C. Sequencing of EGFR, KRAS, BRAF, FISH for ALK, ROS, and IHC for PD-L1

   D. Next generation sequencing

9. You had recently seen a 38-year-old female never smoker with newly diagnosed ALK translocated lung adenocarcinoma. At the time, she was started on crizotinib 250 mg orally twice a day. Two weeks later she is presenting with shimmering, flashing lights in both eyes. These events are short-lived and appear to be more frequent in the evenings. Patient reports no impact on activities of daily living. A quick assessment reveals no problems with visual acuity. What would you recommend?

   A. Hold crizotinib until symptoms resolve and start at a lower dose when symptoms resolve

   B. Switch to a second generation ALK inhibitor

   C. Continue crizotinib and advice caution during driving or operating machinery

   D. Refer to ophthalmology

   E. MRI brain

10. A 66-year-old African-American, male light smoker with EGFR mutated lung adenocarcinoma presents to the emergency room with shortness of breath on exertion since the last 2 weeks. He has minimal nonproductive cough and low-grade fevers. No chest pain or palpitations. Exam reveals a patient in moderate distress with tachycardia, tachypnea, and oxygen saturation of 88%. Auscultation reveals bilateral diffuse crackles. CT scan shows bilateral groundglass infiltrates with more infiltrates on the right than the left lung. He had been on erlotinib over the past 6 months

at a dose of 150 mg daily. At the last restaging CT scan approximately 4 weeks ago, there was an 80% decrease in target lesion measurement from baseline. What is the likely diagnosis and the next best course of action?

    A. Cardiogenic pulmonary edema; diuresis

    B. Bilateral bronchopneumonia; antibiotics

    C. Lymphangitic carcinomatosis; hospice

    D. Drug-induced interstitial lung disease; steroids

11. A 55-year-old light smoker with EGFR-mutated lung adenocarcinoma presents with progressive disease on erlotinib. What is the most likely mechanism of acquired EGFR TKI resistance in this patient's tumor?

    A. A secondary T790M mutation in exon 20 of the EGFR gene

    B. MET amplification

    C. HER2 amplification

    D. Epithelial to mesenchymal transition

    E. Small cell transformation

12. For the patient from question 11, CT scan at the time of progression on EGFR TKI shows bilateral subcentimeter lung nodules. The case was discussed at the tumor board where the pulmonologist and the interventional radiologist agreed that there are no areas that can be safely biopsied in this patient. What is the next best course of action?

    A. Platinum-based chemotherapy

    B. Rociletinib

    C. Osimertinib

    D. Continued observation till one of the tumors are big enough to be biopsied

    E. Blood-based testing for resistance mutation

    F. Immunotherapy

13. For the patient from questions 11 and 12, noninvasive blood-based analysis revealed EGFR T790M mutation. What is the next best treatment course?

    A. Platinum-based chemotherapy

    B. Rociletinib

C. Osimertinib

D. Immunotherapy

---

14. A 65-year-old man presents with cough, hemoptysis, and more than 10% weight loss in the last 6 months. His past medical history includes hypertension, dyslipidemia, coronary artery disease, COPD, and erectile dysfunction. He has 100-pack-year history of smoking and is a current smoker. CT scan of the chest abdomen and pelvis shows 2 cm right lower lobe spiculated mass close to the chest wall with no abnormalities elsewhere. What is the next best step in his management?

    A. Fine-needle aspiration cytology of the right lower lobe mass

    B. Core needle biopsy of the right lower lobe mass

    C. Surgical resection of the right lower lobe mass with mediastinal staging

    D. Bronchoscopy for mediastinal staging

---

15. In the patient from question 14, pathology of the surgically resected tumor shows moderately differentiated lung adenocarcinoma. The tumor was 2 cm in greatest dimension with no evidence of invasion of the main bronchus and surgical margins were negative. No regional lymph node metastasis were identified. Mutational analysis reveals EGFR exon 19 deletion. Based on these findings at surgery, what is the next treatment option?

    A. Chemotherapy

    B. Targeted therapy with EGFR tyrosine kinase inhibitors

    C. Chemoradiation

    D. Observation

---

16. A 45-year-old woman presents to clinic with stage IIA (T1a,N1,M0) lung adenocarcinoma after having undergone a sleeve lobectomy with negative margins. Mutational analysis of her tumor reveals an EML4-ALK translocation. She is a never smoker with an active lifestyle and good performance status. What is the next step in her management?

    A. Chemotherapy

    B. First-generation ALK inhibitor

    C. Second-generation ALK inhibitor

    D. Observation

---

17. A 75-year-old man with multiple medical comorbidities including long-standing chronic obstructive pulmonary disease, poor lung function, and coronary artery disease presents with a right upper lobe lung nodule. Workup reveals stage IA disease. He presents to clinic to discuss available treatment options. What would you recommend?

    A. Sleeve lobectomy

    B. Sublobar resection

    C. Pneumonectomy

    D. Stereotactic body radiation therapy (SBRT)

---

18. A 65-year-old man was diagnosed with stage IV lung adenocarcinoma approximately a year ago. He completed 6 cycles of chemotherapy with a good response and has been under observation ever since. Recently he noted early morning headaches which prompted further workup. He was found to have a right parietal 2 cm mass with minimal peritumoral edema and no mass effect. What would be the best treatment option for this patient?

    A. Whole brain radiation

    B. Surgical resection followed by stereotactic radiosurgery

    C. Stereotactic radiosurgery alone

    D. Palliative doses of dexamethasone

    E. A and B

---

19. A 68-year-old woman with widely metastatic squamous lung carcinoma presents for treatment recommendations. Her diagnosis was made based on fine needle aspirate of a left supraclavicular lymph node. Tissue was not sufficient for testing of additional markers. She is symptomatic with cough, shortness of breath, and chest pain. Her ECOG performance status is 2. What would you recommend?

    A. Core needle biopsy of left supraclavicular lymph node

    B. Excision biopsy of left supraclavicular lymph node

    C. Immune checkpoint inhibitor

    D. Platinum-based combination chemotherapy

    E. Hospice given high tumor burden and poor performance status

20. For the patient in the above question, which of the following do NOT represent an appropriate chemotherapy doublet?

    A. Cisplatin plus paclitaxel

    B. Cisplatin plus pemetrexed

    C. Carboplatin plus gemcitabine

    D. Carboplatin plus albumin bound paclitaxel

21. A 45-year-old patient with EGFR mutated lung adenocarcinoma is now progressing on first-line erlotinib. Although most of the disease sites are stable, there are 2 right upper lobe tumors that appeared to be progressing consistently on the last 2 restaging CT scans, but the patient remains clinically asymptomatic. Which of the following are appropriate treatment recommendations for this patient?

    A. Surgical resection of right upper lobe tumors followed by continuation of erlotinib

    B. Osimertinib

    C. Systemic chemotherapy with platinum-based doublet

    D. Immunotherapy

    E. None of the above

22. Which of the following are not true regarding a newly diagnosed patient with metastatic nonsmall cell lung cancer?

    A. Early palliative care integrated with standard oncologic care improves quality of life, but does not impact survival

    B. Patients who receive early palliative care receive less aggressive end-of-life care

    C. Patients will receive early palliative care have better quality of life

    D. Patients will receive standard care alone have more depressive symptoms than those who receive standard care with early palliative care

23. An 88-year-old man presents with newly diagnosed lung adenocarcinoma. Mutation analysis is negative for EGFR, ALK, and ROS1. PD-L1 expression is found in 10% of tumor cells. His performance status is 2. Which of the following are true regarding his treatment options?

    A. Platinum-based doublet chemotherapy has been shown to improve survival over monotherapy

    B. Platinum-based doublet chemotherapy is associated with more toxic effects than monotherapy

    C. Systemic therapy in elderly patients should be carefully selected to avoid adverse reactions

    D. All of the above

24. Which of the following are not second-line treatment options for a patient with metastatic nonsquamous NSCLC with progression after first-line platinum-based chemotherapy?

    A. Nivolumab

    B. Pembrolizumab

    C. Atezolizumab

    D. Erlotinib

    E. Docetaxel

25. A 65-year-old patient presents with newly diagnosed non-squamous NSCLC. Mutation testing is negative. However, PD L1 expression is found in 60% of tumor cells. Which of the following is the best treatment option?

    A. Nivolumab

    B. Pembrolizumab

    C. Atezolizumab

    D. Durvalumab

    E. Avelumab

26. A patient with NSCLC who was started approximately 6 weeks ago on an immune checkpoint inhibitor presents with increased stool frequency and abdominal pain. Diarrhea has been worsening over the last 3 days. Which of the following is not an appropriate next step?

    A. Colitis diet and oral diphenoxylate

    B. Rule out infectious cause

C. Withhold the immune checkpoint inhibitor

D. Endoscopy and radiologic evaluation

E. Corticosteroids

27. The patient in the previous question was started on oral corticosteroids, but symptoms continue to worsen. Which of the following are recommended to manage this patient?

A. Infliximab

B. Budesonide

C. Cyclosporine

D. Atropine

28. A 62-year-old man was found on screening low-dose CT scan to have a 4 cm right upper lobe mass with atelectasis extending to the hilar region. No hilar or mediastinal adenopathy is noted. A follow-up CT of abdomen and pelvis were unremarkable. Which of the following is the key step in further staging the mediastinum of this patient?

A. Mediastinoscopy

B. FDG/PET

C. Bronchoscopy

D. None of the above

29. A 70-year-old current smoker presents with severe, intractable right shoulder pain radiating to the neck and the ulnar surface of right upper extremity further workup reveals a spiculated, peripherally located, superior sulcus tumor invading into the second and third ribs, and the brachial plexus. A percutaneous needle biopsy confirms adenocarcinoma of lung origin. Mediastinoscopy reveals N1 disease and no evidence of extrathoracic involvement is found on imaging studies. Which of the following is a next appropriate treatment?

A. Chemoradiation followed by surgical resection

B. Chemotherapy followed by surgical resection

C. Surgical resection followed by chemoradiation

D. Surgical resection followed by chemotherapy

30. A 45-year-old woman presents with metastatic nonsquamous NSCLC involving the right lung and left adrenal. CT scan shows a 4 cm right upper lobe mass and a 2 cm left adrenal mass. The tumor is positive for PD L1 expression in approximately 70% of tumor cells and shows an EGFR exon 19 deletion. What is the next best step in her workup/management?

    A. Pemrolizumab

    B. Platinum-based chemotherapy

    C. Left adrenal gland biopsy

    D. Erlotinib

31. A 65-year-old man who is an ex-smoker presents with left shoulder and arm pain and weakness and atrophy of the muscles of the hand. CT shows a tumor arising within the superior sulcus. CT and PET show no mediastinal nodal involvement. What is the next step in management/treatment?

    A. Surgical staging of the mediastinum

    B. MRI or CT scans of the brain

    C. Induction chemoradiotherapy plus surgery

    D. Chemotherapy or chemoradiation

    E. A and B

32. In the patient from question 31, MRI brain shows no evidence of brain involvement and mediastinal staging is negative. What is the next step in management/treatment?

    A. Induction chemoradiotherapy plus surgery

    B. Chemotherapy

    C. Chemoradiation

    D. Surgery

33. Which of the following supplements have been shown to reduce the risk of lung cancer in healthy individuals?

    A. Vitamin D

    B. Selenium

C. Alpha-tocopheral

D. None of the above

---

34. In the United States, lung cancer is the most frequent cause of cancer-related death. What is the most frequent cause of cancer related death worldwide?

   A. Lung

   B. Colorectal

   C. Breast

   D. Liver

---

35. Which of the following is true of KRAS mutations in early stage NSCLC?

   A. KRAS mutated tumors tend to be EGFR mutated also.

   B. KRAS mutation is associated with a better prognosis.

   C. KRAS mutation is associated with a worse prognosis.

   D. KRAS mutation status is not significantly prognostic.

   E. KRAS mutation is predictive of poor response to adjuvant chemotherapy.

ANSWERS TO REVIEW QUESTIONS

1. ANSWER: A. Cisplatin and gemcitabine

The patient with good performance status with newly diagnosed metastatic squamous cell lung cancer would benefit from systemic chemotherapy. Histology of NSCLC is important in treatment selection. Patients with squamous histology have shown showed improved survival with cisplatin/gemcitabine as initial chemotherapy treatment compared with pemetrexed/cisplatin (B is incorrect). Bevacizumab is not recommended in patients who are at increased risk of bleeding: squamous histology, tumor location close to major blood vessels, tumor necrosis, cavitation, or pre-existing hemoptysis (C and D are incorrect).

2. ANSWER: E. None of the above

Randomized trials of screening with chest radiography with or without sputum cytology have shown no reduction in lung-cancer mortality (C and D are incorrect). The National Lung Screening Trial (NLST), a randomized trial compared annual screening by low-dose chest CT scanning with chest x-ray for three years found a reduction in lung cancer–related mortality and all-cause mortality in high-risk patients screened with low-dose CT scan. However, the high-risk population was defined by NLST as individuals between 55 and 74 years of age with at least 30-pack-year cigarette smoking, and former smokers who had quit within the previous 15 years. There is no data to support lung cancer screening in a person with the risk profile described in the question (A and B are incorrect).

3. ANSWER: B. Concurrent chemotherapy and radiation

The patient has stage IIIB disease (T2N3). Stage IIIB lung cancers are not amenable to curative surgical resection unless they are highly selected (A and C are incorrect). For patients with stage IIIB disease with good performance status, combined modality therapy with chemotherapy and radiation is recommended. Concurrent chemotherapy and radiation is superior to sequential therapy (D is incorrect).

4. ANSWER C. Oral erlotinib

Metastatic pleural effusions are considered stage IV disease and thus there is no role for definitive therapy with concurrent chemotherapy plus radiation (B is incorrect). Check point inhibitors with pembrolizumab are used in the first-line and second-line setting of metastatic disease (A is incorrect). Patients with targetable EGFR mutations should have first-line therapy directed toward these driver mutations. This patient fits the profile often seen in EGFR positive patients (female with Asian ethnicity and often light or never smokers) and will benefit from upfront erlotinib (D is incorrect).

5. ANSWER D. Rebiopsy and send for molecular testing

Fifty percent of patients who progress on EGFR-directed therapy will have the "gatekeeper mutation" at T790M. A repeat biopsy to evaluate for this or other resistance mutations is helpful in choosing therapy. Osimertinib is an oral TKI directed against the T790M mutation and would be the next best therapy to consider for this patient. Moving to second-line immunotherapy or cytotoxic chemotherapy should be done after all targeted therapy options have been exhausted (A, B, and C are incorrect).

6. ANSWER A. Immune check point inhibitor

The preferred second-line choice in patients without a targetable mutation and no contraindications would be immunotherapy with check point inhibitors (if they have not received immunotherapy in the first line). In patients with metastatic disease, radiation therapy is reserved for palliation alone generally of a painful bone metastasis or rapidly growing or compressive lymphadenopathy. As he has a good performance status and is motivated for second-line therapy, single agent docetaxel is an option if he has a contraindication to immunotherapy.

REFERENCE:

https://www.ncbi.nlm.nih.gov/pubmed/26412456 and https://www.ncbi.nlm.nih.gov/pubmed/26028407

7. ANSWER: D. This patient has ALK translocated metastatic lung adenocarcinoma. Given the asymptomatic solitary brain metastasis, systemic therapy with ALK inhibitors is the best treatment option. Ceritinib is an orally active tyrosine kinase inhibitor of ALK that has been approved for use for patients with ALK positive NSCLC who have progressed after Crizotinib. Notably, ceritinib is more potent than crizotinib and has shown high overall intracranial response rate of more than 70%.

REFERENCE:

https://www.ncbi.nlm.nih.gov/pubmed/28126333

8. ANSWER: D. Next generation sequencing provides a comprehensive and efficient strategy compared with non-NGS testing to identify actionable genomic alterations in tumors from never or light smokers with lung cancers.

REFERENCE:

https://www.ncbi.nlm.nih.gov/pubmed/25567908

9. ANSWER: C. Visual disturbances are the most common adverse effect of crizotinib. Typically this occurs early during the course of treatment and are usually mild. Patients rarely require dose interruptions or reductions because of visual disturbances. Patients do not require baseline for routine ophthalmologic assessments. If symptoms worsen, ophthalmologic evaluation should be considered.

REFERENCE:

https://www.ncbi.nlm.nih.gov/pubmed/24523601

10. ANSWER: D. EGFR tyrosine kinase inhibitors can cause interstitial lung disease and respiratory failure in patients with NSCLC. All of the above differential diagnoses should be considered in this setting. Given the ongoing tumor response and lack of productive cough, Options C and B are unlikely. Risk factors for EGFR TKI induced interstitial lung disease include pre-existing pulmonary fibrosis and are commonly managed using corticosteroids.

REFERENCE:

https://www.ncbi.nlm.nih.gov/pubmed/15196739

11. ANSWER: A. Lung cancers harboring EGFR mutations respond to EGFR tyrosine kinase inhibitors, but drug resistance invariably emerges. EGFR T790M mutation accounts for approximately 50% to 60% of cases with acquired resistance to EGFR TKI therapy.

REFERENCE:

https://www.ncbi.nlm.nih.gov/pubmed/21430269

12. ANSWER: E. A blood-based testing to identify EGFR T790M mutations in circulating free tumor DNA from plasma was approved in 2016. Patients with positive mutations on blood-based tests are eligible for resistance-based treatment.

REFERENCE:

https://www.ncbi.nlm.nih.gov/pubmed/26446944

13. ANSWER: C. Osimertinib is highly active in NSCLC patients with the EGFR T790M mutation who had had disease progression during prior therapy with EGFR TKI with response rates of approximately 61%. The median progression free survival with osimertinib was 9.6 months compared with 2.8 months in EGFR T790M negative patients.

REFERENCE:

https://www.ncbi.nlm.nih.gov/pubmed/25923549

14. ANSWER: C. In patients with strong clinical suspicion for stage I or II lung cancer (based on risk factors and radiologic appearance), the preoperative biopsy is not required since it adds time, cost, and procedural risks.

Intraoperative diagnosis using needle biopsy or wedge resection is necessary before surgical resection.

REFERENCE:

NCCN guidelines

15. ANSWER: D. The patient has margin negative stage IA tumor. In this setting, observation is recommended. This entails smoking cessation advice, counseling and pharmacotherapy; history and physical and chest CT scan every 6 months for 2 to 3 years, then history and physical and the low-dose noncontrast chest CT annually.

REFERENCE:

NCCN guidelines

16. ANSWER: A. Cisplatin-based doublet is the adjuvant chemotherapy of choice for patients with stage IIA disease. The role of targeted therapies and immunotherapy in the adjuvant setting is under investigation. The Adjuvant Lung Cancer Enrichment Marker Identification and Sequencing Trial (ALCHEMIST) is evaluating the benefit of erlotinib or crizotinib as adjuvant therapy in molecularly selected patients with stage IB–IIIA NSCLC. Several trials are evaluating the role of immune checkpoint inhibitors in the adjuvant setting.

REFERENCE:

http://www.nejm.org/doi/full/10.1056/NEJMoa031644#t=article

17. ANSWER: D. In early-stage nonsmall cell lung cancer, stage I-II, N0 patients with medically inoperable disease and in patients who refuse to have surgery, stereotactic body radiation therapy (SBRT) may be considered after multidisciplinary evaluation. SBRT is also an appropriate option for patients with high surgical risk. When a pooled analysis was conducted of 2 randomized trials that each individually did not complete accrual, SBRT was found to have comparable cancer-specific outcomes and a better toxicity profile compared to surgery.

REFERENCE:

https://www.ncbi.nlm.nih.gov/pubmed/25981812

18. ANSWER: D. Patients with NSCLC and brain metastasis often have long-term survival. Potential neurocognitive issues that may occur with whole brain RT are a concern in these patients. Therefore, in patients with limited brain metastasis, example less than 3 lesions, SBRT alone or surgical resection followed by SBRT may be considered. In these instances, a decision should be based on a multidisciplinary discussion weighing potential benefits over the risk for each individual patient.

REFERENCE:

https://www.ncbi.nlm.nih.gov/pubmed/27458945

19. ANSWER: D. Chemotherapy is recommended for patients with metastatic NSCLC with negative or unknown test results for ALK or ROS1 rearrangements, EGFR sensitizing mutations, or PDL 1 expression. For this patient who has high tumor burden and symptomatic disease with unknown mutation status and PDL 1 expression, chemotherapy is the best intervention.

REFERENCE:

https://www.ncbi.nlm.nih.gov/pubmed/21536661

20. ANSWER: B. Cisplatin and carboplatin are effective in combination with several agents including paclitaxel, pemetrexed, gemcitabine, albumin bound paclitaxel, etoposide, and vinorelbine. However, pemetrexed is recommended only in patients with non-squamous NSCLC based on the survival advantage for pemetrexed in patients with non-squamous histology. If the patient had adenocarcinoma, she would most likely receive a pemetrexed-based regimen (as opposed to a taxine based regimen), which are better tolerated.

REFERENCE:

https://www.ncbi.nlm.nih.gov/pubmed/19221167

21. ANSWER: A. For patients with EGFR sensitizing mutations progressing during or after first-line therapy, all the above are appropriate treatment options. However, in this case with asymptomatic, oligo progressive disease—progressive disease limited in number and organ sites—locally ablative treatment directed to the areas of progressive disease could benefit the patient in terms of protracted progression free interval. Although limited by patient numbers, no improvement in overall survival has been found patients with EGFR sensitizing mutations in phase III trials of immunotherapy agents compared to docetaxel. In a retrospective analysis, objective responses were observed in 3.6% of EGFR mutated or ALK positive patients versus 23.3% of EGFR wild type and ALK negative/unknown patients.

REFERENCE:

https://www.ncbi.nlm.nih.gov/pubmed/23407558 https://www.ncbi.nlm.nih.gov/pubmed/27225694

22. ANSWER: A. In a randomized trial, among patients with metastatic non-small-cell lung cancer, early palliative care led to significant improvements in both quality of life and survival. Despite the fact that fewer patients in the early palliative care group than in the standard care group received aggressive end-of-life care, median survival was longer among patients receiving early palliative care (11.6 months vs. 8.9 months, P = 0.02).

REFERENCE:

https://www.ncbi.nlm.nih.gov/pubmed/20818875

23. ANSWER: D. All of the above are true. Platinum-based doublet chemotherapy was associated with survival benefits compared with vinorelbine or gemcitabine monotherapy in elderly patients with NSCLC. Median overall survival was 10.3 months for doublet chemotherapy and 6.2 months for monotherapy. However, the improvement in survival came at the cost of increased toxic effects which with more frequent in the doublet chemotherapy group.

REFERENCE:

https://www.ncbi.nlm.nih.gov/pubmed/21831418

24. ANSWER: D. All of the above except erlotinib are approved second-line treatment options for patients with metastatic nonsquamous NSCLC. Erlotinib was previously approved as a second line treatment option based on results of BR.21, a phase III trial that randomly assigned unselected NSCLC patients who had received one or 2 prior chemotherapy regimens to erlotinib or placebo. This trial, conducted before the predictive value of EGFR sensitizing mutations were recognized, found improved overall survival in unselected NSCLC patients who received erlotinib. The FDA labeling for this indication was changed based on the results of the IUNO trial which found that survival following treatment with erlotinib was not better than placebo administered as maintenance in patients with metastatic NSCLC tumors not harboring EGFR-activating mutations.

REFERENCE:

https://www.ncbi.nlm.nih.gov/pubmed/16014882 https://www.ncbi.nlm.nih.gov/pubmed/27987585

25. ANSWER: B. Pembrolizumab, a PD 1 inhibitor is the only agent approved for first line therapy for patients whose tumors have PD L1 expression levels of 50% or more with negative EGFR mutations and ALK or ROS1 rearrangements. In the KEYNOTE-024 trial, pembrolizumab was associated with significantly longer progression-free and overall survival and with fewer adverse events than was platinum-based chemotherapy in such patients.

REFERENCE:

http://www.nejm.org/doi/full/10.1056/NEJMoa1606774

26. ANSWER: A. Diarrhea/colitis can occur 6-8 weeks after commencement of immune checkpoint inhibitor therapy. It has been reported in 1% to 3% of cases in studies of anti-PD-1/PD-L1 antibodies. The reported frequencies are higher with CTLA 4 blockade. Worsening or persistent diarrhea for more than 3 days should prompt early investigations to rule out an infectious cause, withholding of the immune checkpoint inhibitor, antidiarrheal medications, endoscopic or radiologic evaluation to confirm the diagnosis and intervention with oral corticosteroids. Mild cases can be managed with colitis diet and antidiarrheal medications.

REFERENCE:

https://www.ncbi.nlm.nih.gov/pubmed/26371282

27. ANSWER: A. In clinically severe cases of immune checkpoint inhibitor associated diarrhea/colitis or those that do not respond to the initial interventions, patients may be admitted to hospital for intravenous corticosteroids (methylprednisolone 1 to 2 mg/kg total daily dose) and additional immunosuppression with anti-TNF agents, such as infliximab.

REFERENCE:

https://www.ncbi.nlm.nih.gov/pubmed/26371282

28. ANSWER: A. Although FDG PET can be used in initial assessment of mediastinal lymph nodes, mediastinoscopy is the gold standard. In this patient, the probability of mediastinal involvement is high based on tumor size and location and warrants a mediastinoscopy even if FDG PET does not suggest mediastinal node involvement.

29. ANSWER: A. The primary modality approach consisting of chemoradiotherapy and surgery is the standard care for patients with superior sulcus tumors. After preoperative concurrent chemotherapy/RT, if there is no evidence of progressive disease, then an attempt at surgical resection is mandated by an experienced thoracic surgeon. For patients who are either unwilling and/or unable to undergo a trimodality approach, then definitive chemoradiotherapy to a total radiotherapy dose of around 60 Gy is recommended.

REFERENCE:

https://www.ncbi.nlm.nih.gov/pubmed/24102007

30. ANSWER: C. Patients suspected of having a solitary site of metastatic disease should have tissue confirmation of that site.

31. ANSWER: E. Accurate staging of superior sulcus (Pancoast) tumors is critical. CT and MRI cannot definitively establish the presence or absence of mediastinal invasion or nodal metastasis, and surgical staging of the mediastinum should generally be undertaken prior to attempts at curative surgery. Because of the high propensity for brain metastasis from NSCLC in this location, brain imaging should be obtained prior to treatment.

REFERENCE:

https://www.ncbi.nlm.nih.gov/pubmed/24102007

32. ANSWER: A. Concurrent chemoradiotherapy as the initial step in management of patients with Pancoast tumors. This is followed by surgical resection if there is no evidence of distant metastases or local progression.

REFERENCE:

https://www.ncbi.nlm.nih.gov/pubmed/24102007

33. ANSWER: D. There is currently no evidence to support recommending vitamins such as alpha-tocopherol, beta-carotene or retinol, alone or in combination, to prevent lung cancer. A harmful effect was found for beta-carotene with retinol at pharmacological doses in people with risk factors for lung cancer.

REFERENCE:

https://www.ncbi.nlm.nih.gov/pubmed/12804424

34. ANSWER: A. Lung cancer is the most frequent cause of cancer-related death worldwide.

REFERENCE:

http://www.who.int/mediacentre/factsheets/fs297/en/

35. ANSWER: D. KRAS mutation status was not significantly prognostic in a pooled analysis of trials of adjuvant chemotherapy for early stage NSCLC.

REFERENCE:

https://www.ncbi.nlm.nih.gov/pubmed/23630215

Small Cell Lung Cancer 3

Christopher E. Wee and James P. Stevenson

REVIEW QUESTIONS

CASE 1

A 60-year-old male with a past medical history of hypertension and tobacco use (50 pack-year) presents to the Emergency Department with chest pain. Acute coronary syndrome and pulmonary embolism were ruled out with EKG, cardiac enzymes, and d-dimer, but a chest x-ray demonstrated a 2 cm right upper lobe mass. CT of chest, abdomen, and pelvis confirmed a 2.1 cm right upper lobe (RUL) mass with no evidence of distant metastases. Bronchoscopy and biopsy of the lung mass reveal small cell carcinoma.

1. What immunohistochemical staining pattern would be most consistent with the above diagnosis?

    A. TTF1 positive, CK 7 positive, keratin positive, chromogranin positive, synaptophysin positive

    B. TTF1 negative, CK 7 negative, keratin negative, chromogranin negative, synaptophysin negative

    C. TTF1 negative, CK 7 negative, keratin positive, chromogranin positive, synaptophysin positive

    D. TTF1 positive, CK 7 negative, keratin negative, chromogranin positive, synaptophysin positive

2. Which of the following staging investigations should be ordered next?

    A. MRI brain with and without contrast

    B. PET/CT including skull base to mid thigh

    C. MRI with and without contrast and PET/CT including skull base to mid thigh

    D. No further imaging

3. You have concluded that the patient has 2 cm tumor with no lymph node involvement. Assuming a good performance status and minimal comorbidities, which of the following treatment options should be considered for this patient?

    A. Chemotherapy alone

    B. Surgery alone

    C. Chemotherapy and sequential radiation

    D. Surgery and chemotherapy

4. In LS SCLC, which of the following chemotherapy regimen(s) is the standard of care?

    A. Cisplatin and irinotecan

    B. Cisplatin and etoposide

    C. Carboplatin and etoposide

    D. B and C

5. A patient with LS SCLC is treated with complete response to front-line therapy. Which is the next best step in management?

    A. Maintenance chemotherapy

    B. Prophylactic cranial irradiation (PCI)

    C. A and B

    D. Surveillance

CASE 2

A 55-year-old woman presented to the Emergency Department with 2 weeks of hemoptysis and shortness of breath. Chest x-ray demonstrates 4 cm right hilar mass with bulky mediastinal lymphadenopathy. CT chest, abdomen, and pelvis shows lesions in the bilateral adrenals and multiple contralateral pulmonary nodules.

6. Which of the following imaging tests are indicated next?

    A. PET/CT

    B. CT brain

    C. MRI brain

    D. No further imaging indicated

7. Extensive stage small cell lung cancer is diagnosed. Which of the following chemotherapy regimens should be given in the front-line setting?

    A. Cisplatin and irinotecan

    B. Carboplatin and etoposide

    C. Carboplatin, etoposide, and bevacizumab

    D. Single-agent topotecan

8. After palliative systemic therapy is initiated, how should response be monitored?

    A. Chest x ray

    B. PET/CT scans

    C. CT scans

    D. No routine imaging; follow clinical symptoms

9. After a complete response to front-line chemotherapy (platinum-based) for ES SCLC, the patient has recurrent disease 8 months later. Assuming good performance status, which palliative regimen should be initiated?

    A. Topotecan

    B. Immunotherapy

    C. Cyclophosphamide, adriamycin, vincristine

    D. Restart platinum plus etoposide chemotherapy

CASE 3

An 80-year-old male with mild cognitive impairment is diagnosed with ES SCLC. He is started on palliative carboplatin and etoposide with progression of disease. He is also undergoing radiotherapy to the spine for symptomatic metastases, but he has no brain metastases.

---

10. What is the role of PCI for this patient?

    A. PCI is recommended

    B. PCI is not recommended

---

11. The patient has progression of disease while on front-line carboplatin and etoposide. He now requires 4L NC of oxygen at rest and requires assistance for nearly all of his activities of daily living. Which of the following treatment decisions is most appropriate?

    A. Single-agent topotecan

    B. Change carboplatin to cisplatin

    C. Immunotherapy

    D. Hospice

ANSWERS TO REVIEW QUESTIONS

1. ANSWER: A. Small cell carcinomas express TTF1 and epithelial markers (CK7 and keratin) most commonly. Neuroendocrine markers (chromogranin and synaptophysin) are often positive in this disease, but can be negative in 10% of small cell carcinoma cases.

2. ANSWER: C. A significant number of patients (10% to 14%) with SCLC have brain metastases at time of diagnosis, so brain imaging, preferably with MRI, is indicated. Patients with suspected LS SCLC should also get a PET/CT to evaluate for distant metastases.

3. ANSWER: D. This patient has limited stage disease, as he has disease that can be confined to one radiation field. Given that the patient has a clinical T1N0 stage and good performance status, surgery should be considered with postoperative chemotherapy. Negative lymph nodes should be pathologically confirmed with mediastinoscopy. Chemotherapy and radiation without surgery is a reasonable option, and could be considered if there are medical comorbidities; however, concurrent chemoradiation, not sequential radiotherapy, is preferred.

4. ANSWER: B. Cisplatin and etoposide is the preferred regimen for LS SCLC, and should be used if there are no contraindications. Carboplatin may be substituted for cisplatin for first-line therapy in ES SCLC since the nature of treatment is inherently palliative and carboplatin is generally better tolerated.

5. ANSWER: B. Prophylactic cranial irradiation has been shown to improve both morbidity and mortality in LS SCLC that responds to chemotherapy. There is no role for maintenance chemotherapy.

6. ANSWER: C. Even though extensive stage disease has already been diagnosed on prior imaging, imaging of the brain is recommended because 10% to 15% patients have CNS metastases on initial presentation, and early evaluation and treatment can decrease morbidity and mortality. MRI, if possible to obtain, is preferred over CT due to its higher sensitivity in detecting parenchymal lesions.

7. ANSWER: B. Carboplatin and etoposide is a first-line regimen for ES SCLC. While irinotecan-containing regimens demonstrated survival benefit in Japanese studies, these results were not reproducible in the United States. At this time, there is no role for bevacizumab in SCLC and topotecan is a second-line agent.

8. ANSWER: C. Response should be monitored with CT Scans. There is no role for PET/CT to monitor disease response. Chest x-rays are not nearly sensitive enough to monitor disease and since radiographic changes often precede clinical changes, treatment decisions should not be based on clinical symptoms.

9. ANSWER: D. Patients who relapse greater than 6 months after completion of chemotherapy, may be re-treated with their platinum plus etoposide. If they relapse within 6 months of front-line treatment, topotecan is the preferred agent. Currently there is no evidence to use cyclophosphamide, doxorubicin, and vincristine, and immunotherapy is currently under investigation.

10. ANSWER: B. The role of PCI in ES SCLC is controversial, as two randomized trials produced conflicting results. This particular patient who already has poor cognitive function, is undergoing radiation elsewhere, and is not responding to chemotherapy; PCI is not indicated.

11. ANSWER: D. The role of treatment in ES SCLC is to prolong survival and maintain quality of life in patients who are candidates for therapy. This patient has a poor performance status and would not benefit from chemotherapy. Initiation of supportive care in the form of hospice is most appropriate.

Esophageal Cancer 4

Megan Greally and Gregory D. Leonard

REVIEW QUESTIONS

1. A 65-year-old Chinese man presents with a 2-month history of progressive dysphagia and weight loss. Upper endoscopy reveals a tumor at 15 cm. Which of the following is the most likely histologic subtype in this patient?

   A. Adenocarcinoma

   B. Adenosquamous carcinoma

   C. Small cell carcinoma

   D. Squamous cell carcinoma

2. A 70-year-old white woman with a history of type 2 diabetes and coronary heart disease is diagnosed with a lower esophageal cancer after endoscopic biopsy. The following is associated with an increased risk of esophageal adenocarcinoma:

   A. Alcoholism

   B. Plummer-Vinson syndrome

   C. Barrett's esophagus

   D. Tylosis

   E. Achalasia

3. A 62-year-old white man is referred to the upper gastro-intestinal surgery clinic following a diagnosis of an esophageal tumor at 32 cm after he undergoes upper endoscopy. Histologic evaluation of tumor biopsies are consistent with a diagnosis of a moderately differentiated adenocarcinoma. Computed tomography of chest, abdomen, and pelvis and endoscopic ultrasound suggest T3N1 disease. The patient has a good performances status and no significant medical co-morbidities. Prior to considering multimodality therapy including surgical resection the most appropriate next staging investigation would be:

   A. Laporoscopy

   B. Positron emission tomography

   C. Barium swallow

   D. Bronchoscopy

   E. Pulmonary function testing

4. A 57-year-old gentleman is investigated for dysphagia and significant weight loss. Upper endoscopy reveals a mid-esophagus tumor which biopsy confirms to be adenocarcinoma. CT thorax and abdomen and EUS imaging suggest T3N1 disease and after multidisciplinary discussion a PET/CT is recommended, which shows no evidence of metastatic disease. Which of the below treatment options would be most appropriate for this patient?

   A. Preoperative chemoradiotherapy followed by surgery

   B. Definitive chemoradiotherapy

   C. Upfront surgery

   D. Esophageal stenting

   E. Surgery and adjuvant chemotherapy

5. A 75-year-old female patient, with a history of chronic obstructive airways disease and coronary artery disease, is investigated for dysphagia and weight loss. She is found to have a SCC of her upper thoracic esophagus, staged as T2N1 by endoscopic ultrasound. PET/CT shows esophageal thickening

with surrounding FDG-avid lymph nodes, but no evidence of metastatic disease. Which therapeutic option would be most optimal for this patient?

A. Esophagectomy

B. Neoadjuvant chemotherapy followed by esophagectomy

C. Esophagectomy followed by adjuvant chemoradiotherapy

D. Definitive chemoradiotherapy

E. Palliative radiotherapy

6. A 70-year-old male is admitted with progressive weight loss and dyspepsia. He is found to have a tumor at the esophagogastric junction, which is causing partial obstruction. CT chest and abdomen shows thickening of the distal esophagus, as well as multiple low-attenuation lesions in his liver, consistent with metastatic disease. Pathologic examination of an endoscopic biopsy reveals poorly differentiated adenocarcinoma. He has an ECOG performance status of 1, and palliative chemotherapy with cisplatin and fluorouracil is planned. What further molecular marker can be used to guide this patient's treatment?

A. Immunohistochemistry (IHC) for VEGFR-1

B. IHC for VEGFR-2

C. EGFR mutational analysis

D. IHC and fluorescent in situ hybridization for HER2

E. ATM protein expression

7. A 58-year-old man with metastatic HER2 negative esophagogastric junction adenocarcinoma attends the oncology clinic for results of restaging evaluation. Following initial diagnosis he was treated with first line Epirubicin/Oxaliplatin/Capecitabine (EOX) and interval imaging showed a partial response to therapy. CT TAP now shows progression of disease with increase in size of liver and nodal metastases. He complains of right upper quadrant pain and has an ECOG performance status of 1. What is the most appropriate second-line treatment option for this patient?

A. FOLFOX

B. Paclitaxel

C. Ramucirumab

D. Irinotecan

E. Paclitaxel plus Ramucirumab

ANSWERS TO REVIEW QUESTIONS

1. ANSWER: D. SCC accounts for approximately 90% of cases of esophageal cancer that occur in high-risk areas of Asia such as China, India, and Iran. Worldwide, SCC is the predominant histologic subtype of esophageal cancer, but since the 1970's ADC has been increasing in incidence in Western countries.

REFERENCE:

Ferlay J, Soerjomataram I, Ervik M, et al. GLOBOCAN 2012 v1.0, Cancer Incidence and Mortality Worldwide: IARC CancerBase No. 11[Internet]. Lyon, France: International Agency for Research on Cancer; 2013. http://globocan.iarc.fr, accessed 09/24/2016

2. ANSWER: C. Barrett's esophagus is the biggest risk factor for ADC and increases the risk of ADC 30-fold over the general population. The annual risk of esophageal cancer is approximately 0.25% for patients without dysplasia and 6% for patients with high-grade dysplasia. Close surveillance and endoscopic eradication therapy is recommended for Barrett's esophagus with low- and high-grade dysplasia.

REFERENCE:

Spechler SJ. Barrett esophagus and risk of esophageal cancer: a clinical review. *JAMA.* 2013;310(6):627.

3. ANSWER: B. Standard treatment for this patient with T3N1 adenocarcinoma and a good performance status is neoadjuvant CRT or pre/perioperative chemotherapy and surgery. PET/CT is more sensitive than CT for detecting distant metastases and is recommended for patients who are surgical candidates. It results in a change in management in up to 20% of this patient group.

REFERENCE:

Flamen P, Lerut A, van Cutsem E, et al. Utility of positron emission tomography for the staging of patients with potentially operable esophageal carcinoma. *J Clin Oncol.* 2000;18:3202.

4. ANSWER: A. The management of locally advanced esophageal cancer has changed significantly over the last 15 years and most patients now undergo combined modality therapy. Several trials provide evidence for use of concurrent trimodality treatment with CRT and surgery. Preoperative CRT results in improved OS and reduced local recurrence rates compared with surgery alone. Because patients with ADC have lower rates of pCR after CRT and some retrospective studies have reported inferior survival with a nonsurgical approach in this group, it is recommended that operable patients with ADC undergo surgery.

REFERENCE:

Van Hagen P, Hulshof MC, van der Gaast A, et al. Preoperative chemoradiotherapy for esophageal or junctional cancer: Results from a multicentre randomized phase III trial. *N Engl J Med.* 2012;366:2074.

5. *ANSWER: D.* The prognosis for patients with SCC has not been shown to differ from those with ADC, but it appears to be a more chemo- and radio-sensitive disease. In addition to this, the operative approach for resection of tumors in the upper esophagus can result in significant morbidity. In light of this, definitive CRT is a reasonable option. Although this approach has not been compared directly to a surgical approach, outcomes appear to be similar and potential operative morbidity is avoided.

REFERENCE:

Bedenne L, Michel P, Bouché O et al. Chemoradiation followed by surgery compared with chemora-diation alone in squamous cancer of the esophagus: FFCD 9102: *Clin Oncol.* 2007;25(10):1160.

6. *ANSWER: D.* Recent advances in understanding the molecular biology of esophagogastric cancer have led to targeted therapies being developed. HER2 is overexpressed in approximately 15% of esophageal ADC, and the ToGA trial demonstrated that the addition of trastuzumab to cisplatin and flu-orouracil chemotherapy results in improved response and OS. Elevated levels of VEGF are associated with poor prognosis in patients with resectable gastric ADC and gastric cancer cell lines with low ATM expression are sensitive to Olaparib but further work is needed to enhance our knowledge of biomark-ers and targets in esophageal cancer.

REFERENCE:

Bang YJ, Van Cutsem E, Kang YK et al. Trastuzumab in combination with chemotherapy versus che-motherapy alone for treatment of HER2-positive advanced gastric or gastroesophageal junction cancer (ToGA): a phase 3, open-label, randomized controlled trial. *Lancet.* 2010;376(9742):687.

7. *ANSWER: E.* This patient has progressed after first-line therapy, has main-tained a good performance status, and is symptomatic with right upper quadrant pain. The combination of paclitaxel and ramucirumab improved objective response rates and OS over paclitaxel alone in the RAINBOW trial. Ramucirumab and paclitaxel is a category 1 recommendation in the NCCN guidelines and is a rational choice for this patient. In addition, the expected higher response rate may provide greater symptomatic benefit.

REFERENCE:

Wilke H, Muro K, Van Cutsem E, et al. Ramucirumab plus paclitaxel versus placebo plus paclitaxel in patients with previously treated advanced gastric or gastro-esophageal junction adenocarci-noma (RAINBOW): a double-blind, randomized phase 3 trial. *Lancet Oncol.* 2014;15:1224.

Gastric Cancers 5

Hiral Parekh and Thomas J. George, Jr.

REVIEW QUESTIONS

1. A 62-year-old male presented to his PCP with abdominal pain, nausea, early satiety, night sweats, and weight loss over the past 3 months. His past medical history include hypertension, hypothyroidism, and chronic gastritis. Physical examination was unremarkable and laboratory studies including CT scans were unremarkable. Upper endoscopy showed gastric mucosal erythema and nodularity. The biopsy showed presence of dense diffuse infiltrate of centrocyte-like cells in lamina propria with prominent lymphoepithelial lesions. *H. pylori* was positive. EUS did not reveal regional lymphadenopathy. What is the best next step before considering the treatment?

   A. Chemotherapy and radiation

   B. Bone scan

   C. Surgery consultation

   D. Florescence in-situ hybridization for t(11:18) translocation

   E. Intraoperative radiotherapy

2. A 56-year-old female was referred to you by her PCP. She has a history of peptic ulcer disease and had undergone partial gastrectomy 5 years ago for peptic ulcer perforation. She does not have symptoms of PUD currently. She has good appetite and stable weight. She wanted to know if she would need screening for gastric cancer as she heard that partial

gastrectomy is one of the risk factors for gastric cancer. Which one of the following statements is TRUE?

A. Because of the high risk of gastric cancer in patients after partial gastrectomy, the recommendation is to perform surveillance upper endoscopy 5 years after partial gastrectomy.

B. There is no sufficient data to recommend surveillance endoscopy after partial gastrectomy for nonmalignant disorders.

C. The risk of gastric stump cancer is three-fold higher than general population 5 years after partial gastrectomy.

D. Because of the low overall incidence of gastric cancer in US, upper endoscopy is not recommended, regardless of risks.

E. Continued acid suppression from the PUD treatment is protective for gastric cancer.

3. A 65-year-old male presented to ER with worsening fatigue, shortness of breath, and black stool for 3 days. He noticed a few pounds weight loss and intermittent epigastric discomfort associated with food for a few months. He has no other major medical problems and has not seen a doctor for many years. Physical examination revealed a thin male with left supraclavicular lymphadenopathy. Other systems examination was unremarkable. Laboratory studies showed microcytic anemia (Hgb = 7.2) and positive heme occult blood in stool. LFT showed elevated AST (90), ALT (75), and alkaline phosphatase (230). EGD revealed nonbleeding ulcer at the gastric antrum with biopsy consistent with gastric adenocarcinoma. CT chest/abdomen/pelvis showed multiple liver lesions with perigastric and celiac lymphadenopathy. CEA was 38. He felt better after blood transfusion and Hgb improved appropriately. He has some limitations in doing strenuous activities but is ambulatory and can do daily activities without problems. Medical oncology was consulted to discuss the treatment options.

Which of the following would you next recommend?

A. Radiation therapy

B. Palliative care alone

C. Trastuzumab in combination with chemotherapy if HER2 overexpressing

D. Chemotherapy and radiation

E. Chemotherapy in combination with bevacizumab

4. A 58-year-old female was recently diagnosed with gastric adenocarcinoma of the distal stomach and underwent subtotal gastrectomy 4 weeks ago. She presented to your clinic today to discuss further treatment options. Pathology showed tumor invading the subserosal connective tissue without invading the visceral peritoneum or adjacent structure and 0/16 lymph nodes were positive with clear margins and without lymphovascular or perinural involvement. She has no other medical problems and was previously healthy until the diagnosis of gastric cancer. She is recovering well from surgery. Physical examination revealed well appearing female, healing abdominal surgical wound with unremarkable exam otherwise. What is the optimal adjuvant treatment option for her?

    A. Repeat resection with more extensive lymph node retrieval (D2)

    B. Infusional fluoropyrimidine for one year

    C. 6 months of ECF (epirubicin, cisplatin, and 5-FU) postoperative polychemotherapy

    D. 5-FU/leucovorin before, during, and after radiation therapy

    E. Observation

5. A 53-year-old male presented with anorexia, epigastric discomfort, and early satiety for 3 months. He did not have significant medical problems and the symptoms were initially thought to be due to acid reflux related to his stressful job. The symptoms did not improve with PPI use. Physical examination was unremarkable and laboratory studies were within normal limits. Upper endoscopy was pursued, which showed 5 cm fungating nonbleeding mass in the gastric body. Subsequent EUS showed tumor invading the muscularis propria with multiple enlarged perigastric lymph nodes. PET/CT showed no other occult sites of disease. Patient wishes to get the most aggressive treatment that would provide the best chance of cure. What would you recommend?

    A. Surgery followed by adjuvant radiation

    B. Neoadjuvant concurrent chemoradiation with cisplatin/5-FU regimen

    C. Perioperative polychemotherapy with ECF (epirubicin, cisplatin, and 5-FU)

    D. Perioperative chemotherapy including bevacizumab

    E. Palliative care

6. A 42-year-old otherwise healthy female presented with dark tarry stools for 2 days, upon further questioning reported loss of appetite, weight loss of 10 lbs in the last 2 months, and progressive fatigue. Her laboratory evaluation confirms hemoglobin of 8 gm/dl but other laboratory studies and physical examination are normal. Upper endoscopy confirms a diffuse gastric cancer with staging revealing three liver lesions. Her performance status is good and she is otherwise healthy. She presents to you for consultation and treatment recommendations. Upon further questioning she reported family history of maternal breast cancer at the age of 35, but no other family history of cancer. Which of the following germline mutations might she carry?

   A. Mutations in E-cadherin (*CDH1* gene)

   B. Mutations in *APC* and *MUTYH* genes

   C. Mutations in folliculin (*FLCN* or *BHD* genes)

   D. Mutations in the *CDKN2A* gene

7. A 72-year-old male is being treated for metastatic gastric adenocarcinoma. He is currently receiving chemotherapy with 5-FU and oxaliplatin. He has received eight cycles of therapy and has developed peripheral neuropathy interfering with his ability to type. He is still active and able to carry out light household work. He presents for follow-up today after restaging scans to evaluate response to chemotherapy. His staging scan reveals progressive disease. After discussion of the results, he reports that he would like to continue to explore additional treatment options. Which of following targeted therapies can be considered at this time?

   A. Bortezomib

   B. Regorafenib

   C. Ramucirumab

   D. Bevacizumab

8. A 62-year-old male is evaluated for iron deficiency anemia with colonoscopy and upper endoscopy. Biopsy of an antral mass confirmed adenocarcinoma and staging work-up was suggestive of metastatic disease to liver. He reports feeling well, denying any symptoms from his diagnosis. He is otherwise healthy and active, walking 2 miles every day. He is being seen for consideration of palliative chemotherapy. When he presents to start chemotherapy, his HER 2 status is reported as 3+ staining in partially

circumferential membrane. Which of the following treatment would be recommended at this time?

A. Cisplatin and infusional 5-FU with radiation

B. Epirubicin, oxalaplatin, and 5-FU

C. Paclitaxel and ramucirumab

D. Trastuzumab, cisplatin, and infusional 5-FU

E. Change plan to supportive care alone

9. A 65-year-old female is diagnosed with gastric adenocarcinoma after she presented with unintentional weight loss and early satiety. Her staging work-up did not show any evidence of metastatic disease and final pathology after a total gastrectomy with D1 lymph node dissection confirms pT2N1 disease. She received postoperative chemotherapy with infusional 5-FU as well as chemoradiotherapy. She completed her therapy 3 years ago. She now presents with new onset fatigue. Complete blood count shows white blood count 2.1 thousand/mm^3, hemoglobin of 9.2 g/dl, and platelets of 70 thousand/mm^3. Her peripheral blood smear demonstrates pancytopenia, macrocytosis, and reduced reticulocytes with hypersegmented neutrophils. What is the next best step in her evaluation?

A. Bone marrow biopsy with cytogenetic evaluation

B. Staging scans with CT chest/abdomen/pelvis

C. Upper endoscopy and colonoscopy

D. Iron profile panel, folate, vitamin B12 levels

E. Empiric treatment for *H. pylori*

10. A 68-year-old female is diagnosed with gastric adenocarcinoma with metastatic disease in the liver and lungs. She is currently undergoing chemotherapy with epirubicin, oxaliplatin, and capecitabine. She is tolerating chemotherapy well and has completed 6 months of therapy. Her first scan after starting therapy suggested a response to therapy with 20% reduction in tumor mass; however, her most recent CT scan confirmed progressive disease with enlarging and new lung and liver lesions. What is the most appropriate targeted combination therapy to consider?

A. Bevacizumab and paclitaxel

B. Ramucirumab and paclitaxel

C. Cetuximab and paclitaxel

D. Panitumumab and paclitaxel

ANSWERS TO REVIEW QUESTIONS

1. ANSWER: D. This patient has an early stage PGL localized to GI tract. Pathology is consistent with extranodal marginal zone lymphoma of mucosa-associated lymphoid tissue tumor (MALT lymphoma) which is typically associated with *H. pylori* infection. Primary gastric lymphoma accounts for 3% of gastric neoplasms and 10% of lymphomas. *H. pylori*-induced gastritis leads to the accumulation of CD4+ lymphocytes and mature B cells in the gastric lamina propria resulting in the activation of T cells with B-cell proliferation and lymphoid follicle formation, which eventually evolve into a monoclonal lymphoma. The treatment of choice for *H. pylori* positive early stage disease (stagey/IIE) is eradication of *H. pylori*. This would provide 50% to 80% histologic complete response and long-term remission. However, patients with the t(11:18) translocation are typically not responsive to *H. pylori* therapy and external beam radiation (RT) is recommended. Local RT (total dose of 25 to 30 Gy) results in high rates of overall and complete responses (100% and 98%, respectively) and 5-year disease-free and overall survival rates of 98% and 77%, respectively. Bone scans are not routinely recommended for MALT lymphoma. Surgery is reserved for patients with obstructive symptoms or bleeding, and chemotherapy is reserved for higher-grade gastric lymphomas.

REFERENCE:

Zucca E, Bertoni F, Roggero E, et al. Molecular analysis of the progression from Helicobacter pylori-associated chronic gastritis to mucosa-associated lymphoid-tissue lymphoma of the stomach. *N Engl J Med.* 1998;338(12):804.

2. ANSWER: B. The risk of gastric cancer increases 15 to 20 years after partial gastrectomy surgery with the relative risk of 1.5 to 3. The mechanism is thought to be due to gastric production of N-nitroso carcinogens in the gastric remnant. These compounds are generated from nitrate and nitrite by gastric bacteria, which have overgrown from postoperative hypochlorhydria. In addition, gastric reflux of bile with increased level of bile acids may play a role. The increasing risk of gastric stump cancer with duration of postoperative period suggests a dose–response relationship and supports this mechanism of carcinogenesis. There are no sufficient data to support routine endoscopic surveillance for patients with previous partial gastrectomy for peptic ulcer disease. However, the threshold should be low to endoscopically evaluate upper GI symptoms. If surveillance is considered, it should be initiated 15 to 20 years postgastrectomy. Routine screening for gastric cancer is not recommended in the United States, where the overall gastric cancer burden is low. Periodic upper endoscopy can be offered to patients who are considered to be at increased risk; however, the benefits and risks are unclear.

REFERENCE:

Leung W, Wu M, Kakugawa Y, et al. Screening for gastric cancer in Asia: current evidence and practice. *Lancet Oncol.* 2008;9(3):279.

3. ANSWER: C. The patient has metastatic gastric adenocarcinoma and the goal of treatment is palliation. He has a reasonable performance status with no major co-morbidities. Therefore, the standard of care is to screen for HER2 expression status by immunohistochemistry (IHC) and gene amplification by florescence in-situ hybridization (FISH) if IHC is equivocal. If HER2 is positive, chemotherapy with trastuzumab is recommended as a first-line treatment. Data from the randomized phase III ToGA study showed the addition of the monoclonal antibody against HER2 (trastuzumab) to cisplatin/fluoropyrimidine provided significantly higher objective response rates (47% vs. 35%) and improved median overall survival compared to chemotherapy alone (13.8 vs. 11.1 months, $P = 0.0046$). Since EGD did not show active bleeding and the patient did not have uncontrolled pain from the tumor, radiotherapy is not indicated at this point. There is no role for concurrent or sequential chemoradiation for metastatic gastric cancer. Bevacizumab with chemotherapy in metastatic gastric cancer did not show a survival advantage in the phase III trial and should not be offered outside of a clinical trial, particularly given the patient's recent bleeding event.

REFERENCE:

Van Cutsem E, Moiseyenko VM, Tjulandin S, et al. Phase III study of docetaxel and cisplatin plus fluorouracil compared with cisplatin and fluorouracil as first-line therapy for advanced gastric cancer: a report of the V325 study group. *J Clin Oncol.* 2006;24:4991–4997.

4. ANSWER: D. The adjuvant treatment options for R0 resected gastric tumor are chemoradiation or potentially chemotherapy if D2 resection is achieved. At least 16 lymph nodes need to be examined for adequate sampling. D2 resection involves removal of extensive lymph nodes including perigastric, hepatic, left gastric, celiac, and splenic arteries; splenic hilar nodes; and +/– splenectomy. D2 resection is not routinely performed in the United States and only performed in the experienced centers because of the significant post op morbidity and mortality. Subjecting the patient to a repeat surgical intervention is not justified given the negative margins and adequate node sampling. INT0116 trial demonstrated a survival benefit with adjuvant chemoradiation (5-FU/leucovorin before, during, and after radiation therapy) as compared to surgery alone in patients who received less than a D2 resection. Oral fluropyrimidine (S-1) for one year adjuvant after D2 resection showed improvement in overall survival and relapse-free survival and is approved for adjuvant therapy in Japan. S-1 is not commercially available in the United States. Perioperative (pre and postop) polychemotherapy using ECF (epirubicin, cisplatin, and infusional 5-FU) is an acceptable standard of care, but the patient did not receive preoperative chemotherapy. Therefore, chemoRT would be the best option to improve relapse-free and overall survival.

REFERENCE:

Macdonald JS, Smalley SR, Benedetti J, et al. Chemoradiotherapy after surgery compared with surgery alone for adenocarcinoma of the stomach or gastroesophageal junction. *N Engl J Med.* 2001;345(10):725–730.

5. ANSWER: C. In a randomized phase III (MAGIC) trial, perioperative chemotherapy with ECF (epirubicin, cisplatin, and 5-FU) given for 3 months before and after surgery was associated with significantly improved 5-year progression-free survival (HR, 0.66; 95% CI, 0.53 to 0.81; $P < 0.001$) and overall survival (36 vs. 23%) compared to surgery alone. After perioperative polychemotherapy, the resected tumors were significantly smaller and less advanced with similar postoperative complications or deaths between two arms. Neoadjuvant concurrent chemoRT is more commonly used for esophageal, GEJ, and gastric cardia cancers than for potentially resectable noncardia gastric adenocarcinomas. There are no randomized trials addressing the benefit of preoperative chemoRT in noncardia gastric cancer. No survival benefit was observed with adjuvant radiation alone after surgery. Preoperative chemotherapy in combination with bevacizumab is still under investigation and should not be used outside the context of a clinical trial.

REFERENCE:

Cunningham D, Allum WH, Stenning SP, et al. Perioperative chemotherapy versus surgery alone for resectable gastroesophageal cancer. *N Engl J Med.* 2006;355:11–20.

6. ANSWER: A. Germline mutations of the E-cadherin gene are associated with hereditary diffuse gastric cancer (DGC). The gene codes for a cell-surface antigen involved in cell–cell adhesion. Based upon data from 75 *CDH1* mutation-positive hereditary diffuse gastric cancer kindred, the lifetime cumulative risk for advanced diffuse-type gastric cancer is up to 70% (95% CI, 59% to 80%) for males and 56% (95% CI, 44% to 69%) for females by the age of 80 years with the median age of onset at 38 years. Women with the germline mutation also have a high risk of developing lobular breast cancer. Given the high mortality associated with invasive disease, prophylactic total gastrectomy at a center of expertise is advised for individuals with pathogenic CDH1 mutations. Breast cancer surveillance with annual breast MRI starting at age 30 for women with a CDH1 mutation is recommended. Guidelines for CDH1 testing take into account cancer in first and second-degree relatives:

(1) families with two or more members with gastric cancer at any age, one confirmed DGC
(2) individuals with DGC before the age of 40
(3) families with diagnoses of both DGC and LBC (one diagnosis before the age of 50)

Other listed mutations do not increase the risk of diffuse gastric cancer. *APC* and *MUTYH* gene mutations are seen in variant forms of familial adenomatous polyposis, frequently referred to as MUTYH-associated polyposis (MAP). Mutations in folliculin gene (also known as the *BHD* gene, Birt-Hogg-Dubé syndrome) increase the risk of kidney cancer. Mutations in *CKDN2A* are associated with familial atypical multiple mole and melanoma (FAMMM) syndrome.

REFERENCE:

Hansford S, Kaurah P, Li-Chang H, et al. Hereditary diffuse gastric cancer syndrome: CDH1 mutations and beyond. *JAMA Oncol.* 2015;1(1):23.

7. ANSWER: C. Ramucirumab is a recombinant monoclonal antibody of the IgG1 class that binds to the VEGFR-2, blocking receptor activation. Trials have shown a survival benefit for therapy with ramucirumab, either as monotherapy or in combination with paclitaxel in patients with previously treated advanced esophagogastric adenocarcinoma. In the phase III REGARD trial, 355 previously treated patients with advanced or metastatic esophagogastric adenocarcinoma were randomly assigned to ramucirumab versus best supportive care. Ramucirumab was associated with significantly improved median progression-free (2.1 vs. 1.3 months) and overall survival (5.2 vs. 3.8 months; HR 0.78; 95% CI, 0.60 to 0.998; $P = 0.047$). Single-agent regorafenib has shown some activity in phase II studies but confirmatory studies are still needed to establish a role. Bevacizumab failed to demonstrate any benefit in a first-line setting when combined with chemotherapy. Bortezomib has no role in esophagogastric adenocarcinoma. Based on the REGARD trial results, ramucirumab monotherapy is FDA-approved for second-line treatment of metastatic gastric carcinoma.

REFERENCE:

Fuchs C, Tomasek J, Yong C, et al. Ramucirumab monotherapy for previously treated advanced gastric or gastro-oesophageal junction adenocarcinoma (REGARD): an international, randomised, multicentre, placebo-controlled, phase 3 trial. *Lancet.* 2014 Jan 4;383(9911):31–39.

8. ANSWER: D. Overexpression of EGF receptor (EGFR)-2 (HER2) is seen in approximately 7% to 22% of esophagogastric cancers. The prognostic significance of HER2 overexpression in esophagogastric adenocarcinoma is unclear. Similar to breast cancer, HER2 overexpression is predictive for response to anti-HER2 therapies. HER2 protein expression is assessed by immunohistochemical (IHC) staining and gene amplification by FISH. HER2 overexpression in esophagogastric cancer is different from that of breast cancer because it tends to spare the digestive luminal membrane. Thus, an esophagogastric cancer with only partially circumferential (i.e., "basolateral" or "lateral") membrane staining can still be categorized as 2+ or 3+. In contrast, a breast tumor must demonstrate complete circumferential membrane staining to be designated as 2+ or 3+. Using breast cancer HER2 interpretation criteria may underestimate expression in esophagogastric cancers. Modified criteria for interpreting HER2 by IHC in esophagogastric cancers were developed and validated with a high concordance rate of HER2 gene amplification and HER2 protein overexpression for IHC 0-1+ and 3+ cases. For an equivocal IHC 2+ expression, FISH analysis is recommended for confirmation.

Therapeutic targeting of HER2 overexpressing esophagogastric adenocarcinoma by a monoclonal antibody, trastuzumab, was studied in combination with chemotherapy in ToGA trial and demonstrated improved median overall survival (13.8 vs. 11.1 months; HR 0.74; 95% CI, 0.60 to 0.91; $P = 0.0046$) in those receiving trastuzumab. This trial established a new standard of care for advanced HER2 overexpressing esophagogastric tumors.

REFERENCES:

Van Cutsem E, Moiseyenko VM, Tjulandin S, et al. Phase III study of docetaxel and cisplatin plus fluorouracil compared with cisplatin and fluorouracil as first-line therapy for advanced gastric cancer: a report of the V325 study group. *J Clin Oncol.* 2006:24:4991–4997.

Van Cutsem E, Bang Y, Feng-Yi, et al. HER2 screening data from ToGA: targeting HER2 in gastric and gastroesophageal junction cancer. *Gastric Cancer.* 2015 Jul;18(3):476–484.

9. ANSWER: D. Following a total gastrectomy, the absence of intrinsic factor leads to the poor absorption of vitamin B12 resulting in megaloblastic anemia. Under normal physiologic conditions, intrinsic factor binds to vitamin B12 and promotes the absorption of this vitamin in the lower portion of the small bowel. When vitamin B12 is poorly absorbed, anemia and neurological deficits can occur. Severe vitamin B12 deficiency can lead to thrombocytopenia and neutropenia (i.e., pancytopenia), mimicking diagnoses such as myelodysplastic syndrome, acute myeloid leukemia, or aplastic anemia; all of which may present with macrocytosis, reduced reticulocyte count, and pancytopenia. Careful evaluation of blood smear for any dysplastic changes or atypical neutrophils as well as determination of serum vitamin B12 levels would help reach the accurate diagnosis. Bone marrow biopsy is generally not indicated if vitamin B12 deficiency is identified. All patients with total gastrectomy should be closely monitored for vitamin B12 and iron deficiency.

REFERENCES:

Hu Y, Kim H, Hyung W, et al. Vitamin B(12) deficiency after gastrectomy for gastric cancer: an analysis of clinical patterns and risk factors. *Ann Surg.* 2013 Dec;258(6):970–975.

Rosania R, Chiapponi C, Malfertheiner P, et al. Nutrition in patients with gastric cancer: An update. *Gastrointest Tumors.* 2016 May;2(4):178–187.

10. ANSWER: B. Ramucirumab is a recombinant monoclonal antibody of the IgG1 class that binds to the VEGFR-2, blocking receptor activation. Trials have shown a survival benefit for therapy with ramucirumab, either as monotherapy or in combination with paclitaxel in patients with previously treated advanced esophagogastric adenocarcinoma. The phase III RAINBOW trial added ramucirumab or placebo to weekly paclitaxel in 665 patients with metastatic esophagogastric adenocarcinoma who had disease progression on or within four months after first-line platinum and fluoropyrimidine-based combination therapy. The combination treatment was associated with an improved median progression-free (4.4 vs. 2.9 months) and overall survival (9.6 vs. 7.4 months; HR 0.807; 95% CI 0.678 to 0.962; $P = 0.017$). Based on this and the REGARD trial, ramucirumab as monotherapy or in combination with paclitaxel is a reasonable treatment option for the second-line treatment of patients with advanced esophagogastric cancer. Bevacizumab, cetuximab, and panitumumab have each failed to demonstrate benefit in similar patients through randomized trials.

REFERENCE:

Wilke H, Muro K, Van Cutsem E, et al. Ramucirumab plus paclitaxel versus placebo plus paclitaxel in patients with previously treated advanced gastric or gastro-oesophageal junction adenocarcinoma (RAINBOW): a double-blind, randomized phase 3 trial. *Lancet Oncol.* 2014 Oct;15(11):1224–1235.

Biliary Tract Cancer 6

Davendra P. S. Sohal and Alok A. Khorana

REVIEW QUESTIONS

1. A 53-year-old woman with a history of hypertension and hypothyroidism presented to the ER with complaints of right upper quadrant discomfort for the past 3 to 4 days. The pain is nonradiating and is described as dull in nature. She stated that there was no correlation with her diet; however, the patient has experienced decreased appetite over the past 2 weeks. She also noted an unintentional 12 lb weight loss. She is afebrile. Physical examination reveals tenderness over the right upper quadrant, and no jaundice or ascites. Labs: WBC 8,600/μL, hemoglobin 14.4 g/dL, Platelet count was 232,000/mL, AST 28 IU/L, ALT 41 IU /L, total bilirubin 1.1 mg/dL, and alkaline phosphatase 77 IU /L. An ultrasound revealed a thickened gallbladder wall. No evidence of cholelithiasis. The bile duct diameter was estimated to be 6 mm. The patient was initially sent home with a short course of antibiotics, however returned within 48 hours with worsening pain and persistent nausea. CT abdomen and pelvis was nonrevealing. MRCP revealed a small polyp within the posterior aspect of the gallbladder wall. The patient underwent a cholecystectomy the following morning. Few gallstones were noted within the gallbladder. A small polyp was seen at the posterior aspect of the gallbladder wall. Pathology revealed a well-differentiated adenocarcinoma consistent with gallbladder cancer. The tumor invaded the muscle layer but not the connective tissue beyond it. Tumor margins were negative. On review of prior CT scan, no lymph nodes were noted within the abdomen or pelvis. What is the next best step in the management of this patient?

   A. Initiate chemotherapeutic treatment with gemcitabine/cisplatin

   B. Observation

    C. Intraoperative staging with possible extended cholecystectomy

    D. Hospice discussion with patient and family

---

2. A 66-year-old man with no significant medical history is admitted to the hospital with right upper quadrant pain, low-grade fevers and worsening jaundice for the past 3 to 4 weeks. On further discussion, the patient states he has unintentionally lost approximately 30 lbs over the past 3 months. Physical examination revealed overt icterus; the patient appeared to be in mild distress secondary to pain. No masses were appreciated in the abdomen; however, there was tenderness to palpation over the right upper quadrant and mid epigastric region. The remainder of the physical examination was unremarkable. Blood work revealed abnormal liver function tests. Alkaline phosphatase was elevated to 381 IU /L. Total bilirubin was 7.2 mg/dL with direct bilirubin 6.6 mg/dL. AST and ALT were both at the upper limits of normal levels. WBC was mildly elevated to 12,000/µL with a normal differential. CEA and CA 19-9 were normal. AFP was normal. An ultrasound revealed the common bile duct to be dilated to 1.8 cm. There was no direct evidence of cholelithiasis. CT scan of the chest, abdomen, and pelvis confirmed the common bile duct dilation but also revealed a distal ductal mass as the likely source of the obstruction. Imaging also revealed diffuse abdominal lymphadenopathy. An ERCP was performed and brush cytology from the distal portion of the common bile duct was consistent with a poorly differentiated adenocarcinoma. During laparoscopic staging, the tumor appeared to involve the head of the pancreas as well as the gallbladder. It also appeared to be wrapped around the base of the celiac axis. The tumor at this time was determined to be unresectable. A biliary stent was placed for symptomatic control. What is the next best step in the management of this patient?

    A. Surveillance

    B. Initiate single-agent chemotherapy with gemcitabine

    C. Begin combination chemotherapy with gemcitabine and cisplatin

    D. Neoadjuvant chemoradiation with gemcitabine

---

3. Which of the following is associated with an increased risk of biliary tract cancer?

    A. Hepatitis C infection

    B. Human immunodeficiency virus infection

C. Tuberculosis

D. Ulcerative colitis

---

4. Which of the following targeted therapies has been shown to be effective in the treatment of biliary tract cancer?

A. Bevacizumab

B. Cetuximab

C. Trastuzumab

D. None of the above

---

5. A 64-year-old man presents with abdominal discomfort. Evaluation includes the ultrasound of the right upper quadrant followed by a CT scan of the abdomen and pelvis, and they demonstrate a 3 cm mass in the left lobe of the liver. Percutaneous biopsy reveals adenocarcinoma. Completion of staging with a CT chest shows no evidence of any other sites of disease. The patient undergoes resection of the left lobe of the liver along with portal node dissection. Final pathology reveals an intrahepatic cholangiocarcinoma, present at resected parenchymal margin, and present in 4 of 5 nodes. What is the next best step in management?

A. Adjuvant chemotherapy with capecitabine

B. Surveillance

ANSWERS TO REVIEW QUESTIONS

1. ANSWER: C. This patient has been diagnosed with a stage I (T1b N0 M0) well-differentiated gallbladder adenocarcinoma, which was incidentally found postsurgical resection. Extended cholecystectomy is recommended. Observation alone is not sufficient as 5-year OS for T1bN0M0 disease is only 50% to 65% (observation may be appropriate for T1aN0M0 disease but only after a careful risk-benefit assessment).

2. ANSWER: C. The patient discussed above appears to have a stage III (T4 N1 M0) poorly differentiated extrahepatic cholangiocarcinoma. Surgical resection (R0) remains the only possibility for cure; however, due to tumor involvement of the blood vessels, the tumor is unresectable. Combination chemotherapy with gemcitabine and cisplatin would be appropriate; this regimen has been shown to improve OS compared with single-agent gemcitabine.

3. ANSWER: D. Ulcerative colitis is associated with primary sclerosing cholangitis (PSC), which increases the risk of biliary tract cancer.

4. ANSWER: D. No targeted therapies have been shown to be effective in the treatment of biliary tract cancer.

5. ANSWER: A. A recent randomized trial demonstrated improvement in overall survival in patients randomized to capecitabine for 6 months, compared to observation alone and this is considered the new standard of care.

Primary Cancers of the Liver 7

Bassam Estfan and Alok A. Khorana

REVIEW QUESTIONS

1. A 57-year-old man with a known history of hepatitis C and cirrhosis presents to ER with abdominal swelling, fatigue, and jaundice. Right upper quadrant ultrasound reveals a 4 cm lesion in the right hepatic lobe, ascites, and no biliary dilation. Laboratory data show a bilirubin of 2.5 mg/dL, albumin of 3.3 g/dL, and low platelets (67,000/mm^3). He was admitted for ascites management. Further workup revealed AFP at 67 ng/mL. CT scan of the liver shows a 3.8 cm lesion in segment 8, which expresses arterial enhancement and venous washout on the background of cirrhosis. Ascites and esophageal varices are noted. What is the appropriate next step in management?

   A. Biopsy of the liver mass

   B. Liver resection

   C. Sorafenib

   D. Referral for liver transplantation

   E. Confirm diagnosis with MRI

2. A 67-year-old woman with no known history of cirrhosis or liver disease presented to her internist with epigastric abdominal pain. A mass was felt on physical exam and a single phase CT scan of the abdomen showed a 7 cm mass in segment II. A biopsy confirmed the diagnosis of HCC. AFP was elevated at 430 ng/mL and further workup showed no evidence of metastatic disease. She was referred to a liver surgeon and underwent a

left hepatectomy. She was referred to oncology for discussion of treatment options given "high risk" features on pathology. Pathology review showed the mass to be 7.5 cm, poorly differentiated with microvascular invasion (pT2Nx). Distance to closest margin was 2 mm. There is no evidence of hepatic cirrhosis or fibrosis. You recommend

  A. Adjuvant sorafenib

  B. Radiation to surgical bed

  C. Surveillance with periodical scans and blood work

  D. Adjuvant doxorubicin

3. A 76-year-old male with a history of chronic HBV infection contracted 15 years ago through needle sharing had a routine follow-up with his hepatologist. Prior to his visit a screening ultrasound of the liver showed new "suspicious" lesions in the liver. AFP was <3 ng/mL. Hepatic function and blood counts were normal. An MRI of the liver showed three lesions in both lobes of the liver measuring 1.8, 2, and 2.2 cm with two of them meeting OPTN class 5 criteria. Two of the lesions are subcapsular close to the hepatic dome near the diaphragm, while the other was in segment V. Other medical problems include diabetes and a history of bypass 10 years ago. His case was presented at tumor board. Which of these is an appropriate next step?

  A. Referral for transplantation.

  B. Chemoembolization with drug eluting beads

  C. Supportive care and hospice

  D. Percutaneous radiofrequency ablation

  E. Start sorafenib

4. A 50-year-old male with known history of HCV presented to ER with symptoms of fatigue, weakness, and anorexia. He has not followed with a healthcare provider for more than 5 years. Initial blood work showed a bilirubin of 1.8 mg/dL and elevated liver enzymes. Abdominal CT showed a mass-like diffuse infiltration in segment VI and VII, without clear evidence of cirrhosis. AFP was 35 ng/mL. A biopsy confirmed a diagnosis of HCC. After discharge he was considered for radioembolization. A planning angiogram with technetium macroaggregated albumin showed a

pulmonary shunt of 22%. He comes back to discuss the next step in management. Which of the following should be advised?

    A. Proceed with right hepatic lobe radioembolization

    B. Switch to chemoembolization

    C. Stereotactic body radiation therapy (SBRT)

    D. Start sorafenib

5. A 46-year-old woman with history of well compensated cirrhosis due to chronic HCV infection was diagnosed with metastatic HCC to the lungs. She was started on sorafenib 400 mg BID. After 4 weeks she developed significant palmar plantar erythema and sorafenib dose was decreased to 200 mg BID. She had stable disease for 7 months after which restaging scans showed progressive disease in the lung and new mild pleural effusion. She continues to be asymptomatic and has a good performance status. Which of the following options you should recommend first?

    A. Clinical trial

    B. Increase dose of sorafenib

    C. Referral to hospice

    D. Systemic doxorubicin

    E. Nivolumab

ANSWERS TO REVIEW QUESTIONS

1. ANSWER: D. This patient has evidence of cirrhosis and portal hypertension with imaging findings characteristic of HCC. An AFP > 400 ng/mL is not a requirement for diagnosis. A biopsy of the mass is not likely to provide further diagnostic advantage and may be associated with needle tract seeding in the future. Furthermore, a confirmatory second-imaging modality is not needed as positive findings on CT scan alone are diagnostic. The presence of portal hypertension and thrombocytopenia makes this patient ineligible for resection due to increased risk of acute hepatic failure after surgery. Based on available information he has a moderately compensating liver function with Child Pugh Class B cirrhosis at least, and his 2-year survival from cirrhosis is less than 60%. This HCC is within Milan criteria for transplantation; according to the American Association for the Study of Liver Disease (AASLD) guidelines and BCLC staging system this patient should be considered for transplantation as a cure from both HCC and cirrhosis. He may be a candidate for transarterial chemoembolization as a "bridging" therapy to transplantation. Furthermore, with the availability of highly effective treatment for HCV infection, this should be managed prior to transplantation. Sorafenib is a systemic therapy for advanced HCC not amenable to curative or locoregional treatment options.

2. ANSWER: C. This patient has a completely resected HCC on the background of a normal liver. She received optimal upfront surgical resection for HCC. While there is an increased risk of recurrence given size, differentiation, and microvascular invasion, there is no evidence that additional treatment would prevent local or systemic recurrence. The phase III STORM trial randomized patients after resection or ablation with curative intent to either sorafenib or placebo for 4 years. There was no difference in time to progression between groups. This patient will need closer follow up with imaging and laboratory testing such as AFP to evaluate recurrence. There is no role for adjuvant radiation especially with a complete resection.

3. ANSWER: B. This patient has an at risk liver due to HBV infection and imaging findings of at least 2 lesions consistent with HCC (OPTN 5 lesion). While the third lesion is not reported as consistent with HCC, it would be highly suspicious of being such. Either way these lesions are within Milan criteria for transplantation. Despite an otherwise unimpressive comorbidities, he would generally be considered old for transplantation. First consideration should be given to potentially curative options. Surgical resection (not listed as an option) is not a good option for multifocal HCC. While RFA can be a reasonable option for smaller lesions like these, a percutaneous approach is not likely to be feasible especially for dome lesions. A laparoscopic approach might be considered. In an otherwise healthy individual with no evidence of advanced or extrahepatic disease sorafenib or supportive care should not be considered upfront options. Of options presented chemoembolization offers a good means of local control that is well tolerated with the use of drug eluting beads.

4. ANSWER: D. This patient has an otherwise relatively preserved liver function with a diffuse type HCC in the right hepatic lobe. A diffuse HCC is not amenable to curative treatment options such as surgery or transplantation. Defining borders of involvement can be challenging. While radioembolization is generally the preferred locoregional treatment option for diffuse type HCC, a pulmonary shunt of 22% is high and puts patients at risk of radiation pneumonitis. Thus proceeding with radioembolization is not advisable. Both SBRT and chemoembolization are not indicated for large diffuse HCC. In the absence of options for locoregional treatment, this advanced HCC should be managed with sorafenib.

5. ANSWER: E. While patients should always be encouraged to participate in clinical trials where available, nivolumab, a checkpoint inhibitor antibody, is approved in the second line setting for the treatment of HCC that has progressed on sorafenib. Increasing the dose of sorafenib is unlikely to be associated with added benefit and likely to cause worsened side effects. There is no evidence that systemic chemotherapy with doxorubicin offers survival advantage in advanced HCC. Of note regorafenib can also be an option in the second line setting. With the current presentation a referral to hospice is premature.

Gastrointestinal Stromal Tumors (GIST) 8

Dale R. Shepard and Alok A. Khorana

REVIEW QUESTIONS

1. A 54-year-old male underwent surgical resection of a gastric mass found on upper endoscopy as part of a workup for anemia. Pathology revealed a 5.8 cm gastrointestinal stromal tumor with >10 mitoses per 50 HPF. The next best step in management is

    A. Observation

    B. Adjuvant radiation therapy

    C. Adjuvant chemotherapy with doxorubicin

    D. Adjuvant imatinib for 1 year

    E. Adjuvant imatinib for 3 years

2. Which of the following best describes the likely origin of GIST?

    A. The serosal layer of stomach

    B. Interstitial cells of cajal

    C. Goblet cells of the endothelium

    D. Lamina propria of the submucosa

3. Which of the following best describes the clinical presentation of patients with GIST?

    A. Many patients are asymptomatic

    B. Most patients have diarrhea and wheezing

C. Some patients have weight loss and jaundice

D. Most patients present with gastrointestinal bleeding.

---

4. Which of the following is true about imaging for patients with GIST?

    A. PET scans should be used to monitor response to treatment

    B. PET scans should be used to determine the duration of treatment

    C. CT of the chest should be obtained every 3 months to monitor for metastatic disease

    D. CT of the abdomen and pelvis should be obtained every 3 to 6 months to assess response.

---

5. A 62-year-old man is found to have a tumor in the duodenum with some nodule in the liver. A biopsy of the liver lesion confirms a diagnosis of GIST with mutational analysis showing a mutation in exon 9. He starts treatment imatinib 400 mg daily. After 6 months, the CT of the abdomen a pelvis shows progressive disease. What is the next best step in management?

    A. Increase the dose of imatinib to 400 mg twice daily

    B. Discontinue imatinib and enroll in a clinical trial

    C. Discontinue imatinib and start treatment with sunitinib.

    D. Discontinue imatinib and initiate therapy with doxorubicin plus ifosfamide

ANSWERS TO REVIEW QUESTIONS

1. ANSWER: E. Adjuvant imatinib for 3 years. The patient has a high risk of recurrence based on the size and mitotic rate of the tumor. There are no data for adjuvant therapy with either radiation therapy or cytotoxic chemotherapy in GIST.

2. ANSWER: B. GIST is thought to originate in the interstitial cells of cajal, which are also dependent on KIT for their activity.

3. ANSWER: A. While some patients with large tumors may have pain or bleeding as symptoms, many patients are asymptomatic. Diarrhea and flushing are characteristic of neuroendocrine tumors, not GIST.

4. ANSWER: D. Patients receiving imatinib for GIST should have a CT of the abdomen and pelvis every 3 to 6 months to assess response. The role of PET scans is not clear and there are not recommendations for monitoring response with this imaging.

5. ANSWER: A. The dose of imatinib should be increased to 400 mg twice daily due to the higher likelihood of resistance to imatinib in patients with a mutation in exon 9. The current recommendation is to increase the dose of imatinib to 800 mg daily if patients are not responding to the standard initial dose of 400 mg daily before changing to a new therapy.

Colorectal Cancer 9

Jason S. Starr and Thomas J. George, Jr.

1. A 50-year-old female is referred after her first routine screening colonoscopy. A 2-cm sessile polyp was identified in the sigmoid colon. The gastroenterologist who did the colonoscopy reports that she "got everything." The biopsy reveals adenocarcinoma invading into the submucosa with a positive margin. What do you recommend as the next step in the management of this patient?

    A. Partial colectomy with removal of regional lymph nodes

    B. Repeat colonoscopy in one year

    C. Repeat colonoscopy with further endoscopic resection

    D. Repeat colonoscopy in 3 months with repeat biopsy

    E. No further follow-up is needed

2. All of the following are correct regarding the revised Bethesda guidelines for identifying patients with possible hereditary nonpolyposis colorectal cancer (HNPCC/Lynch syndrome), except

    A. Colorectal cancer diagnosed in a patient who is less than 40 years of age

    B. Presence of synchronous, metachronous colorectal, or other HNPCC-associated tumors, regardless of age

    C. Colorectal cancer diagnosed in a patient with one or more first-degree relatives with an HNPCC-related tumor, with one of the cancers being diagnosed under age 50

    D. Colorectal cancer diagnosed in a patient with two or more first- or second-degree relatives with HNPCC-related tumors, regardless of age

3. A 48-year-old male presented to his primary care physician with chief complaint of 6 months of progressive fatigue. Labs revealed a hemoglobin of 11 g/dl and a mean corpuscular volume (MCV) of 68. This led to a colonoscopy of revealing a 3 cm friable, fungating mass at the cecum. A biopsy revealed poorly differentiated mucinous adenocarcinoma with increased infiltrating lymphocytes. What is the most likely underlying genomic mechanism resulting in this patient's neoplasm?

    A. Loss of heterozygosity of chromosome 17p

    B. Germline defect in DNA mismatch-repair genes

    C. STK11 gene mutation

    D. Loss of heterozygosity of chromosome 18q

    E. Mutation in APC gene

4. A 50-year-old male presents to you for further recommendations for recently diagnosed colon cancer status post a right hemicolectomy. Pathology revealed poorly differentiated adenocarcinoma invading into the muscularis propria (T3) with perineural and lymphovascular invasion and zero out of thirteen lymph nodes. Adjuvant chemotherapy is being considered; which of the following should be ordered before making a final decision?

    A. CEA

    B. PET/CT

    C. Microsatellite status

    D. Bone scan

    E. EGFR mutation status

5. The 2016 United States Preventive Services Task Force (USPSTF) guidelines include all the following as acceptable methods of colorectal cancer screening in average risk individuals, except

    A. Double barium enema

    B. CT colonography

    C. Colonoscopy

    D. Multitarget stool DNA test

    E. Sigmoidoscopy with fecal immunohistochemical testing (FIT)

6. A 61-year-old male underwent surgical resection 4 weeks ago with end-to-end anastomosis for a sigmoid colon adenocarcinoma. The tumor was 2.5 cm and extended into the muscularis propria, and margins were free of cancer. Fifteen lymph nodes were resected; four were positive for adenocarcinoma. A CT scan of the chest, abdomen, and pelvis showed no evidence of distant metastatic disease. He has healed well and is referred to oncology. Which of the following treatment is recommended after surgery?

    A. Adjuvant chemotherapy with a fluoropyrimidine-based therapy for 6 months

    B. Adjuvant chemotherapy with a fluoropyrimidine-based therapy for 12 months

    C. Adjuvant chemotherapy with a fluoropyrimidine-based therapy with oxaliplatin for 6 months

    D. Postoperative external beam radiotherapy

    E. Observation

7. (FIRST PART) A 63-year-old female was recently diagnosed with Stage IIIC colon adenocarcinoma of the sigmoid. Her oncologist recommended a course of fluoropyrimidine-based adjuvant therapy with oxaliplatin. Two days after beginning treatment the patient developed severe (grade 3) mucositis. The patient was treated with intravenous fluids and local therapies for her mouth pain. The following week the patient reported fever of 102 F. Labs were drawn and revealed hemoglobin 11 g/dl, platelets 20,000/μL, and white blood cell count 700/μL with an absolute neutrophil count of 0. What is the most likely cause of the patient's ongoing toxicity?

    A. UGT1A1 variant

    B. Oxaliplatin toxicity

    C. Serotonin syndrome

    D. Fluorouracil overdose

    E. Dihydropyrimidine dehydrogenase deficiency

8. (SECOND PART) The patient was identified to have dihydropyrimidine deficiency (heterozygous DPYD*2A) 10 days after administration of fluorouracil. Unfortunately, she continued to have profound prolonged neutropenia and died of septic shock with multiorgan failure. What therapy could have potentially been life-saving if given within 96 hours of fluorouracil administration?

    A. Leucovorin

    B. Glucarpidase

    C. Uridine triacetate

    D. Atropine

    E. Methylene blue

9. A 58-year-old male is evaluated for several months of fatigue, abdominal pain, lower back tenderness, and 25-pound unintentional weight loss. Examination is notable for tender hepatomegaly. Laboratory tests reveal a total bilirubin 3 mg/dL, direct bilirubin 2.2 mg/dL, AST 72 units/L, ALT 65 units/L, alkaline phosphatase 212 units/L, creatinine 0.8 mg/dL. CEA is elevated at 478. A CT chest, abdomen, and pelvis shows multiple, hypodense lesions in the right and left hepatic lobes and small bilateral pulmonary nodules. A biopsy of a liver lesion confirms poorly differentiated adenocarcinoma, CK20 positive, CK7 negative, CDX2 positive, supporting the diagnosis of a colorectal malignancy. Molecular mutations in which of the following should be assessed to complete his evaluation?

    A. B-*raf*

    B. K-*ras*

    C. N-*ras*

    D. DNA mismatch repair system

    E. All of the above

10. A 54-year-old female complains of difficulty passing stool and rectal fullness for 2 months. Her medical history is otherwise negative. A colonoscopy shows a 4 cm rectal mass located 8 cm from the anal verge, and biopsy confirms adenocarcinoma. An endoscopic rectal ultrasound shows the lesion penetrates through the muscularis propria and three regional lymph nodes are involved. A CT of chest, abdomen, and pelvis does not

reveal any overt distant metastases. What is the recommended treatment for her rectal cancer?

    A. Surgical resection followed by adjuvant chemotherapy and radiation

    B. Neoadjuvant combined chemotherapy and radiation followed by surgical resection

    C. Definitive chemotherapy and radiation therapy

    D. Neoadjuvant combined chemotherapy and radiation, surgical resection, then postoperative chemotherapy

    E. Transanal microsurgery followed by radiation therapy

11. A 76-year-old male was recently diagnosed with stage IV rectal cancer. His rectal primary tumor is asymptomatic and CT of the chest, abdomen, and pelvis revealed innumerable liver metastasis. Biopsy of a liver metastasis reveals pathologic findings consistent with colorectal adenocarcinoma. Molecular analysis determined a K-*ras* (p. G12V) mutation. The patient is started on treatment with FOLFOX and bevacizumab. After the second cycle of treatment the patient develops severe lower abdominal pain. An abdominal x-ray in the emergency department reveals free air in the abdomen. Which of the following drugs was most likely responsible for these new findings?

    A. Fluorouracil

    B. Bevacizumab

    C. Leucovorin

    D. Oxaliplatin

12. A 59-year-old female with a PMH of hypertension and anxiety was recently diagnosed with stage IIIB colon cancer. Her oncologist recommended she be treated with adjuvant fluoropyrimidine-based chemotherapy. She started her treatment today and 4 hours into her treatment she developed severe crushing chest pain. What is the most likely etiology of this patient's chest pain?

    A. Pulmonary embolism

    B. Coronary vasospasm

    C. Rib fracture

    D. Aortic dissection

    E. Esophageal spasm

13. You are asked to evaluate a 68-year-old female for a second opinion. Patient had a history of stage IIIA colon cancer diagnosed 1 year
ago. She went on to receive 6 months of adjuvant flouropyrimidine-
based chemotherapy. About 3 months ago she developed increasing
diffuse abdominal discomfort. CT of the chest, abdomen, and pelvis
revealed extensive peritoneal disease. Molecular testing of the original
tumor specimen reveals a B-*raf* mutation with mismatch-repair proteins intact. What is this patient's approximate median OS for stage IV
disease?

    A. 36–42 months

    B. 12–18 months

    C. 24–30 months

    D. Less than 6 months

14. A 72-year-old male is being treated for K-*ras* mutated metastatic colon
cancer. The patient has been on FOLFOX with bevacizumab for the last
9 months and has developed progression of liver and lung lesions. Which
of the following targeted therapies would be reasonable to add to FOLFIRI
for second-line treatment?

    A. Ziv-aflibercept

    B. Bevacizumab

    C. Ramucirumab

    D. Any of the above

15. A 75-year-old male with stage IV colon cancer, K-*ras*/N-*ras* wild-type,
presents to start first-line treatment with FOLFIRI and bevacizumab.
Approximately 2 hours into the infusion the patient developed emesis,
abdominal cramping, diaphoresis. On evaluation you recommend which
of the following treatments?

    A. Diphenhydramine

    B. Atropine

    C. Paregoric

    D. Methylprednisolone

    E. Epinephrine

16. A 62-year-old male with stage IV (K-*ras* mutated, B-*raf* wildtype) colon cancer presents with a sigmoid mass and resectable synchronous liver metastasis. The patient reports normal bowel movements and denies hematochezia. He is started on FOLFOX and bevacizumab prior to planned surgery. When should the bevacizumab be stopped prior to surgery?

    A. 1–3 weeks

    B. 4–8 weeks

    C. 9–12 weeks

    D. No need to stop

17. A 78-year-old female is diagnosed with stage IV (K-*ras*/N-*ras*/B-*raf* wildtype) colon cancer. Patient is very functional with an ECOG performance status of 0. Her only past medical history is hypertension and hyperlipidemia. She is started on treatment with FOLFOX and an EGFR antibody. After her fourth cycle she presented to the emergency department because she reported "not feeling right." In the emergency department the patient went into cardiac arrest. Which of the following is the likely abnormality responsible for her cardiac arrest?

    A. Hypokalemia

    B. Hyperkalemia

    C. Hypomagnesemia

    D. Hypocalcemia

    E. Hypophosphatemia

18. A 65-year-old male with refractory metastatic colon cancer (N-*ras* mutation) presents for evaluation and treatment recommendations. The patient's disease progressed through first-line FOLFOX and bevacizumab as well as second-line FOLFIRI and bevacizumab. His ECOG performance status is currently 1. The patient has required granulocyte-colony stimulating factor throughout second-line treatment, and required hospital admission 3 weeks ago for neutropenic fever. Surveillance CT of the chest, abdomen, and pelvis revealed enlarging pulmonary nodules and liver masses. Which of the following third-line treatment options would be optimal for this patient?

    A. Regorafenib

    B. Trifluridine and tipiracil

C. Irinotecan and EGFR antibody

D. Capecitabine

---

19. A 57-year-old female presents for evaluation and discussion of adjuvant therapy. She underwent surgical resection 3 weeks ago for a colon mass at the hepatic flexure. The tumor was a 3 cm poorly differentiated adenocarcinoma with extension through the muscularis propria with margins free of cancer. Fourteen lymph nodes were resected; none were involved with adenocarcinoma. Further molecular analysis of the tumor revealed absence of immunohistochemical staining for *MSH6*. A CT scan of the chest, abdomen, and pelvis showed no evidence of distant metastatic disease. Which of the following treatments is recommended after surgery?

    A. Adjuvant chemotherapy with a fluoropyrmidine-based therapy for 6 months

    B. Adjuvant chemotherapy with a fluoropyrimidine-based therapy for 3 months

    C. Adjuvant chemotherapy with a fluoropyrimidine-based therapy with oxaliplatin for 6 months

    D. Observation

---

20. A 78-year-old male presents for evaluation of recently resected stage IIIA colon adenocarcinoma. CT chest, abdomen, and pelvis showed no evidence of metastasis. The patient's ECOG performance status is 0 and his medical history consists of hypertension, hyperlipidemia, and type II insulin dependent diabetes mellitus. On questioning he reports numbness in his feet. The patient works as a jeweler. He wants to be as aggressive as possible with his treatment plan. What type of adjuvant treatment would you recommend?

    A. Adjuvant chemotherapy with a fluoropyrimidine-based therapy for 6 months

    B. Adjuvant chemotherapy with a fluoropyrimidine-based therapy for 12 months

    C. Adjuvant chemotherapy with a fluoropyrimidine-based therapy with oxaliplatin for 6 months

    D. Observation

21. A 32-year-old female presents for evaluation of ongoing fatigue. Laboratory evaluation reveals a hemoglobin 9.4 g/dl, mean corpuscular volume 68, and a ferritin of 5 ng/ml. On questioning she reports regular menses that last about 4 days. Her medical history is notable for a "bowel obstruction" at age 14 requiring a bowel resection. A colonoscopy is pursued and reveals a 5 cm friable, nonobstructing mass in the ascending colon along with multiple polyps throughout the colon. Biopsies of the ascending colon mass revealed moderately differentiated adenocarcinoma. The polyps were consistent with gastrointestinal hamartomas. You discuss with the patient you have a high suspicion for which of the following genetic syndromes?

    A. Lynch syndrome

    B. Peutz-Jeghers Syndrome

    C. Gardner Syndrome

    D. Li-Fraumeni Syndrome

    E. Turcot Syndrome

22. A 70 year-old female presents with newly diagnosed stage IV colon cancer. She is found to have a cecal mass with multiple peritoneal implants and retroperitoneal lymphadenopathy. Biopsy of the cecal mass reveals poorly differentiated adenocarcinoma. Molecular analysis of the tumor reveals B-*raf* mutation (V600E), K-*ras*/N-*ras* wild-type, and microsatellite instability high on polymerase chain reaction (PCR). Which of the following DNA mismatch-repair proteins would you expect to be absent?

    A. MLH1

    B. MSH2

    C. TP53

    D. MSH6

    E. PMS2

23. A 63-year-old-male was recently diagnosed with stage IV colon cancer (K-*ras*/N-*ras* wildtype, B-*raf* wildtype) presents for evaluation. The patient reports a 10-pound weight loss and mild right upper quadrant pain. He has an ECOG performance status of 0 and no significant past medical history. CT chest, abdomen, and pelvis reveals innumerable liver metastasis. The patient asks you to prescribe the "best stuff you got." After reviewing

the risks of benefits of treatment with the patient, which of the following first-line palliative regimens do you recommend?

    A. FOLFOX and VEGF antibody

    B. FOLFIRI and VEGF antibody

    C. FOLFOX and EGFR antibody

    D. FOLFIRI and EGFR antibody

    E. Any of the above

24. (FIRST PART) A 21-year-old female with a family history of familial adenomatous polyposis (FAP) presents to clinic to discuss her risk of colorectal cancer. She reports her mother was diagnosed with FAP in her 20's. A colonoscopy on the patient reveals innumerable (>100) polyps throughout the colon and rectum. The diagnosis of FAP is confirmed with genetic testing. You recommend the patient undergo a total proctocolectomy. Before committing to the surgery, she would like to know her lifetime risk of developing colorectal cancer. What do you tell her the risk is?

    A. 30%

    B. 60%

    C. 80%

    D. 100%

25. (SECOND PART) On genetic testing, a mutation resulting in functional loss of which gene product would you expect to find for the above patient?

    A. APC

    B. BRCA

    C. TP53

    D. MUTYH

    E. Any one of the DNA mismatch-repair genes

ANSWERS TO REVIEW QUESTIONS

1. ANSWER: A

Rationale:

Patients with unfavorable histologic features (high grade, angiolymphatic invasion, or positive/indeterminate margin) of the malignant polyp should undergo partial colectomy with removal of regional lymph nodes. For a malignant polyp without unfavorable histologic features, it would be reasonable to perform an endoscopic polypectomy followed by observation and repeat colonoscopy in one year.

REFERENCES:

NCCN Clinical Practice Guidelines in Oncology. *Colon Cancer*. https://www.nccn.org/professionals/physician_gls/pdf/colon.pdf. Accessed on September 10, 2016.

Ueno H, Mochizuki H, Hashiguchi Y, et al. Risk factors for an adverse outcome in early invasive colorectal carcinoma. *Gastroenterology*. 2004;127:385–394.

Seltz U, Bohnacker S, Seewald S, et al. Is endoscopic polypectomy an adequate therapy for malignant colorectal polyps? *Dis Colon Rectum*. 2004;47:1789–1797.

2. ANSWER: A

Rationale:

The revised Bethesda guidelines for testing colorectal tumors for microsatellite instability include the following:

1. Colorectal cancer diagnosed in a patient who is less than **50** years of age
2. Presence of synchronous, metachronous colorectal, or other HNPCC-associated tumors, regardless of age
3. Colorectal cancer with MSI-H-like histology diagnosed in a patient who is less than 60 years of age
4. Colorectal cancer diagnosed in a patient with one of more first-degree relatives with an HNPCC-related tumor, with one of the cancers being diagnosed under age 50 years
5. Colorectal cancer diagnosed in a patient with two or more first- or second-degree relatives with HNPCC-related tumors, regardless of age.

The sensitivity and specificity of these guidelines has been reported at 82% and 98%, respectively.

REFERENCES:

Piñol V, Castells A, Andreu M, et al. Accuracy of revised Bethesda Guidelines, microsatellite instability, and immunohistochemistry for the identification of patients with hereditary nonpolyposis colorectal cancer. *JAMA*. 2005;293(16):1986–1994.

Umar A, Boland CR, Terdiman JP, et al. Revised Bethesda Guidelines for hereditary nonpolyposis colorectal cancer (Lynch syndrome) and microsatellite instability. *J Natl Cancer Inst*. 2004;96(4):261–268.

3. ANSWER: B

Rationale:

The patient has histologic and clinical features concerning for hereditary nonpolyposis colorectal cancer (HNPCC). These features include poorly differentiated histology with mucinous features, increased tumor infiltrating lymphocytes, right-sided lesion, and age less than 50. The pathogenesis of malignancy in HNPCC is a germline defect in DNA mismatch-repair genes. Most commonly this involves germline loss of *MLH1* or *MSH2*.

REFERENCE:

Vilar, E, Gruber SB. Microsatellite instability in colorectal cancer – the stable evidence. *Nat Rev Clin Oncol.* 2010;7:153–162.

4. ANSWER: C

Rationale:

Determining microsatellite status would be important before making a treatment decision in this patient with moderate risk stage II colon cancer. Patients with microsatellite instability high (MSI-H), or deficient mismatch-repair system (dMMR), stage II colon cancer do not appear to benefit from adjuvant fluoropyrimidine-based chemotherapy and have an exceptionally good prognosis with surgery alone. A CT scan prior to surgery, not PET/CT, would be indicated for staging purposes. Epidermal Growth Factor Receptor (EGFR) mutational status has no bearing on prognosis or treatment selection in colorectal cancer. Preoperative CEA does have prognostic value but should not influence treatment decision.

REFERENCES:

Benson AB, Schrag D, Somerfield MR, et al. American Society of Clinical Oncology recommendations on adjuvant chemotherapy for stage II colon cancer. *J Clin Oncol.* 2004;22:3408–3419.

Sargent DJ, Marsoni S, Monges G, et al. Defective mismatch repair as a predictive marker for lack of efficacy of fluorouracil-based adjuvant therapy in colon cancer. *J Clin Oncol.* 2010;28: 3219–3226.

5. ANSWER: A

Rationale:

The 2016 USPSTF guidelines for colorectal screening in average risk individuals does not include double barium enema as an acceptable option for screening. The following are acceptable screening options supported by the USPSTF:

- Colonoscopy
- Fecal immunochemical testing (FIT) for occult blood
- Sigmoidoscopy plus FIT
- CT colonography
- Multitargeted stool DNA testing

- Guaiac-based fecal occult blood testing
- Sigmoidoscopy alone

The USPSTF does not support one screening test over another.

REFERENCE:

US Preventive Services Task Force. Screening for colorectal cancer: US Preventive Services Task Force recommendation statement. *JAMA.* 2016;315(23):2564–2575.

6. ANSWER: C

Rationale:

This patient has stage IIIB (pT3N2aM0) colon cancer, and adjuvant chemotherapy is indicated to decrease risk of relapse and improve chances of survival. A fluoropyrimidine (5-FU)-based therapy with oxaliplatin for 6 months would be the most appropriate recommendation based on the results from both the MOSAIC and NSABP C-07 studies.

REFERENCES:

Andre' T et al. Oxaliplatin, fluorouracil, and leucovorin as adjuvant treatment for colon cancer (MOSIAC). *NEJM.* 2004;350:2343–2351.

Kuebler JP, Wieand HS, O'Connell MJ, et al. Oxaliplatin combined with weekly bolus fluorouracil and leucovorin as surgical adjuvant chemotherapy for stage II and III colon cancer: results from NSABP C-07. *J Clin Oncol.* 2007;25(16):2198–2204.

Moertel CG et al. Levamisole and fluorouracil for adjuvant therapy of resected colon carcinoma. *N Engl J Med.* 1990;322:352–358.

7. ANSWER: E

Rationale:

Dihydropyrimidine dehydrogenase deficiency (DPD) is the most likely cause of the patient's current presentation. DPD is the rate-limiting step in 5-FU catabolism. Approximately 3% to 5% of the general population have heterozygous mutations involving the *DPYD* gene. Fluorouracil overdose is certainly possible in this vignette and the medical record should be reviewed as such. UGT1A1 variants portend for toxicity with irinotecan. Acute oxaliplatin toxicity usually results in neurotoxicity, particularly laryngopharyngeal dysesthesia and cold-induced distal dysesthesias.

REFERENCE:

van Kuilenburg AB. Dihydropyrimidine dehydrogenase and the efficacy and toxicity of 5-fluorouracil. *Eur J Cancer.* 2004; 40(7):939–950.

8. ANSWER: C

Rationale:

Uridine triacetate is a pyrimidine analogue and competitively inhibits cell damage and cytotoxicity caused by fluorouracil. This drug was FDA approved for the emergency treatment of adult and pediatric patients following a fluorouracil overdose AND/OR early-onset, unusually severe adverse reactions (i.e., gastrointestinal toxicity, mucositis, neutropenia). The drug must be given within 96 hours of fluoropyrimidine exposure. Leucovorin is a potentiating agent when given with fluoropyrimidines to improve the inhibition of thymidylate synthase. Glucarpidase is an FDA-approved enzyme used to inactivate methotrexate.

REFERENCE:

Ison G, Beaver JA, McGuinn DW, et al. FDA Approval: Uridine triacetate for the treatment of patients following fluorouracil or capecitabine overdose or exhibiting early-onset severe toxicities following administration of these drugs. *Clin Cancer Res*. 2016;22(18):4545–4549.

9. ANSWER: E

Rationale:

Patients with metastatic colorectal should have molecular profiling including assessments of B-*raf*, K-*ras*, N-*ras*, and DNA mismatch repair components as a part of their initial evaluation. K-*ras* and N-*ras* mutations are negative predictors of response to EGFR therapy and thus preclude treatment with anti-EGFR antibodies. B-*raf* mutations portend for a particularly poor prognosis and may necessitate the use of more aggressive cytotoxic chemotherapy. It should be noted that K-*ras*/N-*ras* mutations are mutually exclusive of B-*raf* mutations. DNA mismatch repair system evaluation is important for consideration of hereditary nonpolyposis colorectal cancer (Lynch syndrome). Additionally, DNA mismatch repair system deficient colorectal cancers appear to be sensitive to immunotherapy.

REFERENCES:

NCCN Clinical Practice Guidelines in Oncology. *Colon Cancer*. https://www.nccn.org/professionals/physician_gls/pdf/colon.pdf. Accessed on September 10, 2016.

Karapetis CS, Khambata-Ford S, Jonker D, et al. K-ras mutations and benefit from cetuximab in advanced colorectal cancer. *N Engl J Med*. 2008;359:1757–1765.

10. ANSWER: D

Rationale:

Multimodality treatment is indicated in this patient with stage IIIB (cT3N1M0) rectal cancer. Endoscopic rectal ultrasound and/or MRI of the rectum should be performed for clinical staging. Rectal tumors that are T3 or greater and/or with clinical N1-2 lymph nodes should receive neoadjuvant chemoradiation followed by surgery, followed by chemotherapy (for a total of 6 perioperative months of chemotherapy).

REFERENCES:

NCCN Clinical Practice Guidelines in Oncology. Colon Cancer. https://www.nccn.org/professionals/physician_gls/pdf/colon.pdf. Accessed on September 10, 2016.

Sauer R, Becker H, Hohenberger W, et al. Preoperative versus postoperative chemoradiotherapy for rectal cancer. *N Engl J Med*. 2004;351:1731–1740.

11. ANSWER: B

Rationale:

The patient unfortunately suffered a complication of bowel perforation, which was likely attributable to bevacizumab. The incidence of bowel perforation with bevacizumab is 1% to 2%. The proposed mechanisms for this complication includes vascular disruption of the bowel wall, enhanced chemotherapy delivery to the tumor causing necrosis, and impaired bowel healing. The mortality after bowel perforation in this setting is approximately 25%.

REFERENCES:

Hapani S, Chu D, Wu S. Risk of gastrointestinal perforation in patients with cancer treated with bevacizumab: a meta-analysis. *Lancet Oncol.* 2009;10(6):559–568.

Van Cutsem E, Rivera F, Berry S, et al. Safety and efficacy of first-line bevacizumab with FOLFOX, XELOX, FOLFIRI and fluoropyrimidines in metastatic colorectal cancer: the BEAT study. *Ann Oncol.* 2009;20(11):1842–1847.

12. ANSWER: B

Rationale:

The patient is likely experiencing cardiotoxicity, more specifically coronary vasospasm, from fluoropyrimidine chemotherapy. Anginal chest pain is the most common cardiac symptom related to this class of agents. It should be noted that oral capecitabine has the same potential for cardiotoxicity as the infusional 5-fluorouracil. The other choices of pulmonary embolism, aortic dissection, and esophageal spasm are in the differential; however, the clinical scenario of chest pain shortly after receiving a fluoropyrimidine suggests coronary vasospasm as the most likely answer.

REFERENCE:

Layoun ME et al. Fluoropyrimidine-induced cardiotoxicity: manifestations, mechanisms, and management. *Curr Oncol Rep.* 2016;18(6):35.

13. ANSWER: B

Rationale:

Patients with metastatic colorectal cancer and B-*raf* (V600E) mutations historically have an aggressive tumor biology with a median overall survival of 9 to 14 months. This has recently been improved upon with a more aggressive first-line treatment utilizing FOLFOXIRI and bevacizumab showing a median overall survival of 24.1 months. Patients without B-*raf* mutations have an approximate median overall survival of 30 months in contemporary trials.

REFERENCES:

Loupakis F, Cremolini C, Salvatore L, et al. FOLFOXIRI plus bevacizumab as first-line treatment in BRAF mutant metastatic colorectal cancer. *Eur J Cancer.* 2014; 50(1):57–63.

Samowitz WS, Sweeney C, Herrick J, et al. Poor survival associated with the BRAF V600E mutation in microsatellite-stable colon cancers. *Cancer Res.* 2005;65(14):6063–6069.

Tran B, Kopetz S, Tie J, et al. Impact of BRAF mutation and microsatellite instability on the pattern of metastatic spread and prognosis in metastatic colorectal cancer. *Cancer.* 2011;117(20): 4623–4632.

14. ANSWER: D

Rationale:

Any of the anti-VEGF antibodies listed would be acceptable to combine with second-line chemotherapy for metastatic colorectal cancer. Each of these agents have been shown to improve overall survival in this setting.

REFERENCES:

Grothey A, Sugrue MM, Purdie DM, et al. Bevacizumab beyond first progression is associated with prolonged overall survival in metastatic colorectal cancer: results from a large observational cohort study (BRiTE). *J Clin Oncol.* 2008;26(33):5326–5334.

Tabernero J, Yoshino T, Cohn AL, et al. Ramucirumab versus placebo in combination with second-line FOLFIRI in patients with metastatic colorectal carcinoma that progressed during or after first-line therapy with bevacizumab, oxaliplating, an fluoropyrimidine (RAISE): A randomised, double-blind, multicentre, phase 3 study. *Lancet Oncol.* 2015;5:499–508.

Van Cutsem E, Tabernero J, Lakomy R, et al. Addition of aflibercept to fluorouracil, leucovorin, and irinotecan improves survival in a phase III randomized trial in patients with metastatic colorectal cancer previously treated with an oxaliplatin-based regimen. *J Clin Oncol.* 2012;30(28):3499–3506.

15. ANSWER: B

Rationale:

This patient is experiencing the cholinergic syndrome that can be seen within the first 24 hours after receiving irinotecan. Symptoms of cholinergic syndrome can include diarrhea, emesis, diaphoresis, abdominal cramping, flushing, bradycardia, increased salivation, and rhinorrhea. The exact mechanism for this syndrome is unclear but it is postulated that irinotecan increases anticholinesterase activity causing activation of the parasympathetic system. Atropine is an anticholinergic drug and would be the treatment of choice to help reverse the effects of this syndrome.

REFERENCE:

Hecht JR. Gastrointestinal toxicity of irinotecan. *Oncology* (Williston Park). 1998;12(8 suppl 6):72–78.

16. ANSWER: B

Rationale:

Bevacizumab has a half-life of 20 days and should be stopped at least 28 days prior to planned surgery. It should not be restarted after surgery for at least 28 days and/or the wound is completely healed. Surgical complications exacerbated by bevacizumab include impaired wound healing, fistula formation, bowel perforation, and bleeding.

REFERENCES:

Bevacizumab® [package insert]. San Francisco, CA: Genentech, Inc; 2004.

Scappaticci FA, Fehrenbacher L, Cartwright T, et al. Surgical wound healing complications in metastatic colorectal cancer patients treated with bevacizumab. *J Surg Oncol.* 2005;91:173–180.

17. ANSWER: C

Rationale:

This patient likely suffered a cardiac arrhythmia from hypomagnesemia induced by the EGFR antibody. Both cetuximab and panitumumab can cause hypomagnesemia. The incidence of hypomagnesemia with either agent is approximately 30% (grade 3-4 5-7%). The mechanism for hypomagnesemia is thought to be secondary to a defect in renal magnesium absorption. Patients can also develop secondary hypokalemia and hypocalcemia from the low magnesium. All patients on EGFR antibody therapy should have electrolytes monitored closely.

REFERENCES:

Schrag D, Chung KY, Flombaum C, et al. Cetuximab therapy and symptomatic hypomagnesemia. *J Natl Cancer Inst.* 2005;97(16):1221–1224.

Teipar S, Piessevaux H, Claes K, et al. Magnesium wasting associated with epidermal-growth-factor receptor-targeting antibodies in colorectal cancer: a prospective study. *Lancet Oncol.* 2007;8(5):387–394.

18. ANSWER: A

Rationale:

The optimal third-line therapy for this patient would be regorafenib. The patient's history offers that he had recent issues with neutropenia requiring growth factor support, along with recent hospitalization for neutropenic fever. Trifluridine and tipiracil would not be the best option here because it can also cause clinically relevant myelosuppression. EGFR antibody would be inappropriate for this patient because he has an N-*ras* mutation. The patient has already progressed after two lines of 5-fluorouracil based therapy and would not benefit from capecitabine.

REFERENCES:

Grothey A, Van Cutsem E, Sobrero A et al. Regorafenib monotherapy for previously treated metastatic colorectal cancer (CORRECT): an international, multicentre, randomized, placebo-controlled, phase 3 trial. *Lancet.* 2013;381(9863):303–312.

Mayer RJ, Van Cutsem E, Falcone A, et al. Randomized trial of TAS-102 for refractory metastatic colorectal cancer. *N Engl J Med.* 2015; 372:1909–1919.

19. ANSWER: D

Rationale:

This patient has stage IIA (pT3N0M0) colon cancer with *MSH6* mismatch-repair protein deficiency (dMMR). The poorly differentiated histology would normally be considered a high-risk feature; however, this is an expected finding given the molecular features of the tumor. This patient has an excellent prognosis and the data suggests a lack of benefit from fluoropyrimidine-based chemotherapy. The correct recommendation would be observation with active surveillance. This patient should also be referred to genetic counselors to consider further testing for hereditary nonpolyposis colorectal cancer (Lynch syndrome).

REFERENCES:

Benson AB, Schrag D, Somerfield MR, et al. American Society of Clinical Oncology recommendations on adjuvant chemotherapy for stage II colon cancer. *J Clin Oncol.* 2004;22:3408–3419.

Sargent DJ, Marsoni S, Monges G, et al. Defective mismatch repair as a predictive marker for lack of efficacy of fluorouracil-based adjuvant therapy in colon cancer. *J Clin Oncol.* 2010;28:3219–3226.

20. ANSWER: A

Rationale:

The patient has stage III disease with a good performance status and certainly warrants adjuvant therapy. The most appropriate treatment is a fluoropyrimidine-based therapy for 6 months. Omitting the oxaliplatin would be reasonable given the patient's underlying comorbidities (i.e., neuropathy) and work as a jeweler where worsening neuropathy would be detrimental. Further, the use of oxaliplatin in patients 70 years of age and older is controversial with multiple analyses suggesting lack of benefit.

REFERENCES:

McCleary NJ, Meyerhardt JA, Green E, et al. Impact of age on the efficacy of newer adjuvant therapies in patients with stage II/III colon cancer: findings from the ACCENT database. *J Clin Oncol.* 2013;31:2600–2606.

Yothers G, O'Connell MJ, Allegra CJ, et al. Oxaliplatin as adjuvant therapy for colon cancer: updated results of NSABP C-07, including survival and subset analyses. *J Clin Oncol.* 2011;29:3768–3774.

21. ANSWER: B

Rationale:

This patient has a clinical history and findings consistent with Peutz-Jeghers syndrome (PJS). The patient's bowel obstruction at a young age was likely a result of intussusception of the small bowel caused by hamartomatous polyps. Patients with PJS have approximately a 40% lifetime risk of colorectal cancer. PJS is inherited in an autosomal dominant pattern and a detailed family history should be obtained on this patient. A physical exam should be performed with special attention to the mucosa and skin looking for hyperpigmentation in the areas outlined below. Gardner syndrome is a variant of familial adenomatous polyposis (FAP) with extracolonic manifestations including desmoid tumors, osteomas, epidermal cysts, and fibromas. Turcot syndrome is another variant of FAP that is also associated with medulloblastomas. Li-Fraumeni syndrome is associated with multiple lineage tumors arising from germline loss of p53.

A clinical diagnosis of PJS is made if the patient has two or more of the following features:

- Two or more Peutz-Jeghers-type hamartomatous polyps of the small intestine
- Mucocutaneous hyperpigmentation of the mouth, lips, nose, eyes, genitalia, or fingers
- Family history of PJS

REFERENCES:

NCCN Clinical Practice Guidelines in Oncology. *Genetic/Familial High-Risk Assessment: Colorectal.* https://www.nccn.org/professionals/physician_gls/pdf/genetics_colon.pdf. Accessed on September 10, 2016

Tomlinson IP, Houlston R. Peutz-Jeghers syndrome. *J Med Genet.* 1997;34(12):1007–1011.

22. ANSWER: A

Rationale:

The molecular profile of this patient's colon cancer suggests sporadic loss of MLH1. This is an epigenetic phenomenon resulting from hypermethylation of the CpG island in the MLH1 gene promoter region, effectively silencing the gene. B-*raf* mutations are seen in conjunction with mismatch-repair deficiency approximately 30% of the time. The association of loss of MLH1 with B-*raf* mutations (V600E) is well described but not completely understood. It should be noted that the usual poor prognosis of B-*raf* mutations in metastatic colorectal cancer is attenuated by the presence of the mismatch-repair deficiency. TP53 is not part of the DNA mismatch repair system.

REFERENCES:

Rajagopalan H, Bardelli A, Lengauer C, et al. Tumorigenesis: RAF/RAS oncogenes and mismatch-repair status. *Nature.* 2002;418:934.

Seppala T, Bohm JP, Friman M, et al. Combination of microsatellite instability and BRAF mutation status for subtyping colorectal cancer. *Br J Cancer.* 2015;112(12):1966–1975.

Vilar, E, Gruber SB. Microsatellite instability in colorectal cancer – the stable evidence. *Nat Rev Clin Oncol.* 2010;7:153–162.

23. ANSWER: E

Rationale:

Any of the listed options would be acceptable for first-line treatment of metastatic K-*ras*/N-*ras* wild-type colorectal cancer. This is based on the CALGB 80405 which compared first-line FOLFOX or FOLFIRI with either cetuximab or bevacizumab. This showed a similar median OS for cetuximab and bevacizumab, 32 vs 31.2 months, respectively.

REFERENCE:

Venook A, Niedzwiecki D, Lenz HJ, et al. CALGB/SWOG 80405: Phase III trial of FOLFIRI or mFOLFOX6 with bevacizumab or cetuximab for patients with KRAS wild-type untreated metastatic adenocarcinoma of the colon or rectum. *J Clin Oncol.* 2014;32:5(s).

24. ANSWER: D

Rationale:

Patients with familial adenomatous polyposis have a 100% lifetime risk of developing colorectal cancer. The options for preventative treatment include proctocolectomy or colectomy. If colectomy is performed, endoscopic evaluation of the rectum should be done every 6 to 12 months indefinitely.

REFERENCE:

Galiatsatos P, Foulkes WD, et al. Familial adenomatous polyposis. *Am J Gastroenterol.* 2006; 101:385–398.

25. ANSWER: A

Rationale:

Familial adenomatous polyposis (FAP) is caused by a germline mutation in the APC gene resulting in a loss of function. FAP is inherited in an autosomal dominant fashion. The attenuated form of the disease has a later onset of cancer and fewer adenomatous polyps. Deficiency of the DNA mismatch-repair genes is seen in hereditary nonpolyposis colorectal cancer (Lynch syndrome). MUTYH-associated polyposis (MAP) is an autosomal recessive disease resulting from mutation of the MUTYH gene. The phenotype of this disease includes attenuated adenomatous polyposis and colorectal cancer. BRCA1 or BRCA2 mutation is inherited in an autosomal dominant fashion. Affected individuals are at risk of developing a number of different cancers, namely breast and ovarian cancer.

REFERENCE:

Galiatsatos P, Foulkes WD, et al. Familial adenomatous polyposis. *Am J Gastroenterol.* 2006; 101:385–398.

Pancreatic Cancer 10

Ananth K. Arjunan and James J. Lee

REVIEW QUESTIONS

1. A 62-year-old male presented to his physician with the onset of new jaundice. A CT scan revealed a 3-cm mass in the head of the pancreas without any evidence of metastatic disease. He underwent a Whipple resection. Pathology reveals a moderately differentiated T3 adenocarcinoma of the pancreas. None of 14 lymph nodes showed evidence of malignancy. The patient is recovering well. Which statement is TRUE regarding further management?

   A. Adjuvant chemotherapy is not indicated as the patient's lymph node resection was negative.

   B. Adjuvant chemotherapy is indicated to improve quality of life but it has not been shown to prolong survival in randomized studies.

   C. Adjuvant chemotherapy is indicated based on randomized studies showing a small survival benefit compared to placebo.

2. Which of the following is considered as a standard of care treatment for a patient of good performance status with a newly diagnosed metastatic pancreatic cancer to the liver:

   A. Gemcitabine alone

   B. FOLFIRINOX

   C. Gemcitabine plus nab-paclitaxel

   D. All of the above

3. Which of following statements about CA 19-9 is TRUE?

    A. CA 19-9 is a useful screening tool in pancreatic cancer because it is noninvasive.

    B. CA 19-9 is particularly useful in patients with jaundice who are suspected of having pancreatic cancer.

    C. A rising CA 19-9 following surgery for pancreatic cancer should be treated with early chemotherapy in order to prolong survival, even if the CT scan is negative for metastatic disease.

    D. CA 19-9 has been shown to have prognostic value in both the pre- and postoperative settings.

ANSWERS TO REVIEW QUESTIONS

1. ANSWER: C. Adjuvant chemotherapy has been shown by the CONKO and ESPAC studies to improve survival benefit compared to control. While lymph node positivity does have prognostic relevance, it does not influence the decision about whether to administer adjuvant therapy, perhaps because the vast majority of node-negative patients will still experience disease recurrence.

2. ANSWER: D. While FOLFIRINOX has become the new standard of care for the first-line treatment of metastatic pancreatic cancer, there may be other factors (e.g., comorbid conditions or contraindications such as biliary obstruction) that may preclude this intensive regimen. Gemcitabine plus nab-paclitaxel is an alternative option for the first-line treatment of metastatic pancreatic cancer. Gemcitabine monotherapy is feasible for patients who may not be able to tolerate a combination chemotherapy (FOLFIRINOX or gemcitabine/ nab-paclitaxel).

3. ANSWER: D. CA 19-9 is nonspecific and insensitive for the detection of early-onset disease. Therefore, it has no value as a screening test. Jaundice itself can result in CA 19-9 elevations; therefore, if it is to be used to follow therapy (as an adjunct to, rather than in place of, imaging), the baseline measurement should be post-stent placement. CA 19-9 has been shown to have prognostic value in both the pre- and postoperative settings.

Anal Cancer 11

Chaoyuan Kuang and James J. Lee

REVIEW QUESTIONS

1. A 63-year-old female has been diagnosed with a clinical stage IIIA, T2N1M0 squamous cell carcinoma of the anal canal. She presents with mild rectal bleeding but otherwise is healthy and has a good performance status of ECOG 1. What is the best treatment option for her cancer?

   A. Neoadjuvant chemotherapy with CDDP plus 5-FU followed by concurrent chemoradiation with CDDP plus 5-FU

   B. Concurrent chemoradiation with 5-FU plus MMC

   C. Concurrent chemoradiation with 5-FU plus MMC followed by adjuvant chemotherapy with 5-FU plus CDDP

   D. Concurrent chemoradiation with 5-FU

2. A 63-year-old female has been diagnosed with a clinical stage IIIA, T2N1M0 squamous cell carcinoma of the anal canal. The patient asks about her prognosis. What is her estimated 5-year overall survival?

   A. 75%

   B. 30%

   C. 50%

   D. 15%

3. A 44-year-old HIV+ male with a CD4 count of 630 has been recently diagnosed with a clinical stage II, T3N0M0 squamous cell carcinoma of

the anal canal. The patient is otherwise healthy with a performance status of ECOG 0. What is his best treatment option?

A. Radiation alone

B. Concurrent chemoradiation with 5-FU

C. Chemotherapy with 5-FU plus MMC

D. Concurrent chemoradiation with 5-FU plus MMC

4. A 55-year-old female who was diagnosed with a stage IIIB, T4N1M0 squamous cell carcinoma of the anal canal just completed concurrent 5-FU plus MMC with 59 Gy of radiation (45 Gy to the pelvis + 14 Gy boost to the primary tumor). Ten weeks after completing therapy, a digital rectal examination (DRE) is performed. A small nodule remains within the anal canal. What is the patient's best treatment option now?

A. Abdominoperineal resection (APR)

B. Chemotherapy with 5-FU plus CDDP

C. Reevaluation with repeat DRE, inguinal node palpation, and anoscope 4 weeks later

D. Radiation

5. A 67-year-old male with a newly diagnosed, locally advanced squamous cell carcinoma of the anal canal is having a consultation with the radiation oncologist. He has no significant comorbidity and has a good performance status of ECOG 1. Among his many questions, he inquires the chance of dying from the complications of the recommended chemoradiation therapy

A. 5% to 15%

B. 0% to 5%

C. 10% to 20%

D. 20% to 30%

ANSWERS TO REVIEW QUESTIONS

1. ANSWER: B. The updated RTOG data showed that concurrent 5-FU + MMC with RT was superior to neoadjuvant CDDP + 5-FU followed by concurrent CDDP + 5-FU with RT in terms of overall survival (78% vs. 70%) and DFS (57.8% vs. 67.8%). Thus, answer "A" cannot be correct. The ACT II trial demonstrated that MMC/5-FU + RT was equivalent to concurrent 5-FU + MMC with RT + maintenance chemotherapy. Maintenance therapy did not impact overall survival or DFS. Thus, answer "C" would not be correct. Finally, answer "D" is not correct as 5-FU/MMC + concurrent RT was superior to 5-FU + concurrent RT as demonstrated in RTOG 87-04 in terms of DFS, CFS, and local-regional control.

2. ANSWER: C. The National Cancer Database has provided 5-year survival of anal canal carcinoma patients by stage for both squamous and nonsquamous histologies. The database is based on cases diagnosed from 1998 to 1999 and included 3,598 cases.

For squamous cell histology, the 5-year survival is as follows: stage I = 71.4%, stage II = 63.5%, stage IIIA = 48.1%, stage IIIB = 43.2%, and stage IV = 20.9%.

For nonsquamous histology, the 5-year survival is as follows: stage I = 59.1%, stage II = 52.9%, stage IIIA = 37.7%, stage IIIB = 24.4%, and stage IV = 7.4%.

3. ANSWER: D. Early reports indicated that some HIV-positive patients were receiving less than optimal therapy due to concerns for treatment toxicity. However, patients with a CD4 count of ≥200 have excellent control of their disease with acceptable morbidity. Those with CD4 counts of <200, however, may require a modification in their treatment regimen such as omission of MMC or a reduction in the RT field and/or dose. The University of California San Francisco (UCSF) analyzed 17 HIV-positive patients and documented CD4 counts. All nine patients with a CD4 count ≥200 had control of their disease. Four patients did require a treatment break of 2 weeks, but no hospitalizations occurred. Among the eight patients with CD4 counts <200, four experienced lowered blood counts, intractable diarrhea, or moist desquamation. Four of eight ultimately required colostomies for either treatment-related toxicity or for salvage for disease. Disease, though, was controlled in seven of eight patients. Thus, based on the UCSF experience with HIV-positive patients, one should consider modifying the treatment regimen particularly if CD4 counts are less than 200. Thus, for this patient with a CD4 count >200, he should receive full dose concurrent chemoradiation with 5-FU and MMC.

4. ANSWER: C. After patients have completed definitive chemoradiation therapy, patients should be followed up clinically in 8 to 12 weeks after therapy. Cummings demonstrated that mean time for tumor regression was 3 months but regression of a tumor could occur up to 12 months. Thus, if there is persistent disease at 8 to 12 weeks, patients should be followed up closely (every month) to document regression. As long as there is documented regression on serial examinations, patients may continue to be monitored. However, at any point if there is progression, then biopsy followed by salvage APR should be considered. Thus, answer "C" is correct and "A" is incorrect and immediate APR should not be considered. Answer "B" also is incorrect as chemotherapy alone has not been shown of benefit in this situation. Finally, although option "D" could be considered, as salvage radiation has been attempted, typically salvage APR would be considered in the future if the patient later progresses on future serial examination.

5. *ANSWER: B.* Toxic deaths from CMT have ranged from 0% to 5%. In the UKCCCR study, 6/116 (2%) experienced toxic death, mostly due to septicemia. The EORTC trial reported on 1 toxic death out of 110 patients. In RTOG 8704 study, four patients (3%) experienced death in the MMC arm. More recently, there were no reported toxic deaths in both RTOG 98-11 and ACT II trials. The ACCORD 03 trial, a four-arm randomized trial, showed similar toxic deaths across all four arms (A = 1 [1%], B = 2 [2.6%], C = 3 [3%], D = 1 [1%]).

Breast Cancer 12

Megan Kruse, Leticia Varella, Stephanie Valente, Paulette Lebda, Andrew Vassil, and Jame Abraham

REVIEW QUESTIONS

Epidemiology, Risk Factors, Genetics, Prevention, Screening, and Diagnosis:

1. You are asked to see a 43-year-old premenopausal woman for counseling regarding her risk of developing breast cancer in the future. Her past medical history is remarkable for Hodgkin lymphoma at the age of 22, treated with mantle-field radiation. She has been struggling to lose weight, and her BMI today is 32. She never smoked and drinks 2 glasses of red wine every night. Her last mammogram revealed heterogeneously dense breasts and was otherwise unremarkable. She took oral contraceptive pills for 20 years and has never been pregnant. Which of the following factors in her history is associated with the greatest risk of developing breast cancer?
    A. Dense breasts on mammography
    B. History of radiation to the chest
    C. Nulliparity
    D. Obesity
    E. Oral contraceptive pills

2. What percentage of breast cancers are familial or hereditary?
    A. 5% to 10%
    B. 15% to 20%
    C. 25% to 30%
    D. 45% to 50%
    E. 55% to 60%

3. All of the following patients should undergo genetic risk evaluation, **EXCEPT:**

   A. A 58-year-old woman with stage III ER-negative, PR-negative, HER2-negative breast cancer

   B. A 35-year-old woman with stage I ER/PR-negative, HER2-positive breast cancer

   C. A 52-year-old woman with stage I ER/PR-positive, HER-negative breast cancer and family history of mother with breast cancer at age 45

   D. A 66-year-old woman with stage II ER/PR-positive, HER2-negative breast cancer

   E. A 65-year-old woman with a history of stage II breast cancer at age 47 and a stage I breast cancer in the contralateral breast cancer at age 55

4. A 29-year-old white female of Irish ancestry was seen in the high-risk clinic. Her father was diagnosed with pancreatic cancer at the age of 45, her paternal grandmother was diagnosed with ovarian cancer at the age of 38, and her paternal aunt was diagnosed with breast cancer at the age of 48. There is no other family or personal history of breast cancer. She was referred to Genetic counseling and genetic testing. What is the most appropriate next step in management?

   A. Proceed with bilateral mastectomy and prophylactic oophorectomy

   B. Order a CT/PET scan for ovarian and pancreatic cancer screening

   C. Order a breast MRI and a pelvic ultrasound

   D. Obtain CA-125 and CA 19-9 levels

   E. Wait for the genetic testing results before deciding the next step

5. BRCA 2 mutations are associated with all of the following cancers, **EXCEPT:**

   A. Peritoneal cancer

   B. Prostate cancer

   C. Urinary tract cancer

   D. Pancreatic cancer

   E. Melanoma

6. A 23-year-old woman with unremarkable prior medical history was recently diagnosed with a T2N1M0 invasive ductal carcinoma of the left breast, estrogen receptor positive (ER) 80%, progesterone receptor positive (PR) 20%, and HER2 3+ by immunohistochemistry. Her family history is significant for a brother who had soft tissue sarcoma of the leg at age 9, a paternal uncle with a history of resected adrenocortical carcinoma, and a paternal grandmother who died of breast cancer at age 29. You plan to refer her to genetic counseling. In which of the following genes you expect to find a mutation?
   A. PTEN
   B. TP53
   C. MSH6
   D. PALB2
   E. CDH1

7. A 53-year-old postmenopausal woman with a strong family history of breast cancer comes to clinic to discuss options for chemoprevention of breast cancer. She is a generally healthy woman with well-controlled hypertension. She has no family history of osteoporosis or deep vein thrombosis but is very concerned about the possibility of developing a pulmonary embolus while on treatment. Which of the following would be the most appropriate chemoprevention agent for this patient?
   A. Tamoxifen
   B. Exemestane
   C. Raloxifene
   D. Letrozole
   E. Anastrozole

8. What of the following medications can be considered for risk reduction in a premenopausal woman with elevated risk of breast cancer according to the Gail model?
   A. Raloxifene
   B. Anastrozole
   C. Exemestane
   D. Fulvestrant
   E. Tamoxifen

9. A 24-year-old woman presents to the high-risk breast clinic for an opinion regarding screening for breast cancer. Her 30-year-old sister was found to have a deleterious mutation in the BRCA1 gene after being diagnosed with stage II breast cancer. The patient also underwent genetic testing and was found to have the same BRCA1 germline mutation. She is very concerned about her risk of developing breast cancer in the future. You discuss with her the potential benefits and risks of breast cancer screening. Which of the following screening recommendations should you make?

   A. Annual screening mammogram starting at age 40

   B. Annual screening ultrasound starting at age 25

   C. Annual screening MRI starting at age 30

   D. Annual screening MRI starting at age 25 in addition to annual mammogram starting at age 30

   E. Annual screening mammogram starting at age 25

10. A 32-year-old woman presents to her gynecologist after noticing a lump in her left breast 2 months ago. She has never had a mammogram and does not have a history of breast biopsies. Her family history is significant for prostate cancer in her paternal grandfather at the age of 77. Physical examination confirms a firm, palpable 1.8 cm mass in the outer upper quadrant of the left breast, without nipple discharge. Her gynecologist orders a diagnostic mammogram that reveals heterogeneously dense breasts without evidence of a mass or cyst. What is the most appropriate next step in management?

   A. Given the negative mammography results and her young age, ask her to return for a repeat physical examination in 1 year

   B. Order an ultrasound of the left breast

   C. Order bilateral breast MRI

   D. Repeat mammogram in 1 year

   E. Refer her to genetic counseling

Surgery and Radiation

11. All of the following are contraindications to receiving breast conserving surgery followed by radiation, **EXCEPT:**

   A. Active connective tissue disease

   B. Pregnancy

C. Tumor size 4cm

D. Multifocal tumor occupying >2 quadrants of the breast

E. Diffuse malignant-appearing calcifications

12. Sentinel lymph node biopsy has been shown to improve which of the following side effects compared to complete axillary lymph node dissection?

A. Pain

B. Sensation loss

C. Lymphedema

D. Arm mobility

E. All of the above

13. A 55-year-old postmenopausal woman is seen in the medical oncology clinic after having a lumpectomy and sentinel lymph node dissection for an invasive ductal carcinoma of the breast. The tumor size is 1.8 cm, ER/PR strongly positive and HER2 negative. One of the two sentinel lymph nodes examined was positive for cancer. Which of the following is the best next step in management?

A. She should proceed with complete axillary node dissection for local control, since one sentinel lymph node is positive

B. She should get chemotherapy, because one node is positive

C. She may be a candidate for oncotype, radiation therapy, and endocrine therapy, if she is in the low-risk group

D. Since she has lymph node involvement, she is not a candidate for oncotype, and should proceed with radiation and endocrine therapy

14. Which of the following patients would be more suitable to undergo sentinel lymph node biopsy than axillary lymph node dissection?

A. A 45-year-old woman with triple-negative inflammatory breast cancer

B. A 65-year-old woman with a 1.9 cm breast carcinoma and a positive axillary lymph node by fine needle aspiration scheduled to undergo a lumpectomy

C. A 55-year-old-woman with a clinical T1N0M0 ER/PR-positive, HER2-negative breast cancer

    D. A 60-year-old woman with ductal carcinoma in situ undergoing lumpectomy

    E. A 58-year-old woman with multicentric ER/PR-positive, HER2-negative breast cancer

---

15. A 52-year-old perimenopausal woman is seen in the oncology clinic for an opinion regarding recently diagnosed breast cancer. She initially presented with a palpable mass, and an ultrasound-guided biopsy revealed invasive ductal carcinoma, ER/PR-negative, HER2-negative. She underwent lumpectomy with sentinel lymph node 2 weeks ago, and the final pathologic stage was pT2N0. Which of the following tests should you order to complete her staging?

    A. CT of the chest, abdomen, and pelvis

    B. CT of the chest, abdomen, and pelvis, and a bone scan

    C. CT of the chest, abdomen, and pelvis, bone scan, CA 15-3 and CA 27.29 levels

    D. PET-CT scan

    E. No further staging tests should be ordered

---

16. A 66-year-old postmenopausal woman was recently diagnosed with stage T1cN0M0 invasive ductal carcinoma of the right breast, grade 2, ER/PR-positive and HER2-negative. She was previously healthy. She was seen in the Breast Surgery clinic and was recommended to have a lumpectomy followed by radiation. She read about Intraoperative Radiation Therapy (IORT) and is interested in learning more about it. When compared to whole breast external beam radiation, which of the following statements regarding IORT is correct?

    A. Patients who undergo IORT have a higher chance of having local recurrence

    B. Patients who undergo IORT have worse disease-free survival

    C. Patients who undergo IORT have worse overall survival

    D. Patients who undergo IORT have a lower chance of qualifying for another lumpectomy, if needed in the future

    E. Patients who undergo IORT have a higher chance of developing skin complications

17. A healthy 77-year-old woman was recently diagnosed with a clinical stage I (T1N0) invasive ductal carcinoma of the right breast. The cancer is strongly ER-positive. Which of the following is the LEAST appropriate local control approach?

    A. Bilateral mastectomy

    B. Unilateral mastectomy

    C. Lumpectomy and whole breast radiation

    D. Lumpectomy and Intraoperative Radiation Therapy (IORT)

    E. Lumpectomy

18. A 63-year-old postmenopausal woman with history of breast cancer presents to the emergency department after a motor vehicle accident. She is asymptomatic. Her neurological examination reveals normal cranial nerves function and no focal weakness. A CT scan of the head demonstrates a solitary lesion in the left parietal lobe measuring 1.8 cm, without midline shift. CT scans of the body revealed enlarged mediastinal lymph nodes, a lytic lesion in L4 and L5, and 2 indeterminate small hepatic lesions. She was diagnosed with stage III ER/PR-negative, Her2-positive breast cancer 3 years ago, and was treated with neoadjuvant chemotherapy followed by mastectomy, radiation, and trastuzumab for one year. A fine-needle aspiration of an enlarged mediastinal lymph node confirms ER/PR-negative and HER2-positive breast cancer metastasis. Which of the following is the LEAST appropriate next step in management?

    A. Proceed with stereotactic radiosurgery

    B. Refer her to stereotactic radiosurgery followed by whole brain radiation

    C. Consult Neurosurgery for resection of the brain mass

    D. Proceed with chemotherapy and anti-HER2 therapy

    E. Refer her to Hospice

19. A 51-year-old woman who is being treated for metastatic ER-positive breast cancer with single-agent capecitabine comes to the clinic complaining of severe low back pain for 2 weeks. She states that the pain is progressively worsening, particularly at night and with movement, and intermittently radiates to the lower extremities. She denies bladder or bowel changes.

Her physical examination is significant for mild weakness in the lower extremities flexor muscles. An MRI of the spine with contrast reveals multiple small lytic lesions in the axial skeleton, with a predominant epidural lesion in T11 compressing the thecal sac. What is the best next step in management?

A. Prescribe opioids and recommend bed rest until the pain improves

B. Start dexamethasone, pain management, and continue chemotherapy with single-agent capecitabine

C. Start dexamethasone, pain management, and switch systemic therapy to docetaxel

D. Consult Neurosurgery for surgical decompression

E. Refer to Hospice

20. A 55-year-old woman calls your office to report a new skin rash. She was recently diagnosed with metastatic triple-negative breast cancer after presenting to the Emergency Department with cord compression. She completed palliative radiation to the lower spine 3 weeks ago, and was started on chemotherapy. Her first cycle of adriamycin and cyclophosphamide was given yesterday. When she woke up this morning, she noticed a painful erythematous rash in her lower back. Which of the following is the most likely explanation for her rash?

A. Allergic reaction to cyclophosphamide

B. Allergic reaction to adriamycin

C. Viral infection

D. Radiation recall dermatitis

E. Radiation enhancement

Endocrine therapy:

21. Which of the following options is true regarding tamoxifen therapy following lumpectomy and radiation for ductal carcinoma in situ (DCIS)?

A. Decreases the risk of breast cancer recurrence (ipsilateral and contralateral)

B. Improves disease-free survival

C. Improves overall survival

D. It is effective in both hormonal receptor-positive and negative DCIS

22. A 50-year-old perimenopausal woman presents to medical oncology clinic after having a mastectomy and sentinel lymph node biopsy for invasive ductal carcinoma. Her surgical specimen reveals a 1.5 cm tumor that is ER-positive, PR-negative, and HER-2 negative. Two sentinel lymph nodes were removed and negative for carcinoma. The next best step in her management is

   A. Chemotherapy

   B. Oncotype DX testing

   C. Endocrine therapy

   D. Surveillance consisting of every 3 to 4 months visits including clinical breast exam and annual mammography of unaffected breast

23. A 56-year-old postmenopausal woman with metastatic breast cancer on treatment with exemestane and everolimus presented to the walk-in clinic with new onset fever, cough, and shortness of breath. The chest x-ray showed diffuse patchy infiltrate. Her blood pressure was 134/86 mmHg and heart rate was 84 per minute. Her pulse oxymetry was 94% on room air. Her sites of metastatic disease were L4 and L5 lesions. The patient's last dose of zoledronic acid was about 3 weeks ago. The next best step in management is

   A. Stop exemestane and everolimus and start chemotherapy given that she has lymphangitic spread of breast cancer

   B. Stop everolimus immediately given that she has everolimus-induced pneumonitis, and never rechallenge with everolimus

   C. Interrupt everolimus and restart at a lower dose once the toxicity is improved to grade 1 or less, given that this is only a grade 2 toxicity

   D. Order a bronchoscopy to confirm the diagnosis

   E. Stop zoledronic acid and never rechallenge her again

24. Oncotype DX testing is appropriate for which of the following patients?

    A. 56-year-old-woman with stage I (T1bN0) ER-positive, HER2-positive invasive ductal carcinoma

    B. 62-year-old-woman with stage II (T2N0) ER-positive, HER2-negative invasive ductal carcinoma

    C. 49-year-old-woman with stage I (T1cN0) ER-negative, HER2-negative invasive ductal carcinoma

    D. 67-year-old-woman with stage III (T1cN2) ER-positive, HER2-negative invasive ductal carcinoma

25. A 33-year-old premenopausal woman is seen in the clinic for an opinion regarding a recently diagnosed stage T2N1 invasive lobular carcinoma of the right breast. Her tumor was ER-positive 90%, PR-positive 70%, and HER2 1+ by immunohistochemistry. She underwent a lumpectomy 2 weeks ago and is recovering well. You recommend adjuvant chemotherapy, and discuss the indications for subsequent adjuvant endocrine therapy. Which of the following is her best choice for endocrine therapy?

    A. Tamoxifen for 5 to 10 years

    B. Letrozole for 5 to 10 years

    C. Anastrozole for 5 to 10 years

    D. LHRH agonist in combination with exemestane for 5 to 10 years

    E. Letrozole and palbociclib for 5 to 10 years

26. A 32-year-old woman presents to the fertility clinic after being diagnosed with stage II ER/PR-negative, HER2-negative breast cancer. A recent genetic testing revealed no high-risk gene mutations. She is planned to start neoadjuvant chemotherapy with anthracycline and cyclophosphamide followed by paclitaxel. She recently got married, and would like to have children in the future. Which of the following management options would you recommend?

    A. Proceed with chemotherapy and discuss adoption in the future given that pregnancy is contraindicated after breast cancer

    B. Avoid chemotherapy and proceed with surgery and radiation only

    C. Start a GnRH-agonist for ovarian suppression, and proceed with chemotherapy

D. Avoid in vitro fertilization given that it is contraindicated in patients with a history of breast cancer

E. She would be a candidate for fertility preservation if she is still having menses after chemotherapy

27. A 44-year-old premenopausal woman with a history of stage I ER-positive, PR-positive, HER2-negative invasive lobular carcinoma of the right breast cancer was recently diagnosed with metastatic disease in the bones after presenting with low back pain. She was initially treated with lumpectomy followed by radiation and adjuvant chemotherapy with an anthracycline/taxane-based regimen. She declined adjuvant endocrine therapy with tamoxifen. Her recent bone scan revealed three lytic lesions in the thoracic and lumbar spine, without signs of cord compression. You recommend systemic therapy. Which of the following is the LEAST appropriate treatment option?

A. Anastrozole alone

B. Tamoxifen alone

C. Ovarian suppression in combination with anastrozole

D. Ovarian suppression in combination with fulvestrant

E. Ovarian suppression in combination with letrozole and a cyclin-dependent kinase inhibitor

28. A 65-year-old postmenopausal woman with a history of stage I ER/PR-positive, HER2-negative breast cancer returns to the clinic to review her bone scan results. She was initially treated with lumpectomy followed by radiation and has been taking anastrozole as adjuvant endocrine therapy for the past 4 years. She recently developed a persistent discomfort in the low back and a bone scan showed new bone lesions in T4, L3, and L4. There are no signs of cord compression. Which of the following options is the LEAST appropriate next therapeutic step?

A. Stop the anastrozole and start single-agent fulvestrant

B. Stop the anastrozole and start fulvestrant in combination with a cyclin-dependent kinase inhibitor

C. Stop the anastrozole and start exemestane in combination with everolimus

D. Stop the anastrozole and start tamoxifen

E. Stop the anastrozole and start combination chemotherapy

29. A 68-year-old postmenopausal woman returns to the clinic for follow-up. She was initially diagnosed 4 years ago with a T2N2M0 invasive ductal carcinoma of the left breast, ER/PR-strongly positive, HER2-negative. She was treated with mastectomy, axillary lymph node dissection, anthracycline-based adjuvant chemotherapy, and external beam radiation. She has been taking anastrozole since the completion of radiation, and reports no side effects. Her last bone scan showed no osteopenia or osteoporosis. Her compliance is excellent. Which of the following would you recommend regarding the adjuvant endocrine therapy?

    A. Stop anastrozole after completing 5 years of therapy given that it has been demonstrated to have a detrimental impact in survival beyond 5 years

    B. Stop anastrozole now since she already completed more than 3 years of adjuvant endocrine therapy

    C. Discuss continuing anastrozole for a total of up to 10 years

    D. Stop anastrozole and start tamoxifen given that tamoxifen was shown to improve survival in postmenopausal women who completed 3 years of an aromatase inhibitor

30. A premenopausal woman with ER-positive breast cancer develops bone metastasis 4 years after being started on adjuvant tamoxifen. Which of the following is the LEAST appropriate next treatment option for this patient?

    A. Ovarian suppression plus aromatase inhibitor

    B. Ovarian suppression plus aromatase inhibitor in combination with a cyclin-dependent kinase inhibitor

    C. Ovarian suppression plus single-agent fulvestrant

    D. Ovarian suppression plus fulvestrant in combination with a cyclin-dependent kinase inhibitor

    E. Ovarian suppression plus combination chemotherapy

Chemotherapy

31. A 62-year-old postmenopausal woman presents to the oncology clinic after undergoing a lumpectomy and sentinel lymph node biopsy for a newly diagnosed ER-positive 30%, PR-positive 30%, HER2-negative invasive ductal carcinoma of the left breast. Her breast cancer stage is IA (T1cN0M0) and she is recovering well from her surgery. She is active

and otherwise healthy. Oncotype DX testing was sent and resulted with a Recurrence Score of 32. What is the most appropriate next step in her management?

A. Chemotherapy

B. Radiation

C. Endocrine therapy

D. Surveillance

32. A 57-year-old postmenopausal woman recently had a lumpectomy and sentinel lymph node biopsy done for an invasive ductal carcinoma. On final surgical pathology the tumor was found to be 1.6 cm, strongly ER/PR-positive and HER2-negative. One of three sentinel lymph nodes was involved with carcinoma. Which of the following statements is correct?

A. As she has one sentinel lymph node positive, a complete axillary lymph node dissection should be performed

B. She should have radiation to the axilla due to the positive lymph node

C. She should have chemotherapy due to the positive lymph node

D. Oncotype testing may help to determine if she would benefit from the addition of chemotherapy to breast radiation and endocrine therapy

33. A 65-year-old postmenopausal woman with invasive ductal cancer had a left modified radical mastectomy and 2 lymph nodes were positive for invasive cancer. Her tumor size was 2.7 cm and she was staged as T2 N1 M0 (IIB). ER/PR was 90% to 100% positive and Ki-67 was 5%. HER2 was negative by immunohistochemistry. She is in your office to discuss about adjuvant therapy options. She is otherwise very healthy. Which of the following statements is true regarding her adjuvant therapy?

A. Since she has a IIB tumor, you strongly recommend chemotherapy with docetaxel and cyclophosphamide (TC) for four cycles

B. Chemotherapy may not add much value to her treatment; her maximum benefit will be from endocrine therapy

C. She should receive radiation therapy since she had a 2.7 cm tumor and one lymph node positive

D. It is up to the patient to decide about her therapy since she is older than 65

34. A 52-year-old African American woman is referred to your clinic because of a tenderness and erythema in the right breast that started 1 month ago. Her last mammogram was more than 10 years ago, and her gynecologist has not seen her in the past 15 years. On physical examination, there is skin erythema of the right breast involving half of the breast surface, associated with edema and warmth, as well as multiple palpable lymph nodes in the right axilla. Bilateral diagnostic mammogram revealed asymmetrical increased density throughout the right breast with associated right axillary lymphadenopathy, and no abnormalities in the left breast. A core biopsy of the right breast reveals invasive ductal carcinoma, ER-negative, PR-negative, and HER2 1+ by immunohistochemistry. Fine needle aspiration of the right axillary node confirms ductal carcinoma, and staging scans revealed no distant metastasis. An echocardiogram showed left ventricle ejection fraction of 65%. What is the most appropriate next step in management?

    A. Right lumpectomy with sentinel lymph node, followed by radiation

    B. Right lumpectomy with level I/II axillary lymph node dissection, followed by radiation

    C. Right mastectomy with level I/II axillary lymph node dissection

    D. Bilateral mastectomy

    E. Neoadjuvant chemotherapy, followed by mastectomy with level I/II axillary lymph node dissection, and radiation

35. A 57-year-old woman with metastatic triple-negative breast cancer returns to the clinic to review the results of a PET-CT scan. She was previously treated with docetaxel for 6 months followed by capecitabine for 4 months. The PET-CT shows disease progression in the lungs and liver. You plan to start chemotherapy with eribulin. Which of the following is the LEAST common adverse effect associated with eribulin?

    A. Myelosuppression

    B. Peripheral neuropathy

    C. Hypoglycemia

    D. QTc prolongation

    E. Alopecia

36. A 48-year-old premenopausal woman who was recently diagnosed with stage III triple-negative breast cancer underwent neoadjuvant chemotherapy with an anthracycline/taxane-based regimen, followed by mastectomy. Final pathology analysis revealed T2N1 residual disease. She is planned to receive adjuvant radiation. What is the LEAST appropriate next step in management?

    A. Proceed with surveillance

    B. Discuss the benefits and risks of adjuvant capecitabine

    C. Discuss the benefits and risks of adjuvant neratinib

    D. Refer the patient to a clinical trial

37. A 55-year-old postmenopausal woman with metastatic ER-positive HER2-negative breast cancer returns to the clinic to review the results of her most recent scans. She initially presented with de novo oligometastatic disease 2 years ago, and has been since treated with 3 lines of endocrine therapy. Her new scans reveal progression of disease in the liver, lungs, and bones. Laboratory tests obtained today show normal hepatic and renal function. Her performance status remains excellent. Which of the following is the most appropriate next step in treatment?

    A. Start chemotherapy with capecitabine and docetaxel

    B. Start chemotherapy with gemcitabine and carboplatin

    C. Start chemotherapy with anthracycline and cyclophosphamide

    D. Start chemotherapy with single-agent paclitaxel

    E. Start chemotherapy with cyclophosphamide, methotrexate, and fluorouracil

38. A 41-year-old African American woman was recently found to have a 4 cm palpable mass in the left breast during a routine gynecologic visit. Physical examination also revealed enlarged left axillary lymph nodes. A core biopsy demonstrated invasive ductal carcinoma, grade 3, ER/PR-negative and HER2 1+ by immunohistochemistry. Fine-needle aspiration of one of the left axillary lymph nodes was positive for ductal carcinoma. Bilateral breast MRI confirmed a 4.5 mass in the left breast, at least 3 enlarged lymph nodes in the left axilla, and no abnormalities in the right. Staging CT scans and bone scan had no evidence of distant disease. The

breast surgeon refers the patient to you to start neoadjuvant chemotherapy. Which of the following best describes the rationale for neoadjuvant chemotherapy in this case?

    A. Neoadjuvant chemotherapy may increase her chances to qualify for breast conservation surgery

    B. Neoadjuvant chemotherapy is associated with better disease-free survival

    C. Neoadjuvant chemotherapy is associated with better overall survival

    D. The patient should not receive neoadjuvant chemotherapy given that she has triple-negative disease

    E. Neoadjuvant chemotherapy should not be given outside of a clinical trial

39. You are called by one of the chemotherapy nurses to evaluate a patient who developed facial flushing 6 minutes after starting paclitaxel infusion. The nurse tells you that this is her first dose of paclitaxel and she received pre-medication with dexamethasone, diphenhydramine, and cimetidine. The patient previously underwent lumpectomy for a stage I triple-negative breast cancer, and received four cycles of chemotherapy with adriamycin and cyclophosphamide. On physical examination, there is facial flushing and the lungs are clear to auscultation. Vital signs are normal. What is the most appropriate next step?

    A. Continue paclitaxel infusion and monitor for signs of respiratory distress

    B. Stop paclitaxel infusion temporarily, and monitor for resolution of symptoms

    C. Stop the paclitaxel infusion and never re-challenge her with a taxane again

    D. Stop the paclitaxel infusion and emergently administer subcutaneous epinephrine

HER-2 Targeted Therapies

40. Which of the following is correct regarding the Human Epidermal Growth Factor Receptor 2 (HER2) testing in breast cancer as per the American

Society of Clinical Oncology (ASCO) and College of American Pathologists Clinical Practice 2013 guidelines?

A. HER2 is considered positive if the HER2 copy number is ≥ 6.0 signals/cell by in situ hybridization

B. HER2 is considered positive if the HER2 copy number is ≥ 4.0 and < 6.0 signals/cells and the HER2/CEP17 ratio is < 2.0 by in situ hybridization

C. HER2 is considered equivocal if the HER2/CEP17 ratio is ≥ 2.0 by in situ hybridization

D. HER2 is considered positive if it is 2+ by immunohistochemistry

E. HER2 is considered equivocal if it is 3+ by immunohistochemistry

41. A 44-year-old woman was diagnosed with a stage IIB, ER/PR negative and HER-2 negative breast cancer in 2002. In 2007 the patient presented with chest pain and shortness of breath. Chest x-ray followed by a CT scan of the chest showed a 4 cm left lower lobe lesion, which was biopsied and was confirmed as breast cancer. Repeat ER/PR was negative and HER-2 by immunohistochemistry was 3+. The patient was started on a trastuzumab, pertuzumab, and docetaxel every 3 weeks. She continues to work and has an excellent cardiac function and ECOG performance status. The last restaging scan showed progression of disease. The patient clearly wishes to continue with the treatment. Which of the following would be the best next step in this patient's care?

A. Supportive care only, since she had multiple treatments in the past

B. Continue pertuzumab, trastuzumab, and docetaxel

C. Switch therapy to lapatinib and capecitabine

D. Switch therapy to ado-trastuzumab emtansine (TDM-1)

E. Keep her on trastuzumab and change to a different chemotherapy

42. A 59-year-old-woman with unremarkable past medical history was recently diagnosed with stage II ER/PR-negative, HER2-positive breast cancer. She was treated with mastectomy followed by adjuvant anthracycline, cyclophosphamide and paclitaxel, and has been receiving adjuvant

trastuzumab 6 mg/kg IV every 3 weeks for 6 months. Her left ventricle ejection fraction (EF) on an echocardiogram performed before starting trastuzumab was 60%. She returns today with the result of a follow-up echocardiogram that revealed a left ventricle EF of 43%. She remains asymptomatic. What is the most appropriate next step in management?

    A. Continue trastuzumab at the same dose

    B. Stop trastuzumab and never start it again

    C. Decrease the trastuzumab dose to 2 mg/kg IV every 3 weeks

    D. Stop trastuzumab and start pertuzumab

    E. Hold trastuzumab and repeat echocardiogram in 4 weeks

43. You were asked to see a 57-year-old postmenopausal woman in the Oncology clinic for an opinion regarding her newly diagnosed breast cancer. She recently underwent a screening mammogram and was found to have a mass in the left breast. An ultrasound-guided core biopsy revealed invasive ductal carcinoma, ER-positive, PR-positive, and HER-2 3+ by immunohistochemistry. She underwent a lumpectomy and the final pathology analysis revealed a grade 2 carcinoma measuring 1.9 cm in the largest dimension, and a negative sentinel lymph node. Which of the following is the best next step in treatment?

    A. Refer her to Radiation Oncology to start adjuvant radiation

    B. Start concomitant trastuzumab and lapatinib and complete 52 weeks of therapy

    C. Start weekly trastuzumab for 12 weeks followed by lapatinib for 34 weeks

    D. Start weekly paclitaxel for 12 weeks and trastuzumab for a total of 52 weeks

    E. Start single agent ado-trastuzumab emtansine (T-DM1)

44. A 55-year-old woman is seen in the Oncology clinic for continuation of adjuvant therapy for a recently diagnosed stage II ER-negative, HER2-positive breast cancer. She completed adjuvant chemotherapy and is scheduled to start adjuvant therapy with trastuzumab. Which of the following is the optimal duration of adjuvant therapy with trastuzumab?

    A. 3 months

    B. 6 months

C. 12 months

D. 18 months

E. 24 months

45. A 49-year-old premenopausal woman was recently diagnosed with T2N1 ER-positive, PR-negative, HER2-positive breast cancer. She is scheduled to start adjuvant chemotherapy with doxorubicin and cyclophosphamide given every 2 weeks for 4 cycles, followed by 12 weeks of paclitaxel. Which of the following in the best recommendation regarding anti-HER2 therapy?

   A. Start trastuzumab and pertuzumab in combination with chemotherapy, and continue dual HER2 blockade to complete 1 year

   B. Start single-agent pertuzumab in combination with chemotherapy and plan to complete 1 year of anti-HER2 therapy

   C. Start single-agent ado-trastuzumab emtansine (T-DM1) and plan to complete 1 year of anti-HER2 therapy

   D. Proceed with chemotherapy only, given that anti-HER2 therapy is not indicated in women with hormonal receptor-positive disease

   E. Proceed with chemotherapy only, given that anti-HER2 therapy is not indicated in premenopausal women

46. Which of the following is the best next step in treatment for a patient with metastatic HER2-positive breast cancer who has progressed on first-line therapy with trastuzumab and paclitaxel?

   A. Stop paclitaxel and increase the dose of trastuzumab

   B. Continue paclitaxel and increase the dose of trastuzumab

   C. Stop trastuzumab and paclitaxel and start ado-trastuzumab emtansine (T-DM1)

   D. Stop trastuzumab and paclitaxel and start single-agent pertuzumab

   E. Stop trastuzumab and paclitaxel and start lapatinib plus capecitabine

47. A 62-year-old postmenopausal woman with unremarkable past medical history was recently diagnosed with stage T2N2 ER-positive, PR-negative,

HER2-positive invasive ductal carcinoma of the right breast. She underwent neoadjuvant treatment with anthracycline/taxane-based chemotherapy and trastuzumab, followed by mastectomy with axillary lymph node dissection. Final pathology analysis revealed 2.3 cm residual disease in the breast and 3 lymph nodes involved by carcinoma. Which of the following is the most appropriate next step in management?

   A. Continue trastuzumab every 3 weeks until she completes 52 weeks of treatment

   B. Consider adding adjuvant neratinib after completion of trastuzumab treatment

   C. Consider adding adjuvant lapatinib after completion of trastuzumab treatment

   D. Consider adding adjuvant lapatinib concomitantly to trastuzumab

48. A 55-year-old postmenopausal woman with a history of breast cancer presents to the Oncology clinic for follow-up. She was previously diagnosed with stage T2N1 invasive ductal carcinoma of the right breast, ER/PR-negative, HER2 3+ by immunohistochemistry. She received neoadjuvant chemotherapy in combination with trastuzumab followed by mastectomy and adjuvant radiation. She completed 1 year of adjuvant trastuzumab 3 years ago. A PET-CT now reveals metastatic disease in the thoracic and lower spine, and 3 lung lesions. A biopsy of one of the pulmonary lesions confirms ER/PR-negative, Her2 3+ by immunohistochemistry. What is the most appropriate next step in treatment?

   A. Start combination therapy with trastuzumab, pertuzumab and taxane

   B. Start combination therapy with capecitabine and lapatinib

   C. Start single-agent ado-trastuzumab emtansine (T-DM1)

   D. Start single-agent trastuzumab

   E. Start single-agent neratinib

Novel therapies/Miscellaneous

49. A 55-year-old woman with ER-positive metastatic breast cancer was started on letrozole 2.5 mg PO daily and palbociclib 125 mg PO Days 1

to 21 of 28-day cycle. She returns to the clinic on Day 15 of Cycle 1 and her CBC reveals an absolute neutrophil count of 900/mm3. Which of the following would you recommend?

A. Continue palbociclib at the same dose and repeat CBC in 1 week

B. Decrease palbociclib dose to 100 mg PO Days 1 to 21 of 28-day cycles

C. Decrease palbociclib dose to 75 mg PO Days 1 to 21 of 28-day cycles

D. Hold palbociclib and restart palbociclib in 1 week at 125 mg PO Days 1 to 14 of 28-day cycles

E. Hold palbociclib and repeat CBC in 1 week. If ANC is >1000, restart palbociclib at 100 mg PO Days 1 to 21 of 28-day cycles

50. A 37-year-old woman with BRCA1 mutation and metastatic ER-negative, HER-2 negative breast cancer is interested in participating in a clinical trial with olaparib. Which of the following is NOT correct regarding olaparib?

A. Olaparib is a Poly ADP ribose polymerase (PARP) inhibitor

B. Olaparib was initially approved in the United States in 2014 for patients with advanced ovarian cancer and BRCA mutations

C. Olaparib has been shown to increase progression-free survival in patients with metastatic breast cancer

D. Olaparib has only been approved for use in patients with BRCA mutations

E. Olaparib has been approved for use in maintenance treatment of patients with recurrent ovarian cancer who have achieved a complete or partial response to platinum-based chemotherapy

51. Which of the following tests does NOT need to be monitored during treatment with ribociclib?

A. ECG

B. Echocardiogram

C. Liver function

D. Electrolytes

E. CBC with differential

52. A 66-year-old woman with history of stage I ER-positive breast cancer returns to the clinic to review the results of a bone scan. She recently developed pain in the left shoulder that did not improve with ibuprofen. The bone scan reveals new lytic lesions in the left clavicle, 11th right rib, T6 and L1. Her renal function is normal and she recently had a routine dental examination without any issues. Which of the following is the LEAST appropriate management plan for her bone disease?

    A. Start zoledronic acid 4 mg intravenously and continue it every 4 weeks

    B. Start zoledronic acid 4 mg intravenously and continue it every 12 weeks

    C. Start pamidronate 90 mg intravenously and continue it every 4 weeks

    D. Start denosumab 120 mg subcutaneously and continue it every 4 weeks

    E. She does not need a bone-modifying agent given that she has oligometastatic disease

53. A woman with metastatic breast cancer comes to your office for a second opinion regarding treatment. She was initially diagnosed with stage I triple-negative breast cancer 2 years ago, and was recently found to have metastasis to the bones. Her friend read about immunotherapy, and the patient would like to know more. Which of the following options is correct regarding immunotherapy in breast cancer?

    A. Checkpoint inhibitors are not effective in breast cancer because breast cancer cells do not express programmed cell death protein 1 (PD-1)

    B. Single-agent atezolizumab has been approved for the treatment of metastatic women with triple-negative breast cancer

    C. In phase II trials, patients with metastatic triple-negative breast cancer treated with pembrolizumab had an objective response rate of 40%

    D. The addition of pembrolizumab to standard neoadjuvant therapy has been shown to increase pathologic complete response in ER-positive and triple-negative breast cancer patients

54. A 55-year-old postmenopausal woman presents to the oncologic clinic to discuss adjuvant therapy options for her recently diagnosed breast cancer. She initially presented with a palpable breast mass and was diagnosed with invasive ductal carcinoma, T2N1, ER-positive 40%, PR-negative, HER2-negative. She underwent a lumpectomy and is scheduled to see a radiation oncologist to discuss adjuvant radiation. She has regular visits to the dentist for routine cleaning and her renal function is normal. You recommend adjuvant systemic therapy. Which of the following is correct regarding the use of bone-modifying agents?

    A. Bisphosphonates can be used in metastatic breast cancer to the bones, but have no role in the adjuvant setting

    B. Adjuvant bisphosphonates can substitute for adjuvant chemotherapy in ER-positive patients

    C. Adding zoledronic acid to her adjuvant therapy regimen should be considered

    D. The benefit of adjuvant bisphosphonates is restricted to premenopausal women

    E. Denosumab is the only bone-modifying agent shown to be beneficial in the adjuvant setting

ANSWERS TO REVIEW QUESTIONS

1. ANSWER: B

Explanation

History of thoracic radiation before the age of 30 represents a strong risk factor for the development of breast cancer, with an overall risk up to 55 fold greater than the risk in the normal population. Women with dense breasts on mammogram also have an increased risk of developing breast cancer, with a relative risk of approximately 2.0 to 5.0. High BMI is an independent risk factor for breast cancer, possibly secondary to an increase in estrogen production. Nulliparity has been associated with an increased chance of developing breast cancer, but the magnitude of the risk is much smaller. The use of oral contraceptive pills has not been associated with breast cancer in women without a high-risk genetic mutation.

2. ANSWER: A

Explanation

A minority of breast cancers are hereditary. About 5% to 10% of all women with breast cancer have a mutation in a high-penetrance gene that is passed down in a family, and the most common mutations are those of the genes BRCA1 or BRCA2. Other genes implicated with breast cancer include PTEN, TP53, ATM, CHEK2, NF1, STK11, and CDH1. Although a mutation in a high-penetrance gene can only be found in about 5% and 10% of women with breast cancer, up to 20% of women with breast cancer have a positive family history.

3. ANSWER: D

Explanation

As per NCCN guidelines, patients with breast cancer and one or more of the following features should undergo genetic risk evaluation: early onset breast cancer (age ≤45), triple-negative breast cancer diagnosed age ≤60, ≥2 breast primaries in a single individual or two different individuals from the same side of the family, ≥1 close blood relative (first, second, or third degree relative) with breast cancer at age ≤50, ≥close blood relatives with breast cancer and/or pancreatic cancer at any age, personal history of ovarian cancer or ≥1 close blood relative with ovarian cancer, population at increased risk (ie Ashkenazi Jewish descent), personal or family history of male breast cancer. All patients should undergo genetic counseling prior to having genetic testing sent.

4. ANSWER: E

Explanation

The patient is an unaffected family member with a strong family history. Her family history includes breast cancer, ovarian cancer, and pancreatic cancer and she has a high risk of having a BRCA2 mutation. The next step is to do genetic counseling and testing. Bilateral mastectomy and prophylactic salpingo-oophorectomy are not recommended for every patient with a mutation, and it should be decided case by case. CT/PET scan is not studied for screening in high-risk patients and it should not be used. Breast MRI and pelvic ultrasound can be considered, if she has a mutation. The role of serum markers in mutation carriers is debated. CA-125 may be used in addition to vaginal ultrasound in patients with a BRCA mutation.

5. ANSWER: C

Explanation

BRCA-2 mutations are associated with an increased risk of ovarian, fallopian tube, primary peritoneal cancers, and melanoma. Male patients with BRCA 2 mutations also have an increased risk of prostate cancer.

6. ANSWER: B

Explanation

The patient most likely has Li-Fraumeni syndrome, a rare inherited autosomal dominant disease associated with mutations in the tumor suppressor gene TP53. Li-Fraumeni syndrome is associated with a lifetime risk of developing cancer as high as 100%. The most typical types of cancer in affected families are sarcoma, premenopausal breast cancer, adrenocortical carcinoma, and brain tumors. Mutations in the gene PTEN are characteristic of Cowden syndrome; patients have an increased risk of developing hamartomas and a variety of malignancies including thyroid, breast cancer, and endometrial cancer. Mutations in the MSH6 gene are associated with Lynch syndrome. Although PALB2 and CDH1 genes are associated with an increased risk of breast cancer, this patient's family pedigree is not characteristic of PALB2 or CDH1 mutations.

7. ANSWER: C

Explanation

In the NSABP P-2 study, tamoxifen 20mg daily was compared with raloxifene 60mg daily in postmenopausal women with a high risk of breast cancer. This study demonstrated that the two agents were equivalent in terms of breast cancer risk reduction (approximately 50% with 5 years of therapy) however the side effect profiles were different. There were statistically significantly less pulmonary emboli and deep vein thromboses in patients treated with raloxifene compared to tamoxifen. Raloxifene is also associated with less uterine hyperplasia and fewer cataracts.

8. ANSWER: E

Explanation

Only tamoxifen is approved for prevention of breast cancer in premenopausal women. Tamoxifen and raloxifene can be used in postmenopausal women. While aromatase inhibitors (both steroidal and non-steroidal) have shown benefit in improving outcomes for patients already diagnosed with an invasive breast cancer, these agents are not approved for use in the chemoprevention setting in patients with a high risk of breast cancer but no personal history of breast cancer.

9. ANSWER: D

Explanation

This patient has a BRCA 1 mutation and high risk of developing breast cancer. Screening mammogram should begin at the age of 30. Screening MRI of the breasts has been demonstrated to be beneficial in high-risk in multiple studies. The American Cancer Society (ACS) guidelines recommend screening breast MRI in addition to screening mammograms in patients with BRCA mutations. A common strategy is to schedule the annual mammogram 6 months after the annual MRI.

10. ANSWER: B

Explanation

The patient has a suspicious palpable breast mass and the mammogram revealed dense breasts. Dense breasts decrease the sensitivity of mammograms and are associated with an increased risk of breast cancer. Obtaining an ultrasound in addition to the mammogram increases the detection of breast cancer.

11. ANSWER: C

Explanation

As per the NCCN guidelines, radiation therapy is contraindicated during pregnancy and in the setting of active connective disease. Multifocal tumors occupying >2 quadrants of the breast are not considered amenable to breast conserving surgery due to concerns about ability to achieve negative margins through a single incision with a satisfactory cosmetic result. Generally, tumors <5cm can be managed with breast conserving surgery followed by radiation, with tumor size ≥5cm being a relative contraindication to breast-conserving therapy.

12. ANSWER: E

Explanation

A 2003 study by Veronesi et al demonstrated that patients had less pain, sensation loss, lymphedema, and had better arm mobility following sentinel lymph node biopsy compared to axillary lymph node dissection.

13. ANSWER: C

Explanation

This patient will meet the inclusion criteria for ACOSOG Z0011. In that study, patients with sentinel lymph node-positive (one to two nodes) disease were randomized between complete axillary node dissection and no further axillary surgery. The no further axillary surgery arm had similar progression-free survival and overall survival compared to complete axillary node dissection. Lymph node positivity, by itself, is not a criterion for receiving chemotherapy. She could be in the luminal type A breast cancer group and may very well be treated with endocrine therapy only. Retrospective analysis of the SWOG 8814 study showed that Oncotype can be done in patients with node-positive disease also.

14. ANSWER: C

Explanation

Sentinel lymph node biopsy (SLNB) is recommended for patients with early stage breast cancer with clinically negative lymph nodes. SLNB is contraindicated in patients with inflammatory breast cancer and in patients with clinically positive lymph nodes undergoing surgery upfront. Patients diagnosed with DCIS who are planned for mastectomy should be considered for SLNB given that invasive carcinoma can be found in the final pathology analysis, and a sentinel lymph node biopsy would be compromised after mastectomy. Although multicentric disease is not a contraindication to SLNB, the likelihood of having an additional positive lymph node is higher than in patients with a single focus of disease.

15. ANSWER: E

Explanation

There is no clear evidence that systemic staging tests in early stage breast cancer are beneficial, and they can lead to unnecessary invasive procedures. Both NCCN and ASCO guidelines recommend against systemic staging for early stage breast cancer in the absence of symptoms.

16. ANSWER: A

Explanation

IORT was evaluated in the TARGIT-A and the ELIOT trials. In both trials, there was no difference in survival between IORT and external beam radiation. Skin complications were less common with IORT. Ipsilateral recurrences were more frequent among patients who received IORT.

17. ANSWER: A

Explanation

As per NSABP B-06 and EORTC 10801, no survival difference is seen between patients who are treated with modified radical mastectomy versus lumpectomy and radiation therapy. CALGB 9343 concluded that adjuvant radiation can be safely omitted in women age 70 or older with clinical stage I, ER-positive invasive breast carcinoma who receive lumpectomy and tamoxifen. There was no significant different in overall survival, time to distant metastases, and breast cancer specific survival between groups although there was an 8% difference in locoregional recurrence between groups (10 year freedom from locoregional recurrence 98% in arm receiving radiation v 90% in arm without radiation). Bilateral mastectomy has not been shown to improve survival compared to breast conservation therapy.

18. *ANSWER: E*

Explanation

This patient has not yet received systemic treatment for metastatic disease, and has many therapeutic options available. Her small solitary brain metastasis might be treated with stereotactic radiosurgery followed or not by whole brain radiation. A trial of systemic therapy and no radiation can also be done given that the central nervous system lesion is small and the patient is asymptomatic.

19. *ANSWER: D*

Explanation

Prompt recognition of cord compression is extremely important given that delaying treatment increases the likelihood of permanent neurological deficits. The treatment for cord compression includes immediate administration of glucocorticoids, pain management, and surgical decompression. Radiation therapy is also an option for initial treatment, especially in radiosensitive tumors and in patients who are not a candidate for surgery.

20. *ANSWER: D*

Explanation

Radiation recall dermatitis (RDD) is a rare inflammatory cutaneous reaction that develops in an area of previously irradiated skin after administration of certain medications, most commonly cytotoxic agents. Although RDD is uncommon, doxorubicin is one of the most commonly associated medications. Radiation enhancement occurs when chemotherapy is given concomitantly or within a short interval of time from radiation.

21. *ANSWER: A*

Explanation

As demonstrated in NSABP B-24, tamoxifen reduces the risk of breast cancer recurrence without effecting overall survival. The benefit is limited to ER/PR-positive DCIS.

22. *ANSWER: B*

Explanation

This patient has a Stage I (T1cN0) ER-positive tumor and meets criteria for Oncotype DX testing. This testing provides prognostic information and is also predictive of relative benefit from endocrine therapy and/or chemotherapy based on recurrence score.

23. *ANSWER: C*

Explanation

About 10% of patients receiving everolimus develop pneumonitis. In a majority of patients, after ruling out an infectious cause, the patient can be managed with corticosteroid and discontinuation of the therapy until it is resolved. In grade 1 to 3 pneumonitis, after appropriate supportive therapy, everolimus can be restarted with a dose reduction once the symptoms have resolved to grade 1.

24. ANSWER: B

Explanation

Oncotype DX testing has been prospectively validated in ER-positive, stage I/II lymph node negative breast cancer. There is data from retrospective analyses of the SWOG 8814 and ATAC trials that suggests that the testing provides prognostic information independent of clinical variables in N1 patients also. Results of the SWOG RxPONDER trial (S1007) are awaited to prospectively define the utility of Oncotype DX results in an ER-positive breast cancer population with 1 to 3 lymph nodes involved.

25. ANSWER: D

Explanation

The TEXT (Tamoxifen and Exemestane Trial) and SOFT (Suppression of Ovarian Function Trial) trials evaluated the role of ovarian suppression as adjuvant therapy in premenopausal women with ER-positive breast cancer. Premenopausal women with high-risk features had an improvement in 5-year disease-free survival with exemestane in combination with ovarian suppression, compared to tamoxifen.

26. ANSWER: C

Explanation

Randomized clinical trials have demonstrated that ovarian suppression with a GnRH-agonist given during chemotherapy in premenopausal women increases the likelihood of pregnancy in the future. Resumption of menses is not well correlated with fertility in premenopausal women who undergo chemotherapy.

27. ANSWER: A

Explanation

Aromatase inhibitors are less effective in inhibiting estrogen production by the ovaries, and should not be used alone in premenopausal women. Premenopausal women without previous exposure to anti-estrogen therapy can be treated with a selective estrogen receptor modulator alone, or ovarian suppression in combination with endocrine therapy.

28. ANSWER: E

Explanation

Second-line options for hormone receptor-positive metastatic breast cancer in postmenopausal women include fulvestrant as a single agent, fulvestrant in combination with a cyclin-dependent kinase inhibitor, exemestane in combination with everolimus, and tamoxifen. Combination chemotherapy should not be used in patients with oligometastasis and disease that is still potentially sensitive to endocrine therapy.

29. ANSWER: C

Explanation

Although the MA.17R and the NSABP-B42 trials showed conflicting results in regards to disease-free survival benefit in postmenopausal patients undergoing extended adjuvant endocrine therapy with aromatase inhibitors, it is reasonable to consider extending therapy beyond 5 years for women with high risk of relapse and very good tolerance.

30. ANSWER: E

Explanation

Premenopausal patients with ER-positive metastatic breast cancer can be treated with ovarian suppression plus endocrine therapy as for postmenopausal women. Given that this patient does not have rapidly progressive disease or visceral crisis, she can be continued on endocrine-based therapy.

31. ANSWER: A

Explanation

Patients with a "high risk" Oncotype DX recurrence score (31 or higher) derive benefit from chemotherapy in addition to endocrine therapy while those in the "low risk" group (traditionally defined as 18 or less, now defined more specifically as 10 or less in the TAILORx study by Sparano et al NEJM 2015) do not benefit from the addition of chemotherapy to endocrine therapy. Those with Recurrence Scores that fall between these scores are considered "intermediate risk" and should have treatment decisions made in a personalized manner, taking into account the biology of the tumor and comorbidities.

32. ANSWER: D

Explanation

This patient meets the inclusion criteria for the ACOSOG Z0011 study which demonstrated no difference in overall or disease-free survival in patients who had a complete axillary node dissection or sentinel lymph node biopsy for clinical T1-T2N0 invasive breast cancer and were found to have 1 or 2 sentinel lymph nodes containing metastases. Oncotype DX testing can be used in ER-positive patients with 1 to 3 lymph nodes involved and may identify patients who will not derive additional benefit from chemotherapy.

33. ANSWER: B

Explanation

She has a stage IIB cancer and in the conventional sense she should receive chemotherapy. However, many luminal type A patients (ER/PR positive and Ki-67 less than 14%, as per St. Galen criteria) can be treated with only endocrine therapy and no chemotherapy. She does not meet the criteria for radiation therapy after mastectomy (tumor more than 5 cm, four or more lymph nodes or other poor prognostic features). Even patients older than 65 will benefit from chemotherapy, if indicated.

34. ANSWER: E

Explanation

This patient's clinical presentation is consistent with inflammatory breast cancer (IBC). IBC is an aggressive form of breast cancer that accounts for approximately 1% to 5% of breast cancer cases. It is more frequent in younger and African American women. Breast conservation and sentinel lymph node biopsy are not indicated in the treatment of IBC. In this clinical scenario, chemotherapy before surgery has been demonstrated to have better outcomes than surgery upfront. Radiation therapy is recommended after surgery.

35. ANSWER: C

Explanation

Eribulin was evaluated in the EMBRACE trial, which enrolled breast cancer patients who have received at least 2 chemotherapy agents for metastatic disease. Patients were randomized to receive eribulin or treatment of physician's choice. Eribulin was associated with better overall survival. Eribulin causes myelossuppression, with dose-limiting neutropenia and is also commonly associated with peripheral neuropathy. Patients who are receiving eribulin may develop QTc prolongation, especially if they are concomitantly taking other drugs that prolong the QTc interval. Eribulin has also been associated with hyperglycemia.

36. ANSWER: C

Explanation

Patients with triple-negative breast cancer who have residual disease after neoadjuvant therapy have a higher chance of recurrence compared with patients who achieve complete pathologic response. The CREATE-X trial evaluated the efficacy of capecitabine in patients who have residual cancer after neoadjuvant treatment. Patients with HER2-negative disease who were previously treated with neoadjuvant chemotherapy were randomized to receive standard postsurgical treatment or capecitabine for 6 to 8 cycles. Capecitabine was associated with improved disease-free survival. However, in the subgroup analysis the benefit seemed to be restricted to patients with triple-negative disease. Neratinib is a tyrosine kinase inhibitor of HER2, HER3 and HER4 so it would not be appropriate for this patient has triple-negative disease. Neratinib has been approved for the extended adjuvant treatment of HER2+ breast cancer following the standard year of adjuvant trastuzumab therapy based on the results of the ExteNET study

37. ANSWER: D

Explanation

Combination chemotherapy regimens have not been shown to improve progression-free survival or overall survival in patients with metastatic breast cancer, compared with single chemotherapy agents. Combination therapy has more toxicity than single agent regimens. In the absence of rapidly progressive disease or visceral crisis, patients with metastatic breast cancer should be treated with sequential single agents.

38. ANSWER: A

Explanation

Patients with triple-negative breast cancer who achieve pathologic complete response have better outcomes than patients with residual disease after neo-adjuvant therapy. However, when compared to adjuvant systemic therapy, neoadjuvant therapy has not been demonstrated to improve neither disease-free survival nor overall survival.

39. ANSWER: B

Explanation

The patient's clinical presentation is consistent with a hypersensitive reaction to paclitaxel. Infusion reactions to taxanes usually occur in the initial minutes of an infusion. Although there are patients who develop severe hypersensitive reactions and even anaphylaxis to taxanes, routine premedication with steroids, diphenhydramine and an H2-antagonist has significantly decreased the incidence of infusion reactions. Most patients with minor reactions can be safely re-challenged with a taxane using a reduced infusion rate and/or changing the premedication regimen.

40. ANSWER: A

Explanation

As per the 2013 ASCO/ACP guidelines for HER2 testing, HER2 is considered positive if it is 3+ by immunohistochemistry (IHC). It is considered negative if IHC is 0 or 1+, and equivocal if IHC is 2+. Tumors with a HER2 equivocal by immunohistochemistry should be tested by in situ hybridization before a choice about treatment is made. In regards to in situ hybridization, HER2 is considered positive if either the HER2 copy number is ≥ 6.0 signals/cell or the HER2/CEP17 ratio is ≥ 2.0. If the HER2 copy number is ≥ 4.0 and < 6.0 and the HER2/CEP17 ratio is < 2.0, HER2 should be considered equivocal. If HER2 copy number is < 4.0 and HER2/CEP17 ratio is < 2.0, HER2 is considered negative.

41. ANSWER: D

Explanation

Ado-trastuzumab emtansine is an antibody-drug conjugate composed of trastuzumab linked to a highly potent cytotoxic derivative of maytansine (DM1) by a stable linker. DM1 is a microtubule inhibitor. Ado-trastuzumab emtansine has been found to be active in trastuzumab- and lapatinib-resistant metastatic breast cancer, as well as in trastuzumab-naïve tumors. The phase 3 EMILIA trial that compared trastuzumab emtansine with capecitabine + lapatinib in advanced HER2-positive breast cancer showed a substantial improvement in progression-free survival (PFS) and overall survival with the antibody-drug conjugate.

42. *ANSWER: E*

Explanation

Patients receiving trastuzumab should have an echocardiogram performed as baseline before starting treatment, and every 3 months while receiving trastuzumab. Patients with cardiotoxicity related to trastuzumab are usually asymptomatic and are diagnosed though routine echocardiograms performed during treatment. The decrease in left ventricle ejection fraction is reversible in the majority of the patients, and treatment with trastuzumab may be reinitiated in the future. When the EF decreases 16% from a normal baseline or is below normal limits with ≥10% decrease from baseline, trastuzumab should be held and an echocardiogram should be repeated in 1 month. If the EF remains low, trastuzumab should be discontinued.

43. *ANSWER: D*

Explanation

Patients with stage T1cN0 HER2-positive breast cancer have a significant chance of recurrence and should be considered for adjuvant systemic therapy. In the Adjuvant Paclitaxel and Trastuzumab (APT) trial, published in the *New England Journal of Medicine* in 2015 (Winer et al), patients with small (≤3cm), node-negative and HER2-positive tumors received adjuvant therapy with weekly paclitaxel for 12 weeks and trastuzumab for one year. This regimen was well tolerated and the 3-year invasive-free-survival was 98.7%. In the phase III Adjuvant Lapatinib and/or Trastuzumab Treatment Optimization (ALTTO) trial, dual anti-HER2 adjuvant therapy with trastuzumab and lapatinib either concomitantly or sequentially failed to demonstrate improved disease-free survival as compared with single-agent trastuzumab. T-DM1 is being evaluated in the adjuvant setting in the ATTEMPT trial, however single-agent T-DM1 is not a standard option for adjuvant therapy.

44. *ANSWER: C*

Explanation

The duration of trastuzumab has been studied in the HERA (HERceptin Adjuvant) and the PHARE (Protocol for Herceptin as Adjuvant therapy with Reduced Exposure) trials. Duration shorter than 12 months has not been demonstrated to be noninferior than 12 months. Patients treated with trastuzumab for 24 months had similar survival outcomes than patients treated for 12 months and experienced more side effects.

45. *ANSWER: A*

Explanation

The APHINITY trial evaluated the efficacy of pertuzumab when added to adjuvant trastuzumab and chemotherapy. Patients with high-risk node-negative or with node-positive disease were randomized to receive adjuvant chemotherapy and 1 year of treatment with trastuzumab plus either pertuzumab or placebo. Pertuzumab significantly improved the rates of invasive-disease-free survival however the benefit was small. At 3 years, 93.2% of women who received trastuzumab alone had not developed invasive disease, compared with 94.1% of those who received pertuzumab and trastuzumab. Adjuvant pertuzumab in addition to trastuzumab for one year can be considered in selected high-risk patients, such as those with ER/PR-negative disease or positive lymph nodes.

46. ANSWER: C

Explanation

The phase III trial EMILIA evaluated the efficacy of ado-trastuzumab emtansine (T-DM1) compared with combination of lapatinib and capecitabine in patients with HER2-positive metastatic breast cancer previously treated with trastuzumab and a taxane. Patients who received T-DM1 had a longer progression-free survival and overall survival than patients treated with lapatinib capecitabine. In addition, single-agent T-DM1 was less toxic.

47. ANSWER: B

Explanation

Neratinib in the adjuvant setting was evaluated in the ExteNET phase III trial. Patients with HER2-positive high-risk disease who had completed one year of trastuzumab were randomized to receive either neratinib or placebo. Disease-free survival rate at 2 years was 93.9% in the neratinib group and 91.6% in the placebo group. All-grade diarrhea occurred in approximately 95% of patients treated with neratinib, however the rates of diarrhea significantly decreased with the use of loperamide in the CONTROL trial. The ExteNET study led to neratinib approval by the U.S. Food and Drug Administration (FDA) in July 2017 for extended adjuvant therapy in HER2-positive breast cancer.

48. ANSWER: A

Explanation

Combination of a taxane with trastuzumab and pertuzumab is the preferred regimen for first-line treatment of patients with metastatic HER2-positive breast cancer. In the CLEOPATRA trial, patients were randomized to receive docetaxel in combination with trastuzumab and either pertuzumab or placebo. The addition of pertuzumab significantly improved disease-free survival and overall survival.

49. ANSWER: A

Explanation

Palbociclib is a cyclin-dependent kinase (CDK) 4 and 6 inhibitor that can be used in patients with metastatic ER-positive disease in combination with letrozole or fulvestrant. Although neutropenic fever is rare, palbociclib is associated with low neutrophil counts. A CBC should be monitored every 2 weeks for the initial 2 cycles and on day 1 of each subsequent cycle. No dosage adjustment is required for neutropenia grade 1 or 2 (ANC ≥ 1000). If the CBC on day 1 reveals grade 3 neutropenia (ANC 500 to 1000/mm^3), palbociclib should be held and a CBC should be repeated in 1 week. If the neutropenia improves to ≤ grade 2, palbociclib can be restarted at the same dose. If the CBC on Day 15 of the first 2 cycles reveals grade 2 neutropenia, palbociclib can be continued to complete the cycle and a CBC should be repeated on Day 22. If there is grade 4 neutropenia (ANC <500) on Day 22, palbociclib should be withheld until the neutropenia resolves to ≤ grade 2, and can then be restarted at the next lower dose. If the recovery from grade 3 neutropenia takes more than 1 week or if the patients has recurrent grade 3 neutropenia, dose reduction should be considered. If there is grade 4 neutropenia at any time, palbociclib should be held until neutropenia resolves to ≤ grade 2; after resolution, palbociclib can be resumed at the next lower dose.

50. ANSWER: D

Explanation

Olaparib is a Poly ADP ribose polymerase (PARP) inhibitor that has been approved for the treatment of ovarian cancer patients with and without BRCA mutations. In the phase III OlympiAD trial, patients with previously treated HER2-negative metastatic breast cancer and a germline BRCA mutation were randomized to receive olaparib or standard chemotherapy. Results demonstrated longer median progression-free survival in patients who received olaparib (7 months versus 4.2 months).

51. ANSWER: B

Explanation

Ribociclib is a cyclin-dependent kinase (CDK) 4 and 6 inhibitor that was approved by the FDA in March 2017 in combination with an aromatase inhibitor as initial endocrine therapy for postmenopausal women with hormonal receptor-positive, HER2-negative metastatic breast cancer. Ribociclib can cause QTc prolongation so ECG and electrolytes should be monitored during treatment. In the MONALEESA-2 trial, approximately 3 % of patients treated with ribociclib developed QTc prolongation. Clinicians should be aware of potential interaction with other drugs that are known to prolong the QTc interval. Ribociclib can also cause myelossuppression and elevated liver function tests.

52. ANSWER: E

Explanation

Patients with bone metastasis from breast cancer should receive a bone-modifying agent in addition to endocrine therapy or chemotherapy. Bisphosphonates and rank-ligand inhibitors decrease progression of the bone lesions and decrease the risk of skeletal-related events, including pathologic fractures. Zoledronic acid 4 mg IV has traditionally been given every 4 weeks but the OPTIMIZE-2 trial did not show a difference in incidence of skeletal-related events with 12 weeks intervals. Bone-modifying agents should be accompanied by vitamin D and calcium supplementation.

53. ANSWER: D

Explanation

Programmed cell death protein 1 (PD-1) is expressed in 20% to 30% of breast cancer cells. The KEYNOTE-012 phase Ib study of pembrolizumab in advanced solid tumors included triple-negative breast cancer (TNBC) patients. In this study, the response rate among breast cancer patients was 18.5%. However, in the KEYNOTE-086 phase II trial only 4.7% of metastatic TNBC patients had an objective response to single-agent pembrolizumab. The ISPY-2 phase II trial evaluated the efficacy of pembrolizumab in combination to neoadjuvant chemotherapy in hormone receptor-positive/Her2-negative and TNBC patients. The addition of pembrolizumab increased the pathologic complete response rate in patients with TNBC (60% vs. 20%) and in patients with HR-positive/HER2-negative breast cancer (34% vs. 13%). Although there are multiple ongoing studies evaluating the efficacy of immunotherapy agents in breast cancer, as of August 2017, they have not been approved by the FDA for breast cancer treatment. Should we include something there about the broad approval of pembro with MSI-H cancers?

54. ANSWER: C

Explanation

The Early Breast Cancer Trialists' Collaborative Group (EBCTCG) meta-analysis included data from 18,766 women. In this analysis, bisphosphonates were shown to decrease the risk of bone recurrence (RR 0.83) and to decrease breast cancer mortality (RR 0.91). The benefits however were restricted to postmenopausal patients. The ASCO guidelines published in July 2017 recommend considering adding bisphosphonates to the adjuvant regimen in postmenopausal (or premenopausal women undergoing ovarian suppression) that are deemed to be candidates for adjuvant systemic therapy. Although zoledronic acid 4 mg intravenously every 6 months for 3 to 5 years or clodronate orally at 1,600 mg/d for 2 to 3 years are recommended, the optimal dose and interval of bisphosphonates have not been determined yet. There is not sufficient data to recommend denosumab in the adjuvant setting.

Renal Cell Cancer 13

Ramaprasad Srinivasan, Azam Ghafoor, and Inger L. Rosner

REVIEW QUESTIONS

1. In which of the following patients with metastatic renal cell cancer is cytoreductive nephrectomy most appropriate?

   A. A 50-year-old male with an ECOG performance status of 0, a large 12 cm right renal mass, and four small pulmonary metastases

   B. A 67-year-old female with an ECOG performance status of 0, a 7 cm left renal mass, retroperitoneal adenopathy and hepatic metastases that have doubled in size over 4 weeks

   C. An 81-year-old man with an asymptomatic 6 cm right renal mass, and multiple hepatic metastases who has declined sytemic therapy

   D. A 72-year-old man with an ECOG performance status of 2, a 5 cm right renal mass, and mild dyspnea associated with numerous pulmonary metastases

2. Which of the following regarding interleukin-2 (IL-2) therapy for metastatic RCC is true?

   A. IL-2 has demonstrable efficacy in clear cell as well as papillary RCC

   B. Randomized studies have demonstrated an overall survival benefit associated with high dose IL-2

   C. Low-dose subcutaneous and high-dose intravenous IL-2 have comparable efficacy

D. Durable complete responses are seen in a small proportion of patients receving high-dose IL-2

E. Newer formulations have led to better tolerability of high-dose IL-2

3. A 68-year-old man underwent a right radical nephrectomy for a 12 cm renal mass identified during evaluation of flank pain and unexplained weight loss. Histopathologic evaluation was consistent with clear cell RCC, Fuhrman grade III. Routine surveillance imaging 2 years later revealed multiple bilateral pulmonary nodules and three 2 to 3cm liver masses. Biopsy of a liver lesion was consistent with clear cell RCC and he was referred to a medical oncologist for discussion of systemic therapy options. At the time of referral, he has no symptoms attributable to metastatic disease, and his CBC and chemistry panel are normal. Reasonable treatment options, based on demonstration of clinical benefit in randomized phase 3 trials, include which of the following?

A. Pazopanib

B. Sunitinib

C. Axitinib

D. Temsirolimus

E. Everolimus

4. A 55-year-old woman is referred to you for further management of metastatic type 2 papillary renal cell cancer. She was initially diagnosed at the age of 54 when she underwent a left radical nephrectomy and retroperitoneal lymph node dissection for an 8 cm renal mass and associated regional lymphadenopathy. Complete staging evaluation at the time also revealed extensive mediastinal and hilar adenopathy and multiple bone lesions consistent with metastatic disease. She has received sequential therapy with temsirolimus and then sunitinib with disease progression following brief periods of stability with both agents. Which of the following statements best reflects available treatment options for this patient?

A. Foretinib and other antagonists of the MET pathway are associated with improved survival in this setting.

B. Treatment with axitinib should be considered as this agent has been shown to improve progression-free survival compared to sorafenib.

C. Everolimus has been shown to improve progression-free survival compared to sorafenib in patients with papillary RCC who have failed prior therapy with sunitinib.

D. There are no standard options of proven clinical benefit; appropriate clinical trials could be considered

5. A 31-year-old man presents with a 4-week history of malaise and 2 to 3 episodes of gross hematuria. He has also noticed an unintentional weight loss of approximately 10 lbs over the past 2 to 3 months. His family history is remarkable for kidney cancer in his mother. His physical examination is remarkable for several papular skin lesions, which are very sensitive to touch, temperature changes. A CT of the chest, abdomen, and pelvis reveals a 10 cm left renal mass but is otherwise normal. He is offered a radical left nephrectomy by his urologist, but asks if the procedure can be deferred for at least 4 weeks as he is the sole caregiver for his 24-year-old sister who is undergoing a hysterectomy next week for removal of several large uterine fibroids. Which of the following statements about this patient's condition is most accurate?

A. This presentation is most consistent with hereditary papillary renal cell carcinoma and genetic evaluation will reveal a germline mutation in *MET*

B. Imaging of the CNS in this patient and his sister will likely demonstrate the presence of hemangioblastomas

C. He should undergo genetic counseling and should be evaluated for germline alterations in the *fumarate hydratase* gene

D. His renal tumor will demonstrate loss of heterozygosity affecting the *VHL* gene

6. A 68-year-old man was recently diagnosed with metastatic clear cell RCC. Somatic alterations in which of the following genes in most likely to be found if his tumor genome were to be sequenced?

A. *MET*

B. *PBRM1*

C. *SETD2*

D. *VHL*

E. *BAP1*

7. A 59-year-old woman is seeking therapeutic options for newly diagnosed clear cell RCC with metastases in both lungs and multiple bony lesions. Her medical oncologist proposes to commence therapy with pazopanib. Which of the following statements regarding first line therapy for her condition is true?

    A. Pazopanib is associated with improved overall survival compared to placebo

    B. Pazopanib is associated with improved overall survival compared to sunitinib

    C. Pazopanib is associated with improved overall survival compared to interferon

    D. Pazopanib is associated with improved progression free survival compared to placebo

8. A 69-year-old man undergoes a radical nephrectomy to remove a 9 cm mass. Histopathologic evaluation reveals a high grade clear cell renal tumor (Fuhrman grade IV), with evidence of invasion into the perinephric fat. His urologist is confident that there is no residual macroscopic disease and no evidence of metastatic disease. However, he deems the patient to be at high risk for disease recurrence based on tumor grade and stage and refers the pt to a medical oncologist to discuss adjuvant therapy options. In discussing options for adjuvant therapy, which of the following statements are accurate?

    A. Adjuvant therapy with nivolumab, a PD1 inhibitor, is associated with a survival benefit

    B. At least one study has demonstrated an improvement in PFS with sunitinib compared to placebo in high-risk patients

    C. Sorafenib, but not sunitinib, was shown to be superior to placebo in a randomized study in high risk RCC

    D. Sunitinib, but not sorafenib, was shown to prolong overall survival in high risk RCC when administered in the adjuvant setting

    E. Sunitinib prolongs overall survival in high risk RCC when given for 3 years but not for one year

9. A 55-year-old man was diagnosed 2 years ago with metastatic clear cell RCC. He received sunitinib (50mg/day, 4 weeks on and two weeks off)

at that time and experienced a partial response until recently, when two new metastatic lesions in the liver were identified. Which of the following actions is supported by data from phase III studies?

A. Discontinue sunitinib and start pazopanib

B. Continue sunitinib, but increase the dose to 62.5mg/day with close monitoring for toxicity

C. Discontinue sunitinib and commence therapy with cabozantinib

D. Discontinue sunitinib and commence therapy with everolimus

10. Which of the following statements regarding nivolumab, a PD1 "checkpoint" inhibitor, is true in patients with advanced RCC?

A. Nivolumab was associated with better OS compared to everolimus in patients who had progressed on prior antiangiogenic therapy.

B. Higher PDL1 expression is associated with better outcome in RCC patients receiving nivolumab.

C. Nivolumab is superior to cabozantinib in patients who have progressed on prior antiangiogenic therapy.

D. Nivolumab is superior to pazopanib in patients with untreated metastatic RCC.

11. A 50-year-old athlete in otherwise excellent health was found to have a 10 cm left renal mass and underwent a left radical nephrectomy and ipsilateral retroperitoneal lymph node dissection; histopathologic evaluation was consistent with clear cell renal cancer, with evidence of disease in 4/16 lymph nodes. A metastatic workup revealed no evidence of metastatic disease and the patient was prescribed a surveillance regimen that he followed diligently. Two years later, several pulmonary nodules and two liver lesions were identified on imaging. The patient remained asymptomatic, but had noticed a slight decline in exercise tolerance over the past few weeks. Laboratory evaluation revealed normocytic, normochromic anemia (hemoglobin 9.6 gm/dL), a creatinine of 1.4 mg/dL, an alkaline phosphatase level that was twice the upper limit of normal and a neutrophil count just below the lower limit of normal; all other lab values were within normal limits. He is advised therapy with pazopanib and wishes to understand his prognosis. Based on established prognostic

criteria, which of the following would be considered a risk factor for adverse outcome?

A. Elevated alkaline phosphatase

B. Decreased hemoglobin

C. Elevated creatinine

D. Decreased neutrophil count

12. Which of the following is _not_ true of first-line therapy for patients with metastatic clear cell RCC?

A. Sunitinib and pazopanib appear to have comparable efficacy based on a randomized phase III noninferiority study

B. Pazopanib is generally better tolerated than sunitinib based on quality of life measures and data on patient preference

C. Nivolumab was associated with a better OS compared to pazopanib in a phase III randomized study

D. Sunitinib is superior to interferon-α, and was associated with better PFS and response rates in a randomized phase 3 study

13. A 36-year-old man is diagnosed with papillary RCC following a radical nephrectomy for a 12 cm renal tumor. Six months later presents with multiple metastatic lesions to the liver and bone. He is in otherwise good health. Which of the following statements about his systemic treatment options is true?

A. Sunitinib is associated with a 30% to 40% overall response rate in this subtype of RCC.

B. High dose IL-2 should be considered in this patient given his young age, good performance status, and absence of comorbidities.

C. Pazopanib is associated with improved PFS compared to placebo in patients with metastatic papillary RCC.

D. Enrolment on a well-designed clinical study is a reasonable consideration in this patient.

ANSWERS TO REVIEW QUESTIONS

1. ANSWER: A. Cytoreductive nephrectomy is most likely to benefit patients who are good surgical candidates as well as candidates for postnephrectomy systemic therapy, such as those with a good performance status, a relatively slow rate of disease progression, and those with relatively low metastatic burden (as demonstrated in a randomized phase III study where interferon was offered postnephrectomy). Patients described in b-d are less likely to benefit from this approach as they do not satisfy one or more of the above criteria.

2. ANSWER: D. Complete responses are seen in 7% to 9% of metastatic clear cell RCC patients receiving high-dose IL-2, with the majority of these patients remaining disease-free for long periods. The efficacy of IL-2 has not been adequately evaluated in patients with nonclear cell histologic subtypes and the use of this agent is largely restricted to clear cell RCC patients. There are no randomized phase III studies demonstrating a survival benefit with IL-2.

3. ANSWER: A and B. This patient appears to have "standard" risk metachronous metastatic clear cell renal cell cancer. Sunitinib has been shown to prolong progression-free survival compared to interferon-α in a randomized phase III trial in patients with previously untreated metastatic clear cell RCC, while pazopanib was similarly associated with an improved PFS in a placebo controlled phase III trial. Axitinib and everolimus have both shown clinical benefit in previously treated patients, while temsirolimus is associated with improved overall survival compared to interferon-α in "poor risk" patients. While high dose IL-2 (not listed as a choice in this instance) may be a reasonable option for this patient, there are no randomized studies demonstrating benefit for this agent over other available therapies.

4. ANSWER: D. There are no standard systemic therapy options of proven benefit at this time for most patients with advanced RCC patients with nonclear cell histologies. While foretinib, a MET inhibitor, as well as inhibitors of the VEGF and mTOR pathways have activity in small subsets of these patients, their utility in the majority of patients with nonclear cell RCC remains to be established. Recently, small single arm phase II studies have shown meaningful response rates with bevacizumab based therapies (in combination with either everolimus or erlotinib, respectively), and warrant further study.

5. ANSWER: C. A renal mass in a young man with skin findings suggestive of cutaneous leiomyomata, a family history of kidney cancer and uterine fibroids should arouse suspicion for hereditary leiomyomatosis and renal cell cancer (HLRCC), a familial kidney cancer syndrome characterized by germline mutations in the gene encoding the Krebs cycle enzyme, fumarate hydratase.

6. ANSWER: D. Inactivation of the *VHL* gene by mutation/deletion or promoter hypermethylation is the most common genetic alteration in clear cell renal tumors (seen in up to 90% of tumors in some series). Although alterations in *PBRM1, SETD2,* and *BAP1* have also been seen, they occur less frequently. Mutations in *MET* are seen primarily in a subset of patients with papillary RCC.

7. ANSWER: D. Pazopanib was shown to be superior to placebo in a randomized phase III study in patients who had either received no prior therapy or had received prior interferon-α, with higher response rates and improved median PFS, but no improvement in overall survival. Pazopanib has not been compared to interferon-α and has not been shown to prolong overall survival compared to sunitinib in phase III studies.

8. ANSWER: B. The S-TRAC study has demonstrated a modest improvement in PFS with sunitinib compared to placebo. However, in a second study comparing sunitinib, sorafenib, and placebo (ASSURE), no benefit was discerned with either intervention arm. Differences in study design/ patient population may contribute to some extent to the differences in outcome in these two studies. To date, no randomized study has demonstrated an OS benefit with a VEGF pathway inhibitor in the adjuvant setting. Studies evaluating PD1 inhibitors as well as the impact of duration of therapy with VEGFR-targeted therapy are ongoing.

9. ANSWER: C. In a randomized phase III study (METEOR), cabozantinib was associated with a higher response rate and PFS compared to everolimus in clear cell RCC patients who experienced disease progression on first-line tyrosine kinase inhibitors targeting the VEGFR pathway. Nivolumab (not listed as an option here) is also a reasonable option in this setting based on its superiority over everolimus in a phase III study. Neither pazopanib, nor nonstandard sunitinib dosing regimens have been evaluated in this setting. Although everolimus has demonstrated efficacy in this setting, it has largely been supplanted by cabozantinib as well as nivolumab.

10. ANSWER: A. In a randomized phase III study, nivolumab provided higher response rates as well as improved OS compared to everolimus in patients who had progressed on prior therapy with VEGF pathway antagonists. In this study, the level of PD1 expression in the tumor specimen was not associated with outcome; however, it must be emphasized that there is currently no accepted universal standard for evaluating PD1 expression. Nivolumab has not been directly compared with pazopanib or cabozantinib.

11. ANSWER: B. In patients undergoing antiangiogenic therapy, poor performance status, elevated calcium, anemia, time from original diagnosis to therapy < 1 year, neutrophilia and thrombocytosis were identified as poor prognostic factors by the International Metastatic Renal Cell Cancer Database Consortium (IMDC). This patient would be classified into a good prognosis group based on the presence of only one poor prognostic factor.

12. ANSWER: C. Nivolumab has not been compared directly with pazopanib. All other statements are true.

13. ANSWER: D. There are currently no standard agents of proven benefit in patients with advanced papillary RCC and these patients are often referred to clinical trials. Antiangiogenic agents including sunitinib and pazopanib appear to be associated with modest response rates and PFS in phase II studies. There is no evidence to suggest that high dose IL-2 has activity in nonclear cell RCC variants.

Prostate Cancer 14

Ravi A. Madan and William L. Dahut

REVIEW QUESTIONS

1. A 63-year-old male with a PSA of 9.2 ng/dL has Gleason 4+3 adenocarcinoma of the prostate diagnosed on a biopsy. After surgical resection of his prostate, which of the following findings would not be an indication for adjuvant radiotherapy?

   A. Positive lymph node sampling at surgery

   B. Extracapsular extension

   C. Seminal vesicle involvement

   D. Positive surgical margins

2. A 56-year-old man with a PSA of 21.3 ng/dl was diagnosed 3 years ago with Gleason 5+4 prostate cancer and treated with surgery. After 3 years of follow-up, his PSA is now rising from an undetectable nadir to 12.7 ng/dl and a bone scan and CT scan demonstrated findings consistent with metastatic disease. The CT showed multiple retroperitoneal lymph nodes and the bone scan showed 4 lesions in the spine, pelvis, and one in the scapula. The patient is initiated on androgen deprivation therapy with one month of bicalutamide and goserelin acetate and his PSA has declined to 3.4 ng/dl. Which of the following therapies could be added to this regimen that has demonstrated a survival benefit?

   A. Cabazitaxel

   B. Zoledronic acid

   C. Docetaxel

D. Radium 223

E. Sipuleucel-T

3. A 65-year-old male with mCRPC including metastasis to the pelvis, spine, and ribs has recently started treatment with enzalutamide. His initial PSA on therapy was 46.7 ng/dl. Over the next 6 months the patient's PSA declined to 4.7 ng/dl. After completing 9 months of therapy, his PSA is 16.2 ng/dl. Repeat imaging demonstrates no new areas of disease. He is tolerating the treatment well with some mild fatigue and has no symptoms related to his prostate cancer. What is the most appropriate next step for this patient's treatment regimen based on Prostate Cancer Working Group 3 recommendations?

A. Double the dose of enzalutamide

B. Add abiraterone and continue enzalutamide

C. Discontinue enzalutamide and initiate docetaxel

D. Add docetaxel to the enzalutamide regimen

E. Continue enzalutamide

4. A patient is seeing you in follow-up for his mCPRC including metastasis to the lungs, liver, and spine. He recently had radiographic progression of disease on abiraterone and prednisone after 9 months of therapy. The patient asks about changing to enzalutamide but is also open to other therapies. Which of the following should you tell him?

A. The patient will not respond to enzalutamide because of liver metastasis.

B. Docetaxel is not an effective treatment option for patients who have progressed on abiraterone.

C. Enzalutamide and abiraterone share overlapping mechanisms of resistance that decrease the likelihood enzalutamide will be effective in this patient.

D. Radium 223 is the most appropriate next step because it will decrease the risk of cord compression.

E. The patient should first change his prednisone to decadron.

5. A 61-year-old male with metastatic castration-resistant prostate cancer with metastasis to the pelvis, spine, and pelvic lymph nodes. His PSA

is 56.4 ng/ml and he has minimal pain. He is started on abiraterone 1,000 mg with 10 mg of prednisone daily. He is seen 1 month later and his PSA is now 30.6 ng/ml and his pain has improved. On his next follow-up visit, his PSA is less than 10, his pain has resolved, but he has new bilateral lower extremity edema that was not present previously. What is the most likely cause of the lower extremity edema?

A. Abiraterone

B. Prednisone

C. Deep venous thrombosis

D. Small cell conversion of this patient's prostate cancer

E. Tumor lysis syndrome

6. A 63-year-old male with metastatic castration-resistant prostate cancer (metastatic to the scapula and 3 ribs) is currently being treated with ADT and enzalutamide 160 mg/daily. The patient has been on ADT for 3 years and the enzalutamide was begun 6 weeks ago. He now reports extreme fatigue in the past few weeks. The patient's physical exam is unremarkable including cardiopulmonary assessments. The patient's PSA has declined from 38.1 ng/ml to 4.3 ng/ml. He reports no new medications or herbal agents. What is the most appropriate next step in the evaluation of this patient?

A. Assess immune-related events on the thyroid gland.

B. Evaluate the patient for adrenal insufficiency.

C. Consider reducing enzalutamide dose or holding the enzalutamide for 2 to 4 weeks.

D. Order repeat imaging to evaluate for neuroendocrine differentiation of the tumor and disease progression despite the drop in PSA.

E. Discontinue ADT since ADT can cause fatigue.

7. A 63-year-old male with metastatic castration-resistant prostate cancer has a rising PSA despite ADT. You evaluate the patient and order imaging, which shows multiple bone lesions on bone scan (spine, pelvis, and ribs). The CT scan confirms the bone lesions and shows no visceral disease or lymphadenopathy. The patient is now reporting diffuse bone pain moderately controlled by narcotics in combination with NSAIDs. Which one

of the following therapies is least likely to decrease the pain symptoms reported by this patient?

    A. Sipuleucel-T

    B. Abiraterone

    C. Enzalutamide

    D. Docetaxel

    E. Radium-223

8. Which of the following patients has disease consistent with metastatic castration-resistant prostate cancer?

    A. A 48-year-old patient with newly diagnosed prostate cancer including bone scan findings in the ribs and pelvis who just started ADT 1 month ago and has a declining PSA (0.15 ng/ml)

    B. A 61-year-old patient with a rising PSA (now 4.1 g/ml) after treatment with surgery alone who has never had systemic therapy (testosterone is 450 ng/dl)

    C. A 54-year-old patient with metastatic disease in the spine and just started ADT + Docetaxel and has a declining PSA

    D. A 73-year-old male who develops new metastasis (scapula and 8th rib) while on ADT and enzalutamide

    E. A 55-year-old male with biochemically recurrent prostate cancer who has a rising PSA (doubling time 5 months) and testosterone that is normal (375 ng/dl)

9. A 56-year-old male with biochemically recurrent prostate cancer has been on ADT for 6 months. Which one of the following additional treatments should he consider?

    A. Selenium

    B. Aspirin

    C. Calcium

    D. Calcium and Vitamin D

    E. Monthly zoledronic acid

10. A 54-year-old patient with metastatic castration-resistant prostate cancer is in your office for consultation. He has had previous treatment with

enzalutamide, abiraterone, and docetaxel (given every 3 weeks), but unfortunately has had progressive disease on those therapies. Recent evaluations indicate he has metastatic disease in his pelvis and spine, and liver (a 3-cm lesion). His PSA is 1084 ng/ml and rising. Which one of the following treatment options would be most appropriate?

    A. Cabazitaxel

    B. Retreatment with enzalutamide

    C. Radium-223

    D. Bicalutamide

    E. Weekly docetaxel

11. A 58-year-old male with metastatic prostate cancer in the pelvis, lumbar, and thoracic spine sees you in a follow-up visit in your office. He is currently doing well. His current medications include enzalutamide, zoledronic acid, calcium, vitamin D, and a statin. Which of the following most appropriately describes the role of zoledronic acid in this patient's care?

    A. Zoledronic acid is used primarily to treat hypocalcemia in advanced prostate cancer.

    B. Zoledronic acid is primarily used to delay disease progression in metastatic castration-resistant prostate cancer.

    C. Zoledronic acid has been shown to delay skeletal-related events.

    D. Zoledronic acid improves survival in men with metastatic castration-resistant prostate cancer.

    E. Zoledronic acid improves PSA responses when used with enzalutamide.

12. A 54-year-old male with newly diagnosed prostate cancer was found to have widely metastatic prostate cancer including liver, spine, and pelvis. After consulting with the patient and his family about his newly diagnosed metastatic disease, what is the most appropriate treatment recommendation?

    A. Surgical resection of the primary tumor followed by androgen deprivation therapy

    B. Radiation therapy for the primary lesions, followed by 2 to 3 years of androgen deprivation therapy

    C. Androgen deprivation therapy followed by radium-223

D. Androgen deprivation therapy concurrently with 6 cycles of docetaxel

E. Androgen deprivation therapy followed by additional therapy when PSA starts to rise

13. A 58-year-old male with metastatic castration-resistant prostate cancer has a rising PSA on androgen deprivation therapy alone. His PSA is 10.8 ng/ml and he has 3 metastatic lesions in his lower spine, rib, and pelvis. He asks you about sipuleucel-T therapy. Which one of the following responses is most appropriate?

    A. The treatment has demonstrated the ability to extend survival in phase III studies.

    B. The treatment frequently has 50% declines in PSA within 6 months.

    C. The treatment is associated with nausea, emesis, and neutropenia.

    D. The treatment is most effective if his primary tumor is positive for PDL1 positive.

    E. He is not eligible for this treatment because he has castration-resistant disease.

14. A 63-year-old with metastatic castration-resistant prostate cancer has a rising PSA despite castrate levels of testosterone. He has previously been treated with only androgen deprivation therapy and now seeks additional systemic therapy. His past medical history includes hypertension, hyperlipidemia, and a cerebral vascular accident 8 months ago with minor residual neurological defects. Which of the following therapies is least appropriate for this patient?

    A. Sipuleucel-T

    B. Enzalutamide

    C. Abiraterone

    D. Docetaxel

    E. Denosumab

15. A patient with newly diagnosed localized disease seeks your opinion for optimal therapy for his prostate cancer. He is 62 years old with no significant comorbidities except hypertension controlled by a single medication.

His PSA is 12.1 ng/ml and pathology suggests a Gleason score of 7. Which of the following responses to the patient is most appropriate?

- A. Randomized studies have indicated that surgery is most effective in curing his disease.
- B. Randomized studies have indicated that robotic surgery is most effective in curing his disease.
- C. Randomized studies have indicated that external beam radiation is most effective in curing his disease.
- D. Randomized studies have indicated that proton-based radiation is most effective in curing his disease.
- E. There is limited randomized data comparing radiation and surgery as definitive therapies.

16. A 72-year-old man with newly diagnosed localized prostate cancer has a PSA of 12.2 ng/ml and pathology that indicates Gleason (4+4) 8 disease. He is not willing to have surgery because of personal preference and is not willing to reconsider that opinion. His other comorbidities include hypertension and gout. Based on this patient's disease and preferences, what of the following is the most appropriate recommendation for this patient?

- A. The patient must reconsider surgery because randomized data indicates it has the best overall survival outcomes.
- B. External beam radiation therapy.
- C. External beam radiation therapy with androgen with 6 months of androgen deprivation therapy.
- D. External beam radiation therapy with androgen with 2 to 3 years of androgen deprivation therapy.
- E. Curative therapy should not be recommended because this disease is not likely to be aggressive.

17. A 53-year-old male with newly diagnosed metastatic castration-resistant prostate cancer has bulky lymphadenopathy, liver lesions, and bone disease. A biopsy of his disease has demonstrated BRCA1 mutation. What can you tell the patient about the potential implications of this mutation?

- A. Preliminary data have suggested that PARP inhibitors may be effective in patients with this mutation.
- B. Preliminary data suggest that the chemotherapy with docetaxel is most appropriate as the next treatment.

C. These tumors with this mutation are highlight responsive to AR-directed therapies and enzalutamide should be the next treatment for this patient.

D. The BRCA1 mutation is found in indolent prostate cancer and thus he does not require further disease at this time.

E. These tumors express high levels of PDL1 and thus anti-PD1/PDL1 therapy is the most appropriate next step.

18. A patient has metastatic castration-resistant prostate cancer with a rising PSA on enzalutamide is discussing future therapies with you. He has metastasis primarily in the bone. What is the most likely mechanism of treatment resistance driving this patient's disease?

   A. Changes in the androgen receptor including over expression and splice variants.

   B. De-differentiation into small cell variant.

   C. Selection of anaplastic prostate cancer that have neuroendocrine features.

   D. Increase PSA secretion by prostate cancer cells after treatment with androgen receptor directed therapy.

   E. Androgen receptor directed therapy selects for ductal prostate cancer.

19. A patient with metastatic castration-resistant prostate cancer is currently on his 4th cycle (of 6 planned cycles) of docetaxel and prednisone, with significant symptomatic and biochemical responses. He is currently experiencing minimal paresthesia in his toes, but not in his fingers or elsewhere. It is not functionally impairing his ability to walk. Which of the following is most appropriate next step in his care?

   A. Treat the patient with B12 to reverse potential treatment–related toxicity.

   B. Evaluate the patient with a screening MRI for cord compression.

   C. Discontinue prednisone which can contribute to neuropathy.

   D. Discuss with the patient that docetaxel-related neuropathy is a rare and universally reversible toxicity.

   E. Discuss with the patient that docetaxel can induce irreversible neuropathy and his symptoms need to be monitored closely.

20. A 63-year-old male with metastatic castration-resistant prostate cancer is in your office for follow-up while on docetaxel and prednisone along with androgen suppression therapy. He is reporting some increased back pain and difficult getting out of a chair, but denies incontinence. In fact, he has not urinated in the last 12 hours which is unusual for him. What is your clinical assessment of this patient?

   A. Prednisone can induce proximal muscle weakness and should be reduced.

   B. Cord compression should be ruled out because early presentation may include urinary retention.

   C. Cord compression should not be considered because the patient does not have incontinence.

   D. The back pain should be evaluated by radiation oncology and a routine consult should be requested.

   E. Urinary retention could be induced by docetaxel and the patient should have his chemotherapy held for one cycle and then re-evaluated.

ANSWERS TO REVIEW QUESTIONS

1. ANSWER: A. The indications of adjuvant radiation after RP include T3 disease (such as extracapsular extension or seminal vesicle involvement) or positive surgical margins. The finding of lymph node-positive disease during prostatectomy is not an indication for radiotherapy, although limited data support the use of ADT in such patients.

2. ANSWER: C. Understand the role of chemohormonal therapy in patients with metastatic castration-sensitive prostate cancer. Cabazitaxel, radium 223, and sipuleucel-T all have demonstrated the ability to extend survival in mCRPC (zoledronic acid provides potential decrease in skeletal events), but none have a defined role metastatic castration-sensitive prostate cancer. Based on the designation of the CHAARTED trial, this patient has high volume disease (at least four bone lesions with at least one that is beyond the spine and pelvis; visceral lesions would also put the patient in this category). Based on a randomized trial, adding six infusions of docetaxel 75 mg/m^2 every 3 weeks for 6 infusions (initiated within 120 days of starting ADT) to indefinite ADT extended median OS (57.6 vs. 44.0 months; HR=0.61) (Sweeney CJ et al., *NEJM*. 2015).

3. ANSWER: E. Understand how to implement Prostate Cancer Working Group 3 recommendations in clinical practice (Scher HI et al., *J Clin Oncol*. 2016). This patient had an initial PSA response to enzalutamide but now has a rising PSA despite stable imaging studies and an absence of symptoms. PSA should not be the sole criteria to alter therapy and thus continuing enzalutamide is the most appropriate answer. Progression should be determined primarily based on radiographic imaging or clinical symptoms. There is no data suggesting that doubling the dose of enzalutamide or adding docetaxel or abiraterone will improve clinical response. Although the patient could discontinue enzalutamide and initiate docetaxel, the side effects from chemotherapy are likely to be greater than his current symptom profile and minimal fatigue related to enzalutamide.

4. ANSWER: C. Understand mechanisms of resistance to antiandrogen therapy in mCRPC. The correct answer is that enzalutamide and abiraterone share overlapping mechanisms of resistance that decrease the likelihood of enzalutamide will be effective in this patient. Androgen receptor overexpression and mutations in the androgen receptor (i.e., splice variants) may decrease the likelihood that antiandrogen therapy such as abiraterone and enzalutamide may work sequentially (Antonarakis ES et al., *NEJM*. 2015). Although docetaxel is a rational next step, there is no clear data defining it as the clear next best step. Liver metastasis is contraindication for radium 223 but not enzalutamide. Abiraterone would not be expected to have differential effects in this setting based on the use of decadron as opposed to prednisone.

5. ANSWER: A. Understand the side effects of abiraterone (Ryan CJ et al., *NEJM*. 2013). Although prednisone can cause edema, the most likely answer is Abiraterone. Thrombosis is unlikely to cause bilateral lower extremity edema and small cell conversion of the prostate cancer is a rare event in prostate cancer. Tumor lysis is also a very rare event in prostate cancer and not a likely explanation.

6. ANSWER: C. Understand common toxicity of enzalutamide. Fatigue, sometimes extreme, has been reported with enzalutamide (Beer TM et al., *NEJM*. 2014). Reducing the dose of enzalutamide or holding the medication are appropriate next steps in this patient. Autoimmune-related events and adrenal insufficiency would not be expected with enzalutamide. Neuroendocrine de-differentiation would be a rare occurrence in the management of advanced prostate cancer. While ADT can cause fatigue, it should not be discontinued in advanced disease under routine circumstances and the timing of the fatigue aligns more appropriately with this patient starting enzalutamide.

7. ANSWER: A. While all these options have demonstrated the ability to improve survival in mCRPC, sipuleucel-T does not have immediate effects on disease progression or pain relief (Kantoff PW, *NEJM*. 2010). For that reason, it is indicated in mCRPC patients with minimal or no disease-related symptoms.

8. ANSWER: D. Metastatic castration resistant prostate cancer requires patients to have a rising PSA with castrate levels of testosterone; therefore, patients B and E are not the answer primarily because they are not castrate. Patients A and C have no evidence of progression on ADT based on the case reports provided. Patient D does have progression despite ADT and therefore meets the criteria for metastatic castration-resistant prostate cancer.

9. ANSWER: D. Patients on androgen deprivation therapy are at increased risk for osteopenia and osteoporosis, so the patient would benefit from supplemental calcium and vitamin D. There is little value of calcium in this patient in the absence of vitamin D, because vitamin D increases gastrointestinal absorption of calcium. Zoledronic acid may be indicated annually if the patient has a diagnosis of decreased bone mineral density. Aspirin and selenium have no defined role in the treatment of prostate cancer or as a supportive measure.

10. ANSWER: A. Of the options present, only cabazitaxel has proven potential for a survival benefit in this patient who has already progressed on docetaxel (de Bono JS et al., *Lancet*. 2010). There is no clear data suggesting clinical benefit from retreatment with enzalutamide or docetaxel after progression. Radium-223 is not indicated in patients with visceral lesions (Parker C et al., *NEJM*. 2013).

11. ANSWER: C. Zoledronic acid's primary benefit to this patient is that it has been shown to delay skeletal-related effects of the prostate cancer in a phase III trial. (Saad F et al., *J Natl Cancer Inst*. 2004). There is no clear synergy with enzalutamide on impact on PSA. There is also not randomized data that show this agent delays progression in this population. Zometa can be used to treat hypercalcemia.

12. ANSWER: D. This patient I diagnosed with metastatic castration-sensitive prostate cancer, with a high volume of disease. A randomized phase III study (Sweeney CJ et al., *NEJM*. 2015) demonstrated that docetaxel started within 120 days of ADT and continued for six three-week cycles extend overall survival compared to ADT alone (median 57.6 vs. 44.0 months; HR=0.61). There is no data supporting surgery or radiation in metastatic prostate cancer patients.

13. ANSWER: A. A phase III study of sipuleucel-T (Kantoff PW et al., *NEJM*. 2010) demonstrated that relative to placebo, sipuleucel-T extended survival in metastatic castration-resistant prostate cancer, leading to its FDA approval. Although it was well tolerated with chills, fever, and headache being the most common side effects, PSA declines were not routinely seen during or shortly after therapy. This therapy is a therapeutic cancer vaccine and thus does not require PDL1 expression to potentially have a clinical impact.

14. ANSWER: B. All agents are indicated for metastatic castration-resistant prostate cancer based on a survival advantage (docetaxel, abiraterone, sipuleucel-T) or for supportive measures (denosumab). Enzalutamide may lower the seizure threshold in patients and thus patients with a recent CVA history would preferably be treated with one of the alternatives listed that have a survival advantage in this population (Beer TM et al., *NEJM*. 2014).

15. ANSWER: E. Unfortunately, there is limited and incomplete randomized data comparing surgery and radiation as definitive therapy in prostate cancer. Ideally patients can speak with both surgeons and radiation oncologists, and once informed make decisions tailored to their comorbidities and personal preferences.

16. ANSWER: D. The patient should be treated for his high risk, Gleason 8 prostate cancer. Radiation based therapy is not known to be inferior to surgery based on any randomized study. Adjuvant androgen deprivation therapy for 2 to 3 years has been shown to improve survival and delay recurrence in this population (Horwitz EM et al., *J Clin Oncol*. 2008).

17. ANSWER: A. BRCA1 and other DNA repair defect mutations have been reported in approximately 30% of men with prostate cancer (Robinson D et al., *Cell*. 2015) and PARP inhibition has demonstrated a high probability of clinical benefit in this population (Mateo J. et al., *NEJM*. 2015).

18. *ANSWER: A.* Changes in the AR expression or post-translational modifications that lead to constituently active splice variants are among the more common forms of resistant to enzalutamide (Antonarakis, ES et al, NEJM, 2015). For this reason, sequential AR targeting therapies (i.e., enzalutamide and abiraterone) may not both be effective sequentially in delaying disease in patients who have already progressed on either abirtaerone or enzalutamide.

19. *ANSWER: E.* Docetaxel is an uncommon, but serious side effect seen with docetaxel, even in patients with newly diagnosed castration sensitive prostate cancer (Sweeney CJ et al., *NEJM.* 2015). These symptoms should be closely monitored as they may not be reversible. Considerations should be given for delaying the treatment, dose reduction, or treatment discontinuation.

20. *ANSWER: B.* Understand that back pain, proximal muscle weakness and urinary/fecal incontinence are among the most common presenting symptoms for cord compression. But also realize that incontinence could be preceded by urinary retention. In the setting of metastatic prostate cancer, even single cord compression symptoms should be fully evaluated and appropriate imaging should be considered (Flanagan EP et al, *Handb Clin Neurol.* 2017.)

Bladder Cancer 15

Andrea B. Apolo, Piyush K. Agarwal, and William L. Dahut

REVIEW QUESTIONS

1. A 73-year-old woman presents with gross hematuria. Urine cytology is positive for malignant cells and CT is negative except for thickening of the bladder wall. The patient undergoes an exam under anesthesia. Bimanual assessment reveals no palpable masses, but cystoscopy shows a 3-cm tumor over the dome of the bladder wall. The biopsy of this lesion shows high-grade muscle-invasive urothelial carcinoma. Which of the following is the most appropriate surgery?

   A. Partial cystectomy

   B. Partial cystectomy and sentinel lymph node biopsy

   C. Radical cystectomy and sentinel lymph node biopsy

   D. Radical cystectomy and pelvic lymph node dissection, distal ureterectomy, and removal of the urethra, uterus, fallopian tubes, anterior vaginal wall, and surrounding fascia

2. A 70-year-old man is diagnosed with advanced bladder cancer with liver and bone involvement. He is a construction worker who believes he was exposed to asbestos in the past. He has a history of alcohol abuse and of smoking 50 packs of cigarettes per year. His family history is significant for a brother who developed a germ-cell tumor at age 30. Which of the following risk factors has been shown in clinical studies to have the highest association with the development of bladder cancer?

   A. Asbestos exposure

   B. Alcohol abuse

C. Close relative with a germ-cell tumor

D. History of smoking

---

3. Cystoscopy of a 66-year-old man reveals a 3-cm papillary tumor in the left lateral wall of the bladder, as well as diffuse erythema of the remainder of the bladder wall. An exam under anesthesia demonstrates a mobile bladder. Biopsy of the papillary lesion reveals high-grade papillary carcinoma with no invasion. Biopsy of the erythematous areas reveals diffuse CIS. Muscle is present in the biopsy specimen. Which of the following is the most appropriate therapy for this patient?

A. Intravesical BCG

B. Cystectomy

C. Gemcitabine and cisplatin chemotherapy

D. Intravesical gemcitabine

---

4. A 72-year-old male smoker presents with intermittent, painless, gross hematuria and urinary frequency. Urinalysis is normal except for moderate red blood cells and trace white blood cells. Urine culture is negative. A course of antibiotics does not relieve his symptoms. Complete blood count, electrolytes, and creatinine are normal. Prostate-specific antigen is 0.9. Which of the following would be the next appropriate diagnostic test?

A. Urine cytology and serum carcinoembryonic antigen

B. 18-fluorodeoxyglucose (FDG)-positron emission tomography (PET)

C. CT scan of the chest, abdomen, and pelvis

D. Urine cytology and cystoscopy

---

5. A 68-year-old man presents with gross hematuria. Urine cytology is positive for malignant cells. Cystoscopy reveals a 4-cm ulcerating bladder tumor. TURBT shows high-grade invasive urothelial carcinoma with muscle involvement. A CT scan shows no masses or involved lymph nodes. He has renal impairment with a creatinine clearance of 39 mg/dL. Which of the following treatments should be recommended?

A. Neoadjuvant chemotherapy with a noncisplatin-based regimen followed by radical cystectomy and pelvic lymph node dissection

B. Radical cystectomy and pelvic lymph node dissection

    C. Radical cystectomy and pelvic lymph node dissection followed by adjuvant chemotherapy with a noncisplatin-based regimen

    D. Intravesical BCG

---

6. A 69-year-old man with gross hematuria is found to have a single papillary tumor that is approximately 1 cm in size and attached to the surface of the bladder with a single papillary stalk. Preoperative urine cytology was negative for any high-grade urothelial cancer cells. In addition to tumor resection at TURBT, what other adjunctive therapy is reasonable?

    A. Immediate postoperative instillation of BCG

    B. Immediate postoperative instillation of mitomycin C

    C. Postoperative instillation of BCG at 48 hours

    D. Postoperative instillation of mitomycin C at 48 hours

---

7. A 55-year-old man has high-grade bladder cancer (CIS) and after his tumor is completely resected, he receives an induction course of BCG. His tumor recurs with CIS and is resected and found to be high-grade again. After a second induction course of BCG, his options for treatment with CIS recurrence are all of the following **EXCEPT**

    A. Radical cystectomy

    B. Clinical trial

    C. Intravesical gemcitabine

    D. Intravesical BCG plus interferon

    E. Systemic gemcitabine

---

8. A frail 80-year-old woman has been diagnosed with bladder cancer by the urologist and sent to the radiation oncologist for evaluation for definitive chemoradiotherapy as an alternative to radical cystectomy. All of the following clinical and pathologic features are less than ideal in this patient for successful definitive chemoradiotherapy **EXCEPT**

    A. CIS

    B. Hydronephrosis

    C. Muscle-invasive bladder cancer

D. Impaired renal function

E. Poor performance status

---

9. A 50-year-old woman presents with painful urination and intermittent gross hematuria. Gynecological examination is within normal limits and urinalysis is positive only for red blood cells. Urine culture is negative. However, a urine cytology is positive for malignant cells. A CT scan reveals a mass in the left renal pelvis, with no other masses and no lymph node enlargement. Cystoscopy demonstrates a normal bladder wall. Retrograde pyelogram and ureteroscopy confirm a left renal pelvic mass. Retrograde brushing and urine cytology of the left upper urinary tract are positive for urothelial carcinoma. Biopsy confirms high-grade urothelial carcinoma of the renal pelvis. Which of the following hereditary syndromes is most closely associated with urothelial carcinoma of the renal pelvis?

   A. Inherited mutation in BRCA2 gene

   B. Von Hippel-Lindau (VHL) disease

   C. Hereditary nonpolyposis colorectal cancer (HNPCC)

   D. Multiple endocrine neoplasia type 2 (MEN2)

---

10. A 64-year-old woman presents with gross hematuria. Urine cytology is positive for malignant cells. Cystoscopy reveals a 3-cm bladder tumor. Transurethral resection of bladder tumor shows high-grade invasive urothelial carcinoma with muscle involvement. A CT scan demonstrates multiple bilateral lung metastases, the largest measuring 2 cm. She has renal impairment with a calculated creatinine clearance (CrCl) of 34 mg/dL. Which of the following treatments should be recommended?

   A. Radical cystectomy and pelvic lymph node dissection

   B. First-line therapy with a cisplatin-containing regimen, either gemcitabine and cisplatin or dose-dense MVAC (methotrexate, vinblastine, doxorubicin [Adriamycin], cisplatin)

   C. First-line therapy with a noncisplatin-containing regimen, such as gemcitabine and carboplatin

   D. First-line therapy with atezolizumab or pembrolizumab

   E. C and D

11. Cystoscopy of a 67-year-old man reveals a 2.4-cm papillary tumor in the left lateral wall of the bladder. An exam under anesthesia demonstrates a mobile bladder. Evaluation of the biopsy of the papillary lesion reveals high-grade papillary carcinoma with muscle invasion and prostate involvement. CT of chest/abdomen and pelvis reveals no metastases. Neoadjuvant chemotherapy with cisplatin and gemcitabine x 4 cycles is initiated. Postchemotherapy CT of the chest/abdomen and pelvis (prior to radical cystectomy) reveals multiple new pulmonary nodules and pelvic lymphadenopathy. Biopsy of the largest pulmonary nodule confirms high-grade urothelial carcinoma. Which of the following is the most appropriate subsequent therapy for this patient?

   A. Radical cystectomy followed by adjuvant atezolizumab

   B. Atezolizumab or pembrolizumab

   C. 4 additional cycles of gemcitabine and cisplatin

   D. Nivolumab

   E. Either atezolizumab, pembrolizumab, avelumab, durvalumab, or nivolumab

   F. Switch chemotherapy to dose-dense MVAC (methotrexate, vinblastine, doxorubicin [Adriamycin], cisplatin) for 4 additional cycles

12. A 73-year-old woman presents with intermittent gross hematuria not improved with a course of antibiotics. Urine cytology is positive for malignant cells. Cystoscopy reveals multiple large bladder tumors. Transurethral resection of bladder tumor confirms high-grade invasive urothelial carcinoma. CT scan demonstrates involvement of the bones and pelvic lymph nodes. The patient is initiated on first-line therapy with dose-dense MVAC x 6 cycles. She has a partial response of the pelvic lymph nodes lasting 4 months, but then recurs with multiple new bone metastases. Which of the following treatments should be recommended?

   A. Atezolizumab

   B. Pembrolizumab

   C. Avelumab

   D. Durvalumab

   E. Nivolumab

   F. Either A or B

   G. Either A, B, C, D, or E

ANSWERS TO REVIEW QUESTIONS

1. ANSWER: D. Radical cystectomy and pelvic lymphadenectomy are the gold-standard therapeutic modalities for locoregional MIBC. In men, this includes removal of the prostate, seminal vesicles, and proximal urethra. In women, it includes removal of the urethra, uterus, fallopian tubes, anterior vaginal wall, and surrounding fascia. Nearly one quarter of patients (24%) have unsuspected nodal metastases found upon pelvic lymph node dissection, despite negative preoperative staging. This extensive surgery ensures a low rate of pelvic recurrence, even in lymph node-positive patients, 25% of whom experience long-term survival. A proper lymph node dissection is important. Also, the number of lymph nodes examined in cystectomy specimens has been reported to affect patient outcome.

2. ANSWER: D. Bladder cancer is common around the world. In the United States, cigarette smoking is thought to account for more than half of all cases of urothelial carcinomas of the bladder. It occurs most commonly in patients aged > 50 years, with a marked male predominance. In addition, numerous chemicals have been identified as bladder carcinogens in humans, some relating to occupational exposures to arylamines found in cigarette smoke, permanent hair dyes, and other environmental sources. Treatment with cytostatic drugs, especially cyclophosphamide, is associated with increased risk of bladder cancer, as is radiotherapy. In developing countries, especially in the Middle East and parts of Africa (such as the Nile River Valley), bladder cancer occurs most commonly secondary to schistosomiasis, which is frequently associated with the development of SCC similar to that of other chronic inflammatory processes of the lower urinary tract. Arsenic has been indicated as a bladder carcinogen in Argentina, Chile, and Taiwan.

3. ANSWER: A. Intravesical BCG therapy is indicated for CIS. The presence of muscle in the biopsy allows for an accurate assessment of the invasiveness of the tumor. Cystectomy would be indicated for recurrent or persistent disease only. Other indications for intravesical BCG include treatment of residual nonmuscle-invasive papillary tumor and prophylaxis against recurrence of superficial tumors or progression after tumor resection.

4. ANSWER: D. The most common presenting symptom for patients with bladder cancer is hematuria. Patients may also have urinary symptoms such as frequency and discomfort. In the absence of a urinary tract infection, patients over 50 years of age should be evaluated with cystoscopy and urine cytology. A CT scan of the abdomen and pelvis should be done only if the lesions seen on cystoscopy appear high-grade or suggest muscle invasion. CT of the chest is premature in a patient with hematuria.

5. ANSWER: B. Neoadjuvant chemotherapy with cisplatin combination chemotherapy improves survival in patients with MIBC and good renal function. However, a large proportion of patients are ineligible for cisplatin chemotherapy based on renal function or functional status. There are limited data on the efficacy and survival benefit of noncisplatin-based regimens in the neoadjuvant or adjuvant setting. Therefore, patients with MIBC who are intolerant of or ineligible for cisplatin-based chemotherapy should proceed to cystectomy.

6. ANSWER: B. The patient likely has a low-grade tumor characterized by the presence of a single tumor that is small in size and attached with a simple stalk in the setting of a urine cytology negative for high-grade urothelial cancer. Therefore, a single dose of intravesical chemotherapy such as mitomycin C is reasonable if given within 24 hours after a TURBT to delay recurrence of papillary tumor. BCG is not given for low-grade disease and is never given postoperatively or at 48 hours. Mitomycin C given at 48 hours would not be effective in reducing papillary tumor recurrence.

7. ANSWER: E. This patient has failed two induction courses of BCG and is therefore considered to have BCG-refractory disease. Radical cystectomy is the current standard of care. However, for patients who are unable or unwilling to undergo radical cystectomy, either intravesical gemcitabine or another course of BCG + interferon is reasonable. Clinical trial is also reasonable. Systemic gemcitabine is only given to patients with metastatic disease or to patients with muscle-invasive bladder cancer as part of a neoadjuvant chemotherapy regimen.

8. ANSWER: C. This patient is a common referral for definitive chemoradiotherapy given her poor likelihood of tolerating a radical cystectomy. Chemoradiotherapy is indicated for muscle-invasive bladder cancer and is most successful in patients without accompanying CIS and hydronephrosis. Also, since cisplatin is key to sensitizing the cancer to radiation, poor renal function and performance status make delivery of cisplatin difficult. Therefore, all of the answer choices reflect less than ideal clinical and pathologic features for chemoradiotherapy treatment except for muscle-invasive bladder cancer.

9. ANSWER: C. Hereditary nonpolyposis colorectal cancer syndrome (HNPCC), or Lynch syndrome, is characterized by mutations in many DNA mismatch repair genes and detectable as microsatellite instability. Urothelial carcinoma of the upper urinary tract is less common than urothelial carcinoma of the bladder, occurring in approximately 10% of all urothelial carcinomas, and may develop as a manifestation of HNPCC. Young patients with upper-tract urothelial carcinoma (renal pelvis or ureter) and a family history of cancer, especially colorectal carcinoma, should be referred for genetic counseling and testing.

10. ANSWER: E. A patient with metastatic advanced urothelial carcinoma should be treated with systemic therapy, not radical surgery. Cisplatin-based combination chemotherapy such as gemcitabine and cisplatin or dose-dense MVAC are the standard of care in the first-line treatment of metastatic urothelial carcinoma. However, almost half of patients diagnosed with muscle-invasive urothelial carcinoma have renal insufficiency and are not cisplatin-eligible. Gemcitabine and carboplatin is a good alternative to cisplatin-based combinations in patients with renal insufficiency or who are otherwise ineligible for cisplatin chemotherapy. Atezolizumab and pembrolizumab have both been shown to be active and safe in cisplatin-ineligible patients and are both FDA-approved for this indication.

11. ANSWER: E. This patient's tumor was not responsive to cisplatin-based combination therapy. Therefore, additional chemotherapy with either gemcitabine and cisplatin or dose-dense MVAC will likely not be effective. Patients with metastatic urothelial carcinoma should not be treated with local therapy such as radical cystectomy. Adjuvant checkpoint blockade therapy is being studied in multiple phase III clinical trials in patients with no residual disease postradical cystectomy. Atezolizumab and pembrolizumab are approved for the first-line and second-line treatment of metastatic urothelial carcinoma, but avelumab, durvalumab, and nivolumab are also approved for the second-line treatment of metastatic urothelial carcinoma (and for progressive disease postneoadjuvant or adjuvant chemotherapy). Therefore, any of these 5 agents is an appropriate next treatment option.

12. ANSWER: G. Five checkpoint inhibitors (atezolizumab, nivolumab, durvalumab, avelumab, and pembrolizumab) have demonstrated clinical efficacy in the second-line setting in patients with metastatic urothelial carcinoma, with comparable ORRs of 15% to 20% (Table15.4). Atezolizumab, nivolumab, durvalumab, and avelumab received accelerated FDA approval, while pembrolizumab gained regular approval for the treatment of metastatic urothelial carcinoma or metastatic progression within 12 months of neoadjuvant/adjuvant platinum-based chemotherapy for muscle-invasive disease.

Testicular Carcinoma 16

Kevin R. Rice, Michelle A. Ojemuyiwa,
and Ravi A. Madan

REVIEW QUESTIONS

1. A 30-year-old male with Stage III intermediate nonseminomatous germ cell tumor is presenting to you after completing four cycles of BEP. You recommend post treat imaging and on CT and it displays a 2 cm retroperitoneal lymph node. He undergoes a nerve sparing RPLD and the incidental lymph node pathology was notable for residual embryonal and yolk sac elements. What is your next step in management?

    A. Surveillance monitoring

    B. BEP x 2 cycles

    C. Radiation

    D. EP x 2 cycles

    E. VIP x 4 cycles

2. A 25-year-old male has history of a Stage IIB nonseminomatous germ cell tumor. At diagnosis a CT scan was remarkable for a 4 cm retroperitoneal mass with no evidence of pulmonary or visceral metastasis. His serum markers are notable for an AFP of 65mg/dl, β-HCG of 400, LDH of 235mg dl. He was started on BEP for a goal of three cycles. After two cycles of therapy he presents with symptoms of increasing flank pain. He obtains another CT scan which now displays an increasing retroperitoneal mass of 6 cm. His serum tumor markers are notable for a slight decrease of AFP of 20mg/dl, β-HCG of 200, and LDH of 190 mg dl. What is your next step in management?

A. Continue current management then take patient to surgery for RPLND

B. Switch to VIP for 3 cycles

C. Stop chemotherapy and take patient to surgery for a RPLND

D. Stop chemotherapy and start radiation therapy.

3. A 26-year-old male presents to you with a 3-month history of a painless right testicular mass. You send him for a testicular ultra sound which confirms the presence of a right testicular mass. Tumor markers obtained are notable for an LDH <1.5 ULN, AFP of 75, and β-HCG of 100. The patient undergoes a right orchiectomy in which pathology is notable for a pT2 seminoma with tumor limited to the testis and epididymis without lymphatic or vascular invasion. Post operatively his serum tumor markers normalize. Further staging with a CXR and CT of abdomen and pelvis are unremarkable for metastatic disease. What treatment would NOT be indicated for this patient?

A. Surveillance

B. BEP x 2 cycles

C. BEP x 1 cycle

D. Nerve-sparing RPLND

E. Postoperative radiation

4. What is the most common genetic abnormality in malignant germ cell tumors?

A .c-kit mutation

B. isochomosome of 12p

C. BCR-ABL fusion gene

D. XXY

E. P53 mutation

5. A 23-year-old male presents to you for discussion of adjuvant management of a Stage 1 seminoma. He underwent a left-sided orchiectomy with normalization of tumor makers. His staging imaging demonstrated a normal chest x-ray and CT of abdomen and pelvis. What treatment option do you recommend?

A. BEP x 2 cycles

B. Observation

C. Single dose of carboplatin with an AUC of 7

D. Nerve sparing RPLND

E. Either b or c

6. A 22-year-old man without significant medical history presented with right-sided chest pain and shortness of breath. A chest radiograph showed a mass in the anterior mediastinum. A biopsy of the chest mass reveals nonseminomatous germ cell tumor. Serum β-HCG and AFP levels were elevated but an examination of the testes was unrevealing. Which risk category and treatment option is appropriate for this patient?

A. Poor risk nonseminomatous germ cell tumor; treat with 3 cycles of BEP

B. Poor risk nonseminomatous germ cell tumor; treat with 4 cycles of VIP

C. Intermediate risk nonseminomatous germ cell tumor; treat with 4 cycles of EP

D. Intermediate risk nonseminomatous germ cell tumor; treat with surgical resection

E. Good risk nonseminomatous germ cell tumor; treat with 2 cycles of BEP

7. Which of the following is the greatest risk factor for developing testicular cancer?

A. A young man with a brother has testicular cancer

B. A young man whose father has testicular cancer

C. A male with a history of cryptorchidism

D. A male with history of Lynch syndrome

E. A male whose uncle developed testicular cancer

8. A 25-year-old male was recently diagnosed with intermediate risk Stage IIIC seminoma. His imaging is significant for a 5 cm retroperitoneal mass and multiple pulmonary nodules, and liver metastasis. He was started on BEP with a plan of four cycles. After two cycles of therapy he develops a

progressive nonproductive cough. A subsequent PFT chest CT was notable for ground glass opacities concerning for pulmonary fibrosis, a toxicity of bleomycin. What treatment option do you offer?

   A. Proceed with high-dose chemotherapy followed by ASCT.
   B. Three cycles of etoposide and carboplatin
   C. Four cycles of EP
   D. Four cycles of VeIP
   E. Two cycles of VIP

9. A 37-year-old male with history of Stage II seminoma treated 4 years ago presents for his routine surveillance follow-up. He originally presented with a left testicular mass, and retroperitoneal adenopathy. He was treated with left orchiectomy along with adjuvant etoposide and cisplatin for four cycles. Since therapy he has continued his routine surveillance monitoring, with is most recent labs notable for a slight rise in his β-HCG. LDH and AFP were with in normal limits. He denies history of marijuana use. What is your next step in management?

   A. It is normal for a slight rise in b HCG so continue surveillance monitoring
   B. Start treatment with BEP
   C. Send patient for salvage radiation
   D. Start treatment with EP
   E. Repeat his lab work, this may be result of hypogonadism

10. A 26-year-old male presents with a right testicular mass. Tumor markers obtained are notable for an LDH >1.5 ULN, AFP with in normal limits, and β-HCG of 800. The patient undergoes a right orchiectomy in which pathology is notable for a pT3 seminoma with extension into the epididymis wit lymphatic vascular invasion. Postoperatively his serum tumor markers remain elevated. Further staging with a CXR and CT of abdomen and pelvis are notable for pulmonary and liver lesion. What treatment would be indicated for this patient?

   A. Surveillance
   B. BEP x 4 cycles
   C. BEP x 3 cycle
   D. Nerve-sparing RPLND
   E. Postoperative radiation

ANSWERS TO REVIEW QUESTIONS

1. ANSWER: D. This patient has a partial response to systemic therapy. Residual masses greater then 1cm in NSGCT must be resected. If embryonal, yolk sac, choriocarcinoma, or seminoma elements are found, further systemic therapy is warranted which includes 2 cycles of EP, TIP, VeIP, or TIP.

2. ANSWER: C. This patient has a progressive increase in size of his retroperitoneal mass which is concerning. The increasing mass could be a result of growing teratoma syndrome, which is described as an enlarging mass while receiving appropriate systemic therapy in the setting of normal of declining tumor markers. Histology of those resected lesions revealed benign mature teratomatous elements with no components of viable germ cell tumor. The prevalence of GTS is only 1.9% to 7.6%

3. ANSWER: E. This patient has the diagnosis of NSGCT. Use of radiation is not indicated with nonseminomatous germ cell tumor.

4. ANSWER: B. Isochrome 12p is the genetic abnormality that has been described in all histologic sub types of germ cell tumors.

5. ANSWER: E. Management of Stage I seminoma after orchiectomy and normalization of tumor markers include observation, chemotherapy with carboplatin for 1 to 2 cycles, or radiation. Overall survival of either treatment modality is >95%.

6. ANSWER: B. The primary chemotherapy regimen of choice for patients with advance disease depends of the IGCCCG risk stratification. Primary mediastinal NSCT is in the poor risk category. Therapeutic options for primary mediastinal NSGCT include four cycles of BEP or four cycles of VIP.

7. ANSWER: C. Several risk factors have been discovered in testicular cancer. History of cryptorchidism carries the highest risk, in which individuals with this condition have a 10 to 15 times increased risk of developing testicular cancer. A history of a brother with testicular cancer carries 8 to 10 times relative risk and a father with testicular cancer carries 4 times higher risk.

8. ANSWER: E. Complications of chemotherapy can occur; however, given the curability rate of testicular cancer all therapy should be completed. The most concerning complication of belomycin is pulmonary toxicity to include pulmonary fibrosis. When this occurs in testicular cancer therapy, treatment should be adjusted to include holding bleomycin, and adjusting therapy to complete the remainder of the four cycles of chemotherapy with VIP.

9. ANSWER: E. An elevated serum level of beta hcg has a half life for 1 to 3 days, and may also be present in both seminomatous and nonseminomatous germ cell tumors. Elevation of beta hcg may also be seen in both marijuana use and hypogonadism and can result in a benign elevation of b hcg.

10. ANSWER: B. For patients with seminoma and intermediate risk disease, more intense chemotherapy is recommended which includes BEP x 4 cycles. Disease with nonpulmonary visceral metastasis (i.e., liver, bone, brain) are considered intermediate risk.

Ovarian Cancer **17**

Jung-min Lee and Elise C. Kohn

1. A 54-year-old African-American woman was diagnosed with stage IIIC high-grade serous ovarian 24 months ago. After an exploratory laparotomy resulted in successful resection of all gross disease, she received six cycles of intravenous paclitaxel/carboplatin with a resultant clinical complete remission. She now presents with a rising CA-125 (three successive monthly elevated values with the last value at 360 U/ml). She is asymptomatic. A CT scan of the abdomen/pelvis shows no evidence of recurrent disease. Which of the following would you recommend at this point?

    A. Observation

    B. Exploratory laparotomy and secondary surgical cytoreduction

    C. Insertion of an IP catheter and administration of IP cisplatin

    D. Systemic chemotherapy with a carboplatin-based doublet

    E. Systemic chemotherapy with an active agent to which she has not been previously exposed

2. A 40-year-old woman presents to her gynecologist because her sister, aged 42, was recently diagnosed with serous ovarian carcinoma and she was found to carry a deleterious germline *BRCA1* mutation. The patient reports a strong family history of both breast and ovarian cancer, also including her mother (breast cancer). Testing reveals that she also carries the deleterious *BRCA1* mutation. She has completed child-bearing. Which of the following would you recommend?

    A. Annual screening with transvaginal sonography and CA-125

    B. Pelvic examination every 3 months

    C. Risk-reducing salpingo-oophorectomy

    D. Oral contraceptives

3. A 61-year-old Caucasian woman comes in with a 3 month history of progressive abdominal girth and discomfort. Her gynecologist found her to be in good health with no other significant medical problems other than a slightly distended abdomen, and a 6 cm mass in her left adnexa. Laboratory data showed a CA-125 of 960 U/ml. Computerized tomography of the abdomen showed a 7 cm mass involving the left ovary, ascites, and multiple scattered smaller abdominal masses. She underwent an exploratory laparotomy by a gynecologic oncologist with the identification of stage IIIC epithelial ovarian. There was no visible disease remaining. Which of the following would be the best choice for treatment for this patient?

    A. Intravenous paclitaxel/carboplatin for six cycles

    B. Intraperitoneal/intravenous chemotherapy with paclitaxel and cisplatin or carboplatin for six cycles

    C. Docetaxel/carboplatin (IV) for six cycles

    D. Gemcitabine/carboplatin (IV) for six cycles

    E. Paclitaxel/carboplatin/bevacizumab (IV) for six cycles followed by maintenance bevacizumab until progression

4. A 26-year-old woman comes in with worsening lower abdominal discomfort beginning 6 months prior to seeing her gynecologist. Physical examination observed a slighted distended abdomen and pelvic examination revealed a 7 cm left adnexal mass and chest radiograph was within normal limits. Computerized tomography of the abdomen and pelvis showed the mass involved the left ovary and was associated with one possibly enlarged pelvic lymph node. Preoperative CA-125 measurement was within normal limits and the α-fetoprotein was 10 IU/mL and ßhCG was 800 mIU/mL. She underwent exploratory laparotomy and frozen section indicated embryonal carcinoma; a unilateral oophorectomy was performed due to interest in subsequent child-bearing. At the conclusion of surgery, she had no gross residual disease remaining and pathology review confirmed the diagnosis and indicated high-grade disease. Which of the following are indicated for subsequent therapy?

A. Paclitaxel and carboplatin for 6 cycles

B. Intraperitoneal/intravenous combination chemotherapy with paclitaxel and cisplatin for 6 cycles

C. Cisplatin/etoposide/bleomycin for 3 to 4 cycles

D. Cisplatin/etoposide for 3 to 4 cycles

5. A 53-year-old Asian woman comes in with a 6-month history of progressive abdominal girth and discomfort. She is otherwise in good health with no other significant medical problems other than a distended abdomen, and a palpable 9 cm mass in her right adnexa. Laboratory data showed a CA-125 of 50 U/ml. Computerized tomography of the abdomen confirmed the unilateral mass only. She underwent an exploratory laparotomy by a gynecologic oncologist with the identification of stage IA mucinous tumor. During an exploratory laparotomy, which of the following organs should be carefully assessed to rule out a metastatic mucinous malignancy to the ovary?

A. Adrenal gland

B. Appendix

C. Cervix

D. Uterus

6. A 71-year-old Caucasian woman presents with a 3-month history of progressive abdominal discomfort. She is obese (BMI= 41) and has dyslipidemia and chronic hypertension requiring 3 antihypertensive medications. Laboratory data showed a CA-125 of 840 U/ml and a CEA of 5 ng/ml. Computerized tomography of the abdomen showed a 8 cm mass involving the right ovary, ascites, and multiple scattered peritoneal masses, suspected stage IIIC disease with a high tumor volume. Which of the following would be the best choice for treatment for this patient?

A. Intraperitoneal/intravenous chemotherapy with paclitaxel and cisplatin or carboplatin for six cycles

B. Docetaxel/carboplatin (IV) for six cycles

C. Paclitaxel/carboplatin/bevacizumab (IV) for six cycles followed by maintenance bevacizumab until progression

D. Three cycles of carboplatin/paclitaxel, interval debulking surgery, and then three additional cycles of carboplatin/paclitaxel.

7. A 54-year-old African American woman was diagnosed with stage IIIC high-grade serous ovarian cancer and underwent optimal primary debulking surgery followed by intraperitoneal/intravenous chemotherapy with paclitaxel and carboplatin for six cycles. After a 20-month disease-free interval, she developed a recurrent disease in the lower pelvic area, with a CA-125 of 360 U/ml. Imaging showed pelvic nodes and a posterior cul-de-sac mass with no masses in the upper abdomen or chest. Which of the following treatments would you recommend as most likely to benefit her?

   A. Secondary debulking surgery followed by platinum-based chemotherapy

   B. Platinum-based combination chemotherapy until progression of disease

   C. Secondary debulking surgery followed by observation if her CA125 normalizes after treatment

   D. Nonplatinum-based single agent chemotherapy with bevacizumab

8. A 47-year-old Caucasian woman seeks consultation regarding management of her stage II epithelial ovarian cancer. She reports that her mother had colon cancer at age 52, and her maternal grandmother had endometrial cancer at age 48. The patient has two healthy younger brothers and two daughters. In addition to discussing adjuvant treatments for her stage II ovarian cancer, you recommend:

   A. Genetic counseling, followed by testing for mutations in the *BRCA1* or *BRCA 2* genes

   B. Prophylactic hemicolectomy

   C. Genetic counseling, followed by mutation testing for the four mismatch repair genes

   D. Prophylactic mastectomy

9. A 56-year-old postmenopausal woman was diagnosed with stage II low-grade serous ovarian cancer. She underwent an optimal debulking surgery by a gynecologic oncologist. Mutation testing showed her ovarian tumor to be KRAS mutant, p53 negative and WT-1 negative. Her germline *BRCA* mutation testing showed a *BRCA1* variant

of uncertain significance. Which of following treatments would you recommend?

A. Paclitaxel/carboplatin/bevacizumab (IV) for six cycles followed by maintenance bevacizumab until progression

B. MEK inhibitor, selumetinib

C. BRAF inhibitor, vemurafenib

D. PARP inhibitor, olaparib

E. Paclitaxel and carboplatin IV for six cycles

10. PARP enzyme is important to the function of base excision repair and modulation of nonhomologous endjoining DNA repair. PARP inhibition synergizes with reduction in homologous recombination DNA repair. Patients with which of these genetic syndromes would be most likely to benefit from PARP inhibition?

A. Hereditary breast/ovarian cancer syndrome (HBOC)

B. Hereditary nonpolyposis colon cancer syndrome (HNPCC)

C. Li-Fraumeni syndrome (LFS)

11. A 36-year-old woman who elected to delay getting pregnant comes in with newly diagnosed ovarian cancer. You take her history and find that she has over 6 years of oral contraceptive use, no family history of cancer, and no pelvic pathology in the past. She has recently attempted one cycle of forced ovarian cycling for in vitro fertility (IVF) without conceiving. What in her history may have contributed to her development of ovarian cancer?

A. Age

B. Oral contraceptive use

C. Forced ovarian drive for IVF

D. Delayed attempts at pregnancy

12. A 74-year-old African American woman was diagnosed with stage IC clear cell carcinoma of the ovary and underwent suboptimal primary debulking followed by carboplatin and paclitaxel chemotherapy. She relapsed at just over 5 months and has been referred to you for treatment recommendations. She has short bowel syndrome with ongoing symptoms

from a necessary bowel resection at her debulking surgery and also has some residual marrow suppression, though counts are adequate for current treatment. Current medications include metoprolol for hypertension, digoxin for cardiomyopathy, and metformin for type II diabetes. Which of the following options would be most favorable for both outcome and toxicity for this patient with comorbidities?

A. Pegylated liposomal doxorubicin

B. Bevacizumab

C. Cisplatin

D. Weekly paclitaxel with bevacizumab

E. Tamoxifen with bevacizumab

13. A 63-year-old woman has had a 30 month disease-free interval after completion of carboplatin and weekly paclitaxel for her stage IIIC high grade serous ovarian cancer. She has vague left lower quadrant poster abdominal discomfort, a palpable left inguinal lymph node, a rising CA125 now at 250 U/ml, and confirmatory posterior mesenteric masses and inguino-pelvic lymph nodes on imaging. She is not eager to lose her hair again and wishes to move rapidly into treatment. Her institution does not have an appropriate clinical trial available to her and rather than travel, she has requested standard of care treatment. Which of the following would be the best treatment to initiate?

A. Single agent carboplatin

B. Single agent pegylated liposomal doxorubicin

C. Carboplatin and pegylated liposomal doxorubicin

D. Carboplatin and topotecan

E. Carboplatin and bevacizumab

14. A 36-year-old woman comes to you for a second opinion regarding treatment of her recurrent high grade serous ovarian cancer. She has had prior adjuvant chemotherapy with carboplatin and paclitaxel, carboplatin and paclitaxel again, for her first (platinum-sensitive) recurrence at 2 years, and 6 months later, after subsequent progression, had weekly paclitaxel with bevacizumab. She has a strong family history and genetic testing revealed a deleterious germline *BRCA1* mutation. Her physician is strongly encouraging her to participate in a phase I vaccine clinical trial.

She wishes to have an oral agent. Which of the following is the preferred treatment regimen in this setting?

   A. Gemcitabine 800 to 1000 mg intravenously weeks 1 and 2 of 3

   B. Olaparib tablets 300mg twice daily

   C. Oral etoposide 50 mg alternating with 100 mg daily for 3 of 4 weeks

   D. Tamoxifen 20 mg twice daily.

15. A 48-year-old perimenopausal Hispanic woman comes in to you complaining about abdominal pain and pelvic pressure progressing over the last 4 months. She says that this pain is reminiscent of the endometroisis pain she has with her menstrual periods. She has noted some tightening of her clothes around her middle but no gain of weight over this time frame. A unilateral pelvic mass is palpated on examination and imaging shows abdominal mesenteric disease. She has no family history of gynecologic cancers or colon cancer. A work up leads to a diagnosis of ovarian cancer. Which of these ovarian cancer types is most consistent with her history?

   A. Low-grade serous ovarian cancer

   B. Mucinous ovarian cancer

   C. High-grade serous ovarian cancer

   D. Clear cell ovarian cancer

   E. Transitional cell ovarian cancer

ANSWERS TO REVIEW QUESTIONS

1. ANSWER: A. After initially achieving a clinical complete remission as a result of management of her advanced ovarian carcinoma with the minimum standard of care, this patient presents with a rising CA-125 (based on three successive rising CA-125 with the last value above 100) and no other evidence of disease. She is asymptomatic. This situation was studied in a large phase III trial in Europe. Early versus delayed treatment of relapsed ovarian cancer was examined (MRC OV05/EORTC 55955; a randomized trial; Rustin et al., 2010). There was no difference in overall survival (HR = 1.00) and thus no benefit from earlier initiation of therapy for only a rising CA-125. Furthermore, deterioration of quality of life began a median of 3 months earlier in the early treatment group who also received more cycles and regimens of chemotherapy. These data support *not* treating only a rising CA-125. This is a controversial conclusion in the United States, where many use the Rustin CA-125 criteria (at least doubled and over 100) as an indicator for therapy, even when evaluable disease is observed on examination and/or imaging. When this patient ultimately develops tissue evidence of recurrence, she should be classified as potentially platinum sensitive due to her treatment-free interval of >18 months, substantially greater than the 6 months required for definition, and treated with a carboplatin-based doublet. She should be evaluated for secondary surgical cytoreduction, which should be done if the surgeon feels that he/she can remove all gross disease.

2. ANSWER: D. Risk-reducing salpingo-oophorectomy (RRSO) has been shown to reduce lifetime risk of ovarian/tubal/peritoneal cancer to 5% and is recommended for all women who are at high risk and who have completed childbearing. Optimal time for surgery is upon completion of child-bearing and 10 years prior to the youngest age at cancer presentation in the family, though timing recommendations are not supported by level 1 evidence. Data are not available yet to confirm the safety of salpingectomy without later removal of ovaries. Screening with transvaginal sonography, CA-125, and pelvic examination, alone or in combination, has not been shown to reduce ovarian carcinoma mortality or lead to early detection in the general population or the high-risk population. It is, however, recommended for women who have not completed childbearing or who do not wish RRSO. Oral contraceptives can reduce the risk of ovarian cancer by as much as 50% in the general population; they have not been conclusively shown to be safe and effective in the mutation-carrier population. Oral contraceptives also have a 1.6 RR for the risk of breast cancer.

3. ANSWER: B. This patient has stage IIIC optimally debulked ovarian carcinoma and should receive either neoadjuvant chemotherapy with interval debulking, or in for this set of answers, chemotherapy following surgery. The 2015 Gynecologic Cancer Inter-Group international consensus conference confirms the minimum treatment of choice is six cycles of paclitaxel plus carboplatin. The National Cancer Institute issued a clinical alert in January of 2006, based upon 4 clinical trials demonstrating marked overall survival benefits, declaring combination of intravenous and intraperitoneal therapy to be the treatment of patients with small-volume residual disease (optimal cytoreduction); the alert noted that there was no clear benefit of any one IP regimen. GOG 0252, presented in abstract form in 2016, suggests that intraperitoneal carboplatin can be substituted for intraperitoneal cisplatin without loss of benefit, and with reduced systemic toxicity. Docetaxel/carboplatin has been shown to be noninferior to paclitaxel/carboplatin and is the recommended regimen for women who develop anaphylactoid reactions to paclitaxel/cremophor EL infusion. Gemcitabine/carboplatin has not been studied as a primary doublet regimen and should not be used. GOG 218 showed that the addition of bevacizumab to paclitaxel/carboplatin plus bevacizumab maintenance produced a superior progression-free survival with no benefit in overall survival. A post hoc subset analysis suggested that patients with bulky disease may benefit most from addition of bevacizumab. The use of bevacizumab is not FDA approved for use in newly diagnosed ovarian cancer patients.

4. ANSWER: C. Cisplatin, etoposide, and bleomycin (BEP) treatment is indicated for any advanced grade or advanced stage germ cell cancer. Three cycles of BEP are indicated because this is greater than stage I disease and is grade 3. BEP is used in all but stage I, grade 1 disease, and ≥ stage II dysgerminoma. Paclitaxel and carboplatin, whether all intravenous or a combination of intraperitoneal/intravenous administration are indicated for epithelial ovarian cancers and this is a cancer of germ cell origin. Observation is not done in women generally, and especially when there may be disease outside of the ovary and in this case also high-grade disease. A unilateral oophorectomy is reasonable in young women due to the curative potential of the chemotherapy.

5. ANSWER: B. Mucinous ovarian tumors are rare, representing 2% to 3% of all epithelial ovarian cancer (EOC). Primary mucinous cancer of the ovary has histologic and immunohistochemical features that are more similar to gastrointestinal cancers than other EOC histotypes. Generally stage I mucinous ovarian cancer has an excellent prognosis. A high index of suspicion is required to prevent misdiagnosis, missing a metastatic neoplasm, most often from appendiceal cancer, and also from gastric cancer. A thorough pathologic inspection of the appendix should be performed in patients with a mucinous ovarian tumor with or without borderline features (Elias KM, *Gynecol Onc.* 2014).

6. ANSWER: D. All women with suspected stage IIIC or IV invasive epithelial ovarian cancer should be evaluated by a gynecologic oncologist prior to initiation of chemotherapy. The primary clinical evaluation should include a CT of the abdomen/pelvis, and chest. Women with a high perioperative risk profile or a low likelihood of achieving cytoreduction to < 1 cm of residual disease (ideally to no visible disease) are recommended to receive neoadjuvant chemotherapy. Primary cytoreductive surgery is preferred if there is a high likelihood of achieving cytoreduction to < 1 cm (ideally to no visible disease) with acceptable morbidity. Published studies (CHORUS, JGOG 0602, EORTC 55971) suggest that for selected women with stage IIIC or IV epithelial ovarian cancer, neoadjuvant chemotherapy and interval cytoreduction are noninferior to primary cytoreduction and adjuvant chemotherapy with respect to overall and progression-free survival and are associated with less perioperative morbidity and mortality. Intraperitoneal therapy is contraindicated with bulky disease either at presentation or as residual after primary debulking surgery. Docetaxel may be substituted for paclitaxel in women with a contraindication to paclitaxel treatment, most commonly those having had an anaphylactoid reaction to paclitaxel/cremophor. It has not been examined in neoadjuant treatment. Bevacizumab has not been approved in the United States for use in treatment of newly diagnosed ovarian cancer. It is approved in Europe for patients with stage IV and bulky stage IIIC disease, such as this patient.

7. ANSWER: A. This patient has a platinum-sensitive ovarian cancer recurrence, as defined by recurrence more than 6 months after completion of primary treatment. Although two prospective randomized clinical trials are still maturing, the standard of care for women with long primary disease free intervals (>12 to 18 months) is secondary debulking surgery. This is focused to women with disease assessed on imaging and examination to be resectable to ≤1 cm (R1) or no visible disease (R0). Adjuvant platinum-based chemotherapy is then commenced for up to 6 cycles. This may include carboplatin with either paclitaxel, pegylated liposomal doxorubicin, or gemcitabine. Platinum-based chemotherapy is generally given for a defined number of cycles postsurgery. If the patient was assessed to not be a surgical candidate, 6 to 8 cycles may be given, with the recognition that the risk of allergic reaction (anaphylactic) to platinum agents increases with the total body exposure over time. The standard of care is to use platinum-based combination therapy in platinum-sensitive recurrence, and single agents in platinum-resistant recurrences. It is not incorrect to use nonplatinum-based chemotherapy with bevacizumab; however, there are no data supporting this direction.

8. ANSWER: C. Lynch syndrome is an autosomal dominant inherited disorder caused by germline mutations in DNA mismatch repair genes (MLH1, MSH2, MSH6, PMS2) or the EPCAM gene. Hereditary nonpolyposis colorectal cancer (HNPCC) refers to patients and/or families who fulfill the Amsterdam criteria for Lynch syndrome. Genetic counseling should be done prior to any germline analysis. Mutation carriers are at substantially increased risk of developing cancers of the colorectum, endometrium, ovary, or breast, among other sites. Evaluation methods consist of 1) immunohistochemistry for the MMR proteins MLH1, MSH2, MSH6, and PMS2, followed by DNA methylation analysis for cases with deficiency in MLH1 and PMS2 and/or 2) microsatellite instability testing using polymerase chain reaction. Colon cancer and endometrioid endometrial cancers are not notable components of hereditary breast and ovarian cancer syndromes in which mutations in the *BRCA1* or *BRCA 2* genes are found. Patients with HNPCC have the higher risk of colon cancer and, if/when done, would undergo a sphincter-sparing complete colectomy. Prophylactic mastectomy is not recommended for Lynch syndrome.

9. ANSWER: E. Carboplatin and paclitaxel for 6 cycles remains the standard of care adjuvant therapy for newly diagnosed low-grade serous cancers, including those with KRAS or BRAF mutations. Low-grade serous ovarian tumors are genetically stable in contrast to high grade serous ovarian cancers. Somatic mutations in the KRAS (up to 50%) or BRAF (up to 20%), and rarely ERBB2 (<5%), genes have been reported in low-grade serous ovarian cancer. The mitogen-activated protein kinase kinase (MEK) inhibitor selumetinib had modest single agent activity in recurrent low-grade serous cancers and response did not correlate with the presence of BRAF or KRAS mutation (Farley, *Lancet Onc.* 2013). It has been reported that mutation in KRAS or BRAF are associated with better survival and recurrence outcome than wild type cancers (Grisham, *Cancer.* 2013).

10. ANSWER: A. HBOC is associated with deleterious germline mutations in the *BRCA1* or *2* genes. These genes are necessary for proper function of the high fidelity double stranded DNA repair homologous recombination repair program. Loss of this pathway defaults to base excision repair and nonhomologous end-joining repair. Base excision repair requires functional PARP enzyme; whereas, the poor fidelity nonhomologous end-joining repair, which can introduce new mutations, is kept in check by normal PARP function. Loss of PARP enzyme function is thus clinically synthetically lethal with deleterious germline mutations in the *BRCA1* or *2* leading to homozygous loss in the ovarian cancers. All high grade ovarian cancers and those with deleterious germline mutations in the *BRCA1* or *2* genes have loss of normal function of p53. LFS is associated with loss of function p53 mutations but is not associated with increased risk of development of ovarian cancers. HNPCC, or Lynch Syndrome, is associated with abnormalities in single stranded DNA mismatch repair. Ovarian cancer is part of HNPCC, although a rare component. There are limited data to demonstrate benefit of PARP inhibition in HNPCC ovarian cancers.

11. ANSWER: D. Infertility, primary and secondary and elective (nonfertility), have all been found to be associated with the risk of ovarian cancer. Thus, her elective delay of child-bearing and lack of conception with the one cycle of IVF can be considered infertility. The median age of diagnosis of ovarian cancer in women who do not have a deleterious germline mutation in the *BRCA1* or *2* genes is 63 years in the United States. Risk of ovarian cancer in carriers is considered to start rising approximately 10 years prior to the earliest age of onset of ovarian cancer within the kindred. This patient has no family history. Oral contraceptive pills (OCP) have been shown to be associated with a prevention of ovarian cancer, especially when used for over 5 years. That benefit has been shown to persist for up to 10 years after completion of OCP use.

12. ANSWER: D. The best treatment would be weekly paclitaxel with bevacizumab. This combination does not contribute to her residual marrow toxicity, and is unlikely to complicate her cardiomyopathy. It may cause reversible sensory neuropathy. The recent AURELIA study of topotecan, pegylated liposomal doxorubicin, or weekly paclitaxel +/- bevacizumab demonstrated added benefit of PFS for all 3 combinations. Unplanned post hoc subset analysis suggested that the greatest benefit and fewest toxicities were observed in the weekly paclitaxel/bevacizumab arm. The FDA licensed the 3 combinations with bevacizumab for use in platinum-resistant ovarian cancer in 2015. With this new standard of care and no contraindications, use of single agent pegylated liposomal doxorubicin or bevacizumab are no longer preferred regimens. The patient recurred within less than 6 months from prior carboplatin treatment making single agent cisplatin contraindicated. Tamoxifen, while used, has not been shown to have activity in clear cell cancer of the ovary and there are no data for a tamoxifen/bevacizumab combination. Clotting risks would be of significant concern for this combination due to overlapping risks.

13. ANSWER: C. The international standard of care for treatment of recurrent platinum-sensitive ovarian cancer is combination platinum-based chemotherapy. Three standards of care are available: carboplatin with paclitaxel, gemcitabine, or with pegylated liposomal doxorubicin. Carboplatin with paclitaxel would be associated with hair loss. The CALYPSO trial examined carboplatin and paclitaxel v. carboplatin and pegylated liposomal doxorubicin, showing noninferiority of the carboplatin and pegylated liposomal doxorubicin combination (HR 0.8 favoring carboplatin and pegylated liposomal doxorubicin) and an improved quality of life. Carboplatin and topotecan would result in hair loss and other toxicity and is not considered a standard of care combination. There are no data to support the use of carboplatin with bevacizumab. The OCEANS study examined carboplatin/gemcitabine with or without bevacizumab showing a PFS benefit with no OS benefit. It has not been licensed in the United States for use.

14. ANSWER: B. The FDA approved oral olaparib, a PARP inhibitor for the treatment of recurrent ovarian cancer in 4th or later line for women with deleterious germline *BRCA1/2* mutations in December 2014. While current clinical trials are using tablet formulation, approval was for capsules. The FDA has now approved tablets for all olaparib indications; capsules will be phased out of production. Olaparib in platinum-sensitive deleterious germline *BRCA1/2* mutation carriers can result in a response rate of up to approximately 50%; its activity as a single agent in carriers with platinum-resistant ovarian cancer is approximately 25% to 30%. It also has activity in nonmutation carriers approximating 35% in platinum-sensitive women and 10% to 15% in platinum-resistant women. The next best choices would be gemcitabine, approved as a single agent and in combination with cisplatin for platinum-resistant women. Oral etoposide has approximately a 40% response rate in platinum-sensitive ovarian cancer and 18% to 20% in platinum-resistant ovarian cancer. While often used, tamoxifen has a response rate of <10% in recurrent ovarian cancer and is not recommended. The functionality of the expressed estrogen receptor on ovarian cancer has not been determined.

15. ANSWER: D. A unilateral, advanced stage presentation in a woman with prior endometriosis and no family history is most consistent with clear cell cancer of the ovary. Transition zones between endometriosis and clear cell cancers have been identified to link the diseases. Further, data demonstrate that the adjacent endometriosis often has the same somatic *ARID1a* mutation as is seen in the clear cell ovarian cancer (up to 40% mutation incidence). Low-grade serous cancers are most commonly bilateral, whether early or advanced stage. High-grade serous cancers, also predominantly bilateral at presentation, have associated family history in up to a third of cases and deleterious germline *BRCA1/2* mutations seen in approximately 20% and have not been linked to endometriosis. Mucinous cancers are now not diagnosable with advanced stage disease unless all other gastrointestinal potential primaries, especially appendiceal, are ruled out. Transitional cell ovarian cancers are rarely advanced stage at presentation.

Endometrial Cancer 18

Kristen P. Zeligs and Christina M. Annunziata

REVIEW QUESTIONS

1. A 56-year-old-female with a history of obesity and type II diabetes presents for follow-up 18 months after completion of surgery and for stage IIIC, grade 3 endometrioid endometrial cancer. The tumor was strongly ER and PR positive and lymphovascular space invasion was present. She also received adjuvant RT (50 Gy EBRT along with vaginal irradiation with vaginal cylinder to bring the vaginal surface dose to 90 Gy). On review of symptoms she complains of cough with mild shortness of breath on going up two flights of stairs, and 3 kg weight loss over the past 2 months. CXR reveals three lung nodules measuring between 1.2 and 2.3 cm—one on the left and two on the right. CT scan also shows a 1.4 cm para-aortic LN. She is in good health otherwise and is able to carry out all other activities of daily living. What is the most appropriate therapeutic option?

    A. External beam radiotherapy to lungs and para-aortic LNs

    B. Chemotherapy with TAP (doxorubicin 45 mg/m^2, cisplatin 50 mg/m^2 on day 1; paclitaxel 160 mg/m^2 on day 2) for six cycles with G-CSF support

    C. Medroxyprogesterone acetate 200 mg PO daily

    D. TAM 20 mg PO twice daily

    E. Bevacizumab 10 mg/kg IV every 2 weeks

2. A 40-year-old premenopausal woman with no significant comorbidities presents for her 6-month routine oncology follow-up. One year ago she underwent wide local excision for a stage II ER-positive, PR-positive, HER-2-negative ductal carcinoma of the breast. She completed chemotherapy and radiotherapy. Her menses returned postchemotherapy. She commenced TAM 20 mg PO daily 6 months ago. She is concerned about the increased risk of uterine cancer while taking TAM and asks your advice about how she should be monitored for the occurrence of endometrial cancer. Which of the following is the *correct* advice for surveillance for endometrial cancer in patients taking TAM:

    A. Annual transvaginal ultrasound while on TAM

    B. Annual pelvic ultrasound and pelvic examination while on TAM

    C. Screening hysteroscopy and biopsy every 2 years while on TAM

    D. Annual pelvic examination and routine age-appropriate Papanicolaou smear with symptom-directed investigations should symptoms of endometrial cancer arise

    E. MRI of pelvis every 2 years while on TAM

3. A 37-year-old woman presents to her primary care physician for routine health maintenance examination. Her father died from metastatic colon cancer at age 49. She reports that in the past year her brother aged 30 and a paternal cousin aged 33 were both diagnosed with colon cancer. She has seen a gastroenterologist and is scheduled for a screening colonoscopy. What further advice would you give her regarding her gynecologic health?

    A. No additional gynecologic health screening is required beyond routine annual pelvic examination and age-appropriate Papanicolaou smear

    B. She should immediately have a hysterectomy

    C. Consultation with a genetic counselor is advised

    D. Annual pelvic examination and endometrial biopsy after age 35

    E. C and D

4. A 40-year-old African-American woman presents with a 3-week history of low back pain, abdominal swelling, serosanguinous vaginal discharge, and early satiety. CA125 is 120 units/L. Serum albumin is 2.5 mg/dL. CBC is normal. Serum chemistries reveal mildly elevated LFTs <2× upper limit of normal. CT scan shows a mass in the uterus, enlarged pelvic LNs, large volume ascites, peritoneal metastases, bilateral pleural effusions, and numerous liver lesions suspicious for metastases. She has a suboptimal debulking surgery including a TAH, BSO, omentectomy, pelvic and para-aortic LN dissection, and peritoneal stripping. Pathology reveals a grade 3 uterine papillary serous carcinoma. Peritoneal cytology is positive. Her disease is classified as FIGO stage IVB. What would you recommend next?

   A. Clinical trial

   B. Medroxyprogesterone acetate

   C. Vaginal brachytherapy

   D. Chemotherapy with cisplatin, irinotecan, and 5-FU

   E. None of the above

5. A 50-year-old woman with stage 2 endometrioid endometrial adenocarcinoma underwent TAH-BSO, followed by vaginal brachytherapy. She returned 2 years later for a routine follow-up visit and reported new right upper quadrant discomfort. CT scan shows disease in the liver capsule and biopsy reveals recurrent endometrial cancer. Which of the following histologies would make her a candidate for hormonal therapy with progestational agents?

   A. Carcinosarcoma

   B. Papillary serous carcinoma

   C. Low-grade endometrioid carcinoma

   D. Clear cell carcinoma

ANSWERS TO REVIEW QUESTIONS

1. ANSWER: C. Hormonal therapy is preferred as first-line intervention for recurrent or metastatic endometrial cancer due to its lower toxicity profile and response rate similar to chemotherapy. Hormonal therapy produces responses in 15% to 30% of patients and is associated with survival twice as long as in nonresponders. On average, responses last for 1 year. TAM is reserved for second-line hormone therapy. Currently, NCCN guidelines recommend the use of bevacizumab only after progression on prior cytotoxic chemotherapy. External beam radiotherapy is used in the metastatic setting if it can be directed to a particular tumor site. In this case the patient has bilateral lung nodules so systemic therapy is preferred.

2. ANSWER: D. There is currently insufficient evidence to recommend routine surveillance with MRI, ultrasound, or hysteroscopy for detection of endometrial cancer in patients on TAM. Women taking TAM should have a gynecologic evaluation according to the same guidelines for women not taking TAM. The presence of symptoms such as abnormal vaginal bleeding should trigger prompt investigation.

3. ANSWER: E. The patient's strong family history of colon cancer diagnosed in family members at a young age is strongly suggestive of HNPCC also known as Lynch syndrome. Lynch syndrome is caused by an autosomal dominant disorder characterized by a germline mutation in mismatch repair genes and is associated with tumors exhibiting microsatellite instability. Lynch syndrome is associated with increased risk of cancers of the colon, endometrium, ovary, stomach, small intestine, hepatobiliary tract, urinary tract, brain, and skin. The ACS recommends that women with HNPCC undergo annual endometrial biopsy after age 35, since the lifetime risk of endometrial cancer in patients with HNPCC is 40% to 60%. Prophylactic hysterectomy and BSO is a risk-reducing option that should be considered by women who have completed childbearing, since the lifetime risk of ovarian cancer in patients with Lynch syndrome is 10% to 20%.

4. ANSWER: A. In stage III and IV metastatic papillary serous endometrial cancer referral for clinical trials is strongly recommended as there is no FDA-approved standard of care. A reasonable first-line treatment is chemotherapy, for example, with a triplet regimen such as cisplatin, doxorubicin, and paclitaxel, or carboplatin and paclitaxel doublet. Hormone therapy with medroxyprogesterone acetate is only recommended for endometrioid subtype and is not recommended for papillary serous and clear cell subtype. Vaginal brachytherapy alone is generally reserved for localized disease (stage I disease and stage II grade 1).

5. ANSWER: C. Hormonal therapy is only used in low-grade endometrioid histology. It is not appropriate for high grade (grade 3) endometrioid, serous, clear cell, or carcinosarcoma. Women with these histologies should receive multiagent chemotherapy preferably with carboplatin or cisplatin, or single agent chemotherapy if unable to tolerate combination regimens. Clinical trial participation is also strongly encouraged for women with high-risk histologic subtypes.

Cervical Cancer 19

Sarah M. Temkin and Charles A. Kunos

REVIEW QUESTIONS

1. A 36-year-old woman has been diagnosed with uterine cervix cancer. She is now in your office and after discussing her particular case, she asks about uterine cervix cancer in the broader population. You tell her that all the following epidemiologic factors are true, EXCEPT:

   A. Worldwide, uterine cervix cancer is the fourth leading cause of cancer death in women.

   B. Simian virus 40 (SV40) is thought to be a causative agent in the majority of the cases.

   C. Incidence of uterine cervix cancer is higher in American black women and Hispanic women of any race compared to American women of white race.

   D. During the past 50 years, death rates from uterine cervix cancer have declined because of routine screening with Papanicolaou (Pap) smears.

2. A 49-year-old woman is diagnosed with squamous cell uterine cervix cancer after physical examination and biopsy. All of the following risk factors are associated with extrapelvic metastatic disease EXCEPT:

   A. Presence of uterine cervix microinvasion

   B. Depth of uterine cervix stromal invasion

   C. Uterine cervix tumor size

   D. Presence of lymphovascular space invasion (LVSI)

3. A 40-year-old woman presents with a one-year history of bleeding after sexual intercourse. She has not had a Papanicolaou (Pap) smear in eight years. During a pelvic speculum examination, a 3 cm lesion of the uterine cervix is observed and then biopsied. The result of the biopsy shows uterine cervix adenocarcinoma. In regard to her clinical staging all of the following are true EXCEPT:

   A. If hydronephrosis is seen on abdominopelvic CT scan, she would be stage IIIB.

   B. MRI is the best imaging modality for determining parametrial tissue involvement.

   C. Staging for uterine cervix cancer is clinical, involving, at minimum, pelvic examination.

   D. If enlarged lymph nodes are seen on CT scan, she would be at least stage III.

4. A 50-year-old woman with history of abnormal Papanicolaou (Pap) smears presents with bleeding after sexual intercourse. On pelvic speculum examination, she has a 2 cm visible lesion on her uterine cervix. A rectovaginal examination reveals no evidence of parametrial tissue spread. After lesion biopsy and further evaluation, she is diagnosed with stage IB1 squamous cell uterine cervix cancer. The best treatment option for her includes the following:

   A. Simple hysterectomy

   B. Radical hysterectomy with pelvic lymph node dissection

   C. Radical trachelectomy

   D. Cervical conization

5. A 44-year-old woman with stage IIIB uterine cervix cancer develops a central pelvic recurrence less than 2 years from the completion of her initial treatment. She had received primary radiochemotherapy at the time of her initial diagnosis. Current imaging shows only a central pelvic tumor with no extrapelvic metastatic disease. The only treatment option that has a chance for cure in this setting is

   A. Chemotherapy with combined cisplatin and topotecan

   B. Chemotherapy with combined cisplatin and paclitaxel

    C. Referral back to radiation oncology for consideration of further radiation

    D. Referral to gynecologic oncology for consideration of pelvic exenteration

6. A 36-year-old woman with 3 children, 2 of them girls, has been diagnosed with early stage uterine cervix cancer in follow-up of an abnormal cervical smear. The girls are now 14 and 15 years old. She comes to your office to ask how she can protect her family from this diagnosis. Which of the following is the best recommendation?

    A. There are no hereditary risks of cervical cancer, thus nothing needs to be done.

    B. All three of her children should receive HPV vaccination if they have not yet done so.

    C. Her daughters should go immediately for baseline cervical smears.

    D. Her son has no risk of HPV infection.

7. A 49-year-old woman is diagnosed with squamous cell uterine cervix cancer after physical examination and biopsy. Her bimanual examination identifies a 1 cm cervical lesion with no palpable lymph nodes. Biopsy shows invasion, and positive lymphovascular space invasion (LVSI). Which additional test may provide key information to guide treatment planning?

    A. Barium enema

    B. HPV typing

    C. MRI brain

    D. FDG-PET CT scan

8. A 40-year-old woman presents with a one-year history of bleeding after sexual intercourse. She has not had a Papanicolaou (Pap) smear in eight years. During a pelvic speculum examination, a 4.5 cm lesion of the uterine cervix is observed and then biopsied. The result of the biopsy shows uterine cervix adenocarcinoma. Abdominopelvic CT scan reveals

unilateral hydronephrosis and pelvic lymph nodes. Which most accurately describes preferred treatment?

A. A simple hysterectomy

B. Radical hysterectomy with pelvic and para-aortic nodal dissection

C. Radical hysterectomy with sentinel lymph node testing

D. Definitive chemoradiation

ANSWERS TO REVIEW QUESTIONS

1. ANSWER: B. Uterine cervix cancer is caused by exposure to high-risk strains of HPV not SV40. The rest of the epidemiologic information is correct. The higher incidence of uterine cervix cancer among minorities in the United States is thought to be due to barriers in screening secondary to lack of insurance, low income, and immigration from low-screening regions.

2. ANSWER: A. Major prognostic factors are stage, lymph node involvement, tumor size, depth of cervical stroma invasion, lymphovascular space invasion (LVSI), and to a lesser extent histologic type and grade. Spread is usually orderly starting from the cervix to the pelvic nodes, along lymphovascular planes to the iliac (pelvic) lymph nodes and finally to the paraaortic lymph nodes. Spread by blood-borne mechanisms are typically a late occurrence. Women with microinvasive uterine cervix cancer have minimal risk (1% or less) of metastatic disease and are adequately treated with a cervical conization or simple hysterectomy.

3. ANSWER: D. Because of the global burden of uterine cervix cancer, mostly distributed among low-resource regions where abilities to surgically stage are limited, uterine cervix cancer is clinically staged. Imaging may include CT or combined PET/CT and MRI when available, for treatment planning purposes only. Hydronephrosis seen on intravenous pyelogram represents stage IIIB disease. If hydronephrosis is noted on CT scan or CT-IVP, this is also acceptable to determine stage IIIB disease, because the same finding would likely be apparent on traditional IVP.

4. ANSWER: B. Although radiochemotherapy is superior to surgical therapy for advanced-stage disease, both treatments have comparable survival for early-stage disease. Radiochemotherapy avoids a surgical procedure, while the benefits of radical hysterectomy include preservation of ovarian function, avoidance of acute and chronic radiation–induced changes to the genitourinary and gastrointestinal systems, and obtaining a surgical specimen characterizing prognosis. Cervical conization or simple hysterectomy would not be appropriate for this woman, since she has clinically visible disease. If future fertility is desired, radical trachelectomy with pelvic lymph node dissection could be considered. Since this woman is near or at menopause, a fertility-sparing procedure would not be appropriate.

5. ANSWER: D. The woman has an isolated central pelvic recurrence after radiochemotherapy. Since she has already undergone pelvic radiation, additional delivery of radiation would be challenging. Any chemotherapeutic regimen would only be palliative; however, pelvic exenteration performed for a centrally recurrent disease provides a 5-year survival of approximately 50%.

6. ANSWER: B. Uterine cervix cancer is caused by infection with high-risk strains of human papilloma virus (HPV). There are now 3 approved vaccinations against risk of HPV infection. Current guidelines recommend vaccination of all children and teens over the age of 9, and up to age 26 if not infected and not previously vaccinated. There are no hereditary risks of cervical cancer; however, vaccination can be done to prevent infection and thus risk of cancers. Initiation of cervical smear testing (Pap and/or HPV testing) is recommended to start around age 21 unless sexually active and with multiple partners. HPV infection is a risk for males as well as females. Infection is spread sexually and thus is a risk to males; penile cancer, while rare, has up to a 50% HPV positivity rate.

7. ANSWER: D. Major prognostic factors of cervical cancer include clinical stage, lymph node involvement, tumor size, depth of cervical stroma invasion, lymphovascular space invasion (LVSI), and to a lesser extent histologic type and grade. Spread is usually orderly starting from the cervix to the pelvic nodes, along lymphovascular planes to the iliac (pelvic) lymph nodes and finally to the paraaortic lymph nodes. Spread by blood-borne mechanisms are typically a late occurrence. Thus, FDG-PET/CT to examine lymph nodes, especially in the face of +LVSI, could change treatment decision to allow surgical treatment. Women with positive lymph nodes would more likely be treated with chemoradiation or radical surgery rather than cervical conization or simple hysterectomy. While useful to do and preoperative standard of care, it is extremely unlikely that a barium enema or MRI of the brain would identify disease that would change treatment planning. HPV typing has no bearing on treatment decisions.

8. ANSWER: D. Because the global burden of uterine cervix cancer, mostly distributed among low-resource regions where abilities to surgically stage are limited, uterine cervix cancer is clinically staged. Imaging may include CT or combined PET/CT and MRI when available, for treatment planning purposes only. Hydronephrosis seen on a dye study (IVP or CT, CT/IVP) represents stage IIIB disease. Such disease is treated with definitive chemoradiation. A simple hysterectomy is used only for stage IA1 disease, negative margins on biopsy, no LVSI, and microinvasion at greatest. Patients with pelvic lymph nodes without organ compromise may be treated with radical hysterectomy with pelvic nodal dissection. Paraaortic lymph node dissection should be done if there is a high risk of high nodal involvement in a setting without organ compromise. Sentinel node examination is not a worldwide cervical cancer standard of care, nor is it yet a US SOC.

Vulvar Cancer 20

Kristen P. Zeligs and Christina M. Annunziata

REVIEW QUESTIONS

1. A 74-year-old woman presents to her primary care physician with an 18-month history of vulvar pruritus, difficulty with urination, and hard left inguinal mass. Pelvic examination reveals an erythematous ulcerating lesion on the labia majora extending on to the urethral orifice and labia minora bilaterally. On vaginal examination there is a hard mass palpable anteriorly. CT scan reveals extension into the lower posterior bladder and wall and involvement of the left inguinal and pelvic LNs. Biopsy of the vulvar lesion reveals a poorly differentiated SCC arising from the vulva. She has a history of depression and mild hypertension. What is the most appropriate treatment?

    A. Tamoxifen

    B. Pelvic exenteration

    C. Chemoradiation to vulva and inguinal area followed by resection of any residual disease on the vulva

    D. Vaginal brachytherapy

    E. A and B

2. A 72-year-old female with a history of stage IVB SCC of the vulva treated 1 year ago with chemoradiation followed by resection of residual disease on the labia minora now presents to the ER with urinary retention, reduced appetite, and hard mass in the right lower abdomen. Serum chemistries and CBC are normal. Urethral catheterization is performed to relieve her urinary retention. On CT scan she has recurrence of her disease in the

pelvis with involvement of the urethra causing a stricture and right-sided pelvic LN mass within the radiation port. She lives alone and was working as a secretary until her admission. She has no other significant comorbidities. What is the most appropriate next step?

A. Repeat external beam radiotherapy to the pelvis

B. Referral for a clinical trial

C. Carboplatin plus bevacizumab

D. Aromatase inhibitor

E. None of the above

3. A 69-year-old female with a history of stage I screen-detected ER- and PR-positive breast cancer treated 5 years ago with lumpectomy and adjuvant radiation therapy followed by 5 years of anastrozole presents for routine follow-up. On review of systems she reports a 6-month history of itching of the vulva. On examination there is a 0.5 cm erythematous raised lesion. Colposcopy and biopsy reveal VIN with no evidence of invasive disease. What is the most appropriate treatment?

A. Radical vulvectomy

B. Cisplatin 50 mg/m^2 IV every 3 weeks

C. No therapy. Observation only is required

D. Vaginal brachytherapy

E. Laser ablation

4. An 84-year-old woman status post prior total abdominal hysterectomy and bilateral salpingo-oophorectomy with multiple medical co-morbidities presents for evaluation of a large vulvar mass. On exam the patient is found to have a large vulvar mass and gross inguinal lymph node enlargement. Imaging findings are concerning for tumor involvement invading the bladder. Biopsy results are consistent with squamous cell carcinoma likely of vulvar origin. The recommended treatment for this patient includes

A. Neoadjuvant cisplatin concurrently with radiation therapy

B. Hospice consultation

C. Immediate surgical exploration

D. 5-FU treatment

E. imiquimod

5. A 72-year-old woman undergoes an excisional biopsy of a 1-cm diameter pigmented lesion on the lateral side of her right labia majora. Pathology findings are consistent with malignant melanoma, nodular type, with a thickness of 0.9 mm. The lateral margin is positive for melanoma. The biopsy site is healing well, and a complete physical examination is unremarkable. You advise the patient that the most appropriate next step in management is

   A. wide re-excision of the surgical site

   B. radical left hemivulvectomy with ipsilateral inguinal and pelvic lymphadenectomies

   C. radiation of the vulva and left groin

   D. interferon alfa

   E. observation

ANSWERS TO REVIEW QUESTIONS

1. ANSWER: C. The patient has stage IVB disease. Pelvic exenteration is a radical surgery with significant morbidity and uncertain survival benefit. Chemoradiation may allow less extensive resection. There are no data for tamoxifen in the management of SCC of the vulva. Brachytherapy would be inadequate treatment for stage IVB disease.

2. ANSWER: B. There is no proven standard of care for relapsed stage IV SCC of the vulva. Since the patient appears to have a good performance status, referral for a clinical trial is appropriate. Repeat radiation to the pelvis would not be recommended given that the treatment was <2 years ago and is unlikely to give benefit.

3. ANSWER: E. In patients in whom invasive disease is not suspected or seen on biopsy, laser ablation is an appropriate therapy. Radical vulvectomy is reserved for invasive disease. Observation is not appropriate since invasive disease may develop.

4. ANSWER: A. Neoadjuvant chemoradiation may improve operability and should be considered in patients with extensive disease, including those with anorectal, urethral, or bladder involvement, disease fixed to the bone, and gross inguinal or femoral lymph node involvement. This particular patient has multiple medical co-morbidities in the setting of extensive tumor involvement including involvement of the bladder, making neoadjuvant chemoradiation the best treatment option.

5. ANSWER: A. Vulvar melanoma is the second most common vulvar malignancy following squamous cell carcinoma. The disease is most frequently observed in postmenopausal women, and a pigmented lesion is the most common finding on physical exam. Tumor thickness, stage, and age of patient are all prognostic factors for patients with vulvar melanoma. Historically, vulvar melanomas were treated with radical excisions and regional lymph node dissections. This has largely been replaced by more limited operations as no survival advantage was found with more extensive excisions. Lesions less than 1mm thick can be treated by wide local excision alone. A surgical margin of at least 1 cm is desirable for lesions less than 1 mm thick. Given that this patient did not have tumor-free margins with her initiation excisional procedure, it is most advisable that she undergo a wide re-excision of the operative site in order to obtain 1-cm tumor-free margins. Lymphadenectomy is not necessary in patients with lesions less than 1mm thick as the risk of lymph node metastasis is less than 5%.

Sarcomas and Malignancies of the Bone 21

Dale R. Shepard

REVIEW QUESTIONS

1. A 9-year-old boy is seen by a pediatric oncologist for a mass identified during an evaluation by his pediatrician for pain in his left femur that is worse during soccer practice. He has a needle biopsy of the mass. What finding would indicate a Ewing family tumor (EFT)?

   A. A *EFTR1-FL1* mutation

   B. A t(8;22) mutation

   C. Presence of a BCR-ABL oncogene

   D. A *EWSR1-FL1* mutation

2. A 65-year-old man presents with a mass on the right chest wall. Imaging studies show numerous nodules in his lungs measuring up to 2 cm and three lesions in his liver. A biopsy is positive for a high-grade liposarcoma. Which of the following chemotherapy regimens is associated with an overall survival benefit as first-line treatment?

   A. Doxorubicin and olaratumab

   B. Doxorubicin and ifosfamide

   C. Trabectedin

   D. Gemcitabine and docetaxel

3. Which of the following correctly describes the incidence of soft tissue sarcoma?

    A. About 5% of adult cancers are sarcomas with 95% of these soft tissue sarcoma.

    B. About 1% of adult cancers are sarcomas with 25% of these soft tissue sarcoma.

    C. About 1% of adult cancers are sarcomas with 20% of these bone sarcoma.

    D. Sarcomas represent about 1% of cancers in both adults and children.

4. A 19-year-old female has a painful mass in her leg and is found to have a mass associated with the bone on an x-ray. She is seen by an orthopedic oncologist and after an MRI of the leg confirms the presence of a mass, she undergoes an open biopsy that is positive for a high-grade osteosarcoma. A PET/CT shows no evidence for metastatic disease. Which of the following best describes the role of chemotherapy for osteosarcoma?

    A. Osteosarcomas are not very sensitive to chemotherapy and it should only be given for metastatic disease.

    B. Patients with high-grade osteosarcoma should receive neoadjuvant chemotherapy, wide excision of the tumor, and additional chemotherapy after resection.

    C. Patients with high-grade osteosarcoma should only receive chemotherapy after surgical resection.

    D. Patients with low-grade and high-grade osteosarcoma benefit from chemotherapy prior to, but not after surgical resection.

5. Which of the following correctly describes the most common location of soft tissue sarcomas?

    A. Groin/thigh/buttock > torso > upper extremity = retroperitonium

    B. Torso > groin/thigh/buttock > upper extremity > retroperitoneum

    C. Retroperitoneum > upper extremity > groin/thigh/buttock > torso

    D. Upper extremity >retroperitoneum > torso > groin/thigh/buttock

6. A 14-year-old girl has a 4-month history of pain in her pelvis that has been becoming more intense over the past 2 weeks, particularly at night. She has also noted some increase in fatigue. She is seen by her pediatrician who orders an x-ray that shows a mass in the pelvis. She is sent to an orthopedic oncologist with concern for Ewing Family Tumor (EFT) based on her age and the presentation. Which of the following is true about the management of this sarcoma?

   A. The pediatrician should arrange a needle biopsy prior to referral to the orthopedic oncologist to determine the diagnosis and expedite surgery.

   B. Patients with EFT rarely have metastatic disease and surgery alone is usually curative.

   C. EFT is very sensitive to doxorubicin-based chemotherapy and patients rarely need surgery.

   D. Patients should receive chemotherapy before surgery and additional chemotherapy after surgery to minimize risk for recurrence.

7. A 15-year-old boy is seen by his dentist for a persistent ache in his mandible, thought to be due to a wisdom tooth, and is found to have a mass in the mandible. He is referred to an otolaryngologist who does a biopsy that is positive for a nonpleomorphic rhabdomyosarcoma. Which of the following is correct about the treatment of this sarcoma?

   A. Surgical resection alone is appropriate due to the low likelihood for metastatic disease.

   B. Radiation therapy should not be used for patients with rhabdomyosarcoma due to the resistance of this tumor to radiation.

   C. Patients with resected rhabdomyosarcoma require a very long course of chemotherapy and radiation.

   D. Nonpleomorphic sarcoma should be treated like a soft tissue sarcoma.

8. Which of the following best describes the epidemiology of osteosarcoma?

   A. Osteosarcoma represents about 9% of all cases of cancer diagnosed in the United States annually.

B. Osteosarcoma is the second most common type of bone cancer in children and adolescents behind Ewing sarcoma.

C. There is a bimodal distribution for osteosarcoma with a peak in infants and again in adolescents.

D. In adults, osteosarcoma is often not a primary malignancy and has been linked to Paget's disease.

9. A 55-year-old man with pain in his left shoulder is seen by his primary care physician and found to have a palpable mass. An MRI shows a 4.5 cm mass on the left scapula. He is seen by an orthopedic oncologist and has a complete resection of a low-grade undifferentiated pleomorphic sarcoma. He is referred to a medical oncologist for discussion of adjuvant chemotherapy. What is the best guidance for this patient?

A. Undifferentiated pleomorphic sarcoma is not likely to be responsive to chemotherapy and it should not be given.

B. There are conflicting data from primary trials and meta-analyses and, ideally, adjuvant chemotherapy would be given in a clinical trial.

C. Due to very high response rates, adjuvant chemotherapy should be given to all patients with soft tissue sarcoma.

D. Adjuvant chemotherapy should only be given in combination with radiation therapy for patients with soft tissue sarcoma.

10. A 71-year-old female with a history of breast cancer previously treated with a right mastectomy, radiation therapy, and chemotherapy is seen in clinic with a painful right clavicle. Evaluation with a chest x-ray and subsequently a PET scan shows a 2.3 cm lesion in the right clavicle and 1.6 cm and 2.3 cm nodules in the right upper and left lower lobes of the lungs, respectively. A biopsy of the mass in the clavicle is positive for osteosarcoma. Which of the following best describes the management of this patient?

A. Sites of metastatic osteosarcoma should be evaluated for resection prior to starting chemotherapy.

B. Osteosarcomas become metastatic quickly and she should undergo immediate chemotherapy.

C. There is no role for chemotherapy for osteosarcoma and all three lesions should be removed surgically.

D. There is no role for chemotherapy for osteosarcoma and all three lesions should be treated with definitive radiation.

ANSWERS TO REVIEW QUESTIONS

1. ANSWER: D. Ewing family tumors are characterized by the presence of an *EWSR1* mutation with *EWSR1-FL1* being the most common mutation.

2. ANSWER: A. The combination of doxorubicin and the platelet-derived growth factor receptor inhibitor olaratumab was studied as first-line therapy in patients with soft tissue sarcoma compared with doxorubicin alone. The combination therapy showed an improvement in overall survival of 11.8 months. [Tap WD, Jone RL, Van Tine BA, et al. Olaratumab and doxorubicin versus doxorubicin alone for treatment of soft-tissue sarcoma: an open-label phase 1b and randomized phase 2 trial. *Lancet.* 2016;388:488–497]

3. ANSWER: C. The incidence of sarcoma is about 1% of all cancers diagnosed annually with about 80% of these sarcomas in the soft tissues. In 2017, the estimated number of soft tissue sarcomas is 12,390 with 3,260 cases of cancer of the bone or joints. The total number of new cases of cancer is 1,688,780. [Siegel RL, Miller KD, and Jemal A. Cancer Statistics, 2017. *CA Cancer J Clin.* 2017;67:7–30]

4. ANSWER: B. Patients with a low-grade osteosarcoma can proceed directly to a wide excision. Patients with a high-grade osteosarcoma should receive neoadjuvant chemotherapy followed by restaging prior to resection by wide excision. [Biermann JS, Adkins DR, Agulnik M. Bone Cancer. *J Natl Compr Canc Netw.* 2013;11:688–723]

5. ANSWER: A. The pattern of occurrence of soft tissue sarcomas is that about half are in the groin, thigh, or buttock, about 20% are in the torso and about 15% are in the retroperitoneum and the upper extremities. [Lawrence W, Jr., et al. Adult soft tissue sarcomas. A pattern of care survey of the American College of Surgeons. *Ann Surg.* 1987;205(4):349–359]

6. ANSWER: D. There is a high incidence of micrometastatic disease in patients diagnosed with EFT and all patients should have initial chemotherapy for 12 weeks, restaging and resection of the primary tumor in the absence of metastatic disease. After resection, patients should have adjuvant chemotherapy with addition of radiation therapy if there are positive resection margins. [Biermann JS, Chow W, Reed DR. Bone Cancer. *J Natl Compr Can Netw.* 2017;15:155–167]

7. ANSWER: C. Nonpleomorphic rhabdomyosarcoma is rarely treated successfully with surgical resection as the only treatment modality. These tumors are sensitive to radiation therapy. Treatment for patients with all clinical risk groups are likely to benefit from a long postoperative course of chemotherapy with inclusion of radiation therapy. [NCCN Clinical Practice Guidelines in Oncology. Soft Tissue Sarcoma. V.1.2018. https://www.nccn.org/professionals/physician_gls/PDF/sarcoma.pdf]

8. ANSWER: D. Osteosarcoma is the most common type of cancer of the bone in children and adolescents and has an incidence of about 1% of all cancers in the United States. In older adults, osteosarcoma is often associated with Paget's disease and not a primary malignancy. The bimodal distribution is in adolescents and again in older adults. [Mirabello L, Troisi RJ, Savage SA. Osteosarcoma incidence and survival rates from 1973 to 2004: Data from the survellance, epidemiology, and end results program. *Cancer.* 2009;115:1531–1543]

9. ANSWER: B. Unlike some sarcomas, like rhabdomyosarcoma, osteosarcoma or EFT, there is no clear role for adjuvant chemotherapy for patients with most soft tissue sarcomas. While there are some positive meta-analyses that suggest a benefit, there are many primary clinical trials that fail to show a benefit. Until there is more evidence for benefit, patients interested in adjuvant chemotherapy for a soft tissue sarcoma should enroll in a clinical trial. [Le Cesne A, Ouali M, Leahy MG. Doxorubicin-based adjuvant chemotherapy in soft tissue sarcoma: pooled analysis of two STBSG-EORTC phase III clinical trials. *Ann Oncol.* 2014;25:2425–2432; Woll PJ, Reichardt P, Le Cesne A, et al. Adjuvant chemotherapy with doxorubicin, ifosfamide, and lenograstim for resected soft-tissue sarcoma (EORTC 62931): a multicentre randomized controlled trial. *Lancet Oncol.* 2012;13;1045–1054].

10. ANSWER: A. Patients with metastatic osteosarcoma may still achieve a cure from resection of the metastatic sites and subsequent therapy with chemotherapy. Assessing patients with metastatic osteosarcoma for metastatectomy is in the treatment guidelines. [Biermann JS, Adkins DR, Agulnik M. Bone Cancer. *J Natl Compr Can Netw.* 2013;11:688–723]

Skin Cancers and Melanoma 22

Upendra P. Hegde and Sanjiv S. Agarwala

REVIEW QUESTIONS

1. A 47-year-old Caucasian male presents to his primary care provider with a pigmented lesion of left arm that has increased in size over last 6 months and appears to exhibit change in colors. An evaluation by his dermatologist reveal an asymmetric pigmented lesion on left arm that measures about 8 mm in diameter with irregular margins and variegate colors. A clinical suspicion of melanoma led to an incisional biopsy of the lesion. Histology findings confirm a diagnosis of cutaneous melanoma with a depth of 1.8 mm, without ulceration and 2 to 3 mitosis/mm^2 without lympho-vascular invasion and regression. A wide excision of this tumor is performed with negative margins and a lymphoscintigraphy revealed two sentinel lymph nodes in the left axilla negative for metastasis. A chest x ray is negative for any abnormalities and peripheral blood is normal for liver functions and LDH. Cutaneous melanoma is staged as AJCC T2aN0M0 IB and patient is scheduled for a counseling session to discuss future follow-up and risk stratification as well as any need for adjuvant treatment. Which of the following statement is not true?

    A. Evidence of lymph-vascular invasion and regression increase recurrence risk

    B. Absence of ulceration reduce risk of recurrence

    C. The patient's risk of recurrence is low since his stage is IB

    D. Diagnosis of cutaneous melanoma increase risk of new primary cutaneous melanoma

2. A 45-year-old Caucasian male reports a pigmented mole on his right upper back that is pruritic and bleeds intermittently. He is seen by a dermatologist who suspects cutaneous melanoma and performs a biopsy of this mole. Histologic findings confirm cutaneous melanoma 4.5 mm deep, ulceration, mitosis $8/mm^2$, Clark level V, lympho-vascular invasion present, and nonbrisk tumor infiltrating lymphocytes. Clinical examination also reveal a 1.5 cm lymph node in the right axillary region biopsy of which shows metastasis from cutaneous melanoma. A wide excision of this tumor is performed along with a complete lymph node dissection from right axilla that confirms one lymph node with multiple foci of melanoma metastasis while one additional lymph node out of 14 lymph nodes reveal microscopic metastasis. A whole body imaging study with positron emission tomogram (PET scan) and a brain MRI reveal no evidence of systemic metastasis. The melanoma is staged as AJCC T4bN2bM0, stage IIIC and he has referred to you melanoma education, risk stratification, and counseling for adjuvant treatment to improve long-term outcome. The patient is very anxious about his melanoma diagnosis and wants the best treatment options available to him. Which is the best option available to this patient?

   A. Risk of recurrence is low, recommend clinical follow-up every 4 to 6 months

   B. Recommend adjuvant therapy with high dose interferon alfa-2b (HD IFN-alfa) for one year

   C. Discuss the risk and benefits of anti CTLA-4 antibody ipilimumab treatment for 3 years

   D. Recommend four cycles of biochemotherapy

3. You are seeing a 36-year old Caucasian woman with astrocytoma of the brain undergoing radiation therapy with concurrent Temozolomide treatment following surgical resection of the brain tumor. The patient report a previous history of invasive cutaneous melanoma of the right leg at age of 26 that was completely excised while a biopsy of a pigmented lesion noted on her right parietal scalp confirms invasive cutaneous melanoma. The family history includes surgical treatment of cutaneous melanoma of right leg in her 17-year-old son and a cutaneous melanoma of the right shoulder in her father when he was 47 years of age. The patient who has multiple cutaneous moles of the trunk and extremities is alarmed of the risk of melanoma in her children and inquires if her melanoma is

associated with genetic predisposition. Select one correct answer related to her clinical condition

    A. Patient has a low risk of inherited melanoma and no further work up is necessary

    B. Refer the patient to a genetic counselor because you think she might have an inherited melanoma

    C. Order genetic testing to identify a gene mutation responsible for causing predisposition to develop melanoma

    D. Germinal mutation of BAP-1 gene is the most common cause of inherited melanoma

4. A 78-year-old male with history of hypertension and type II diabetes mellitus, presents with a lump on right upper lateral chest wall of one month duration. The mass is a 2.5 cm in two dimension, painless, and increasing in size. His past medical history is significant for surgical treatment of a cutaneous melanoma of the right upper chest wall (stage IIIB) followed by close surveillance. A biopsy of the right lateral chest wall mass is consistent with metastatic melanoma and stage workup with a whole body PET scan revealed 1.5 cm x 1.4 cm enhancing mass in right lower lobe of the lung. A biopsy of the chest wall and the lung mass revealed features consistent with metastatic melanoma. Genetic testing for BRAF gene showed the tumor to be BRAF wild type while the tumor tested positive for PD-L1 ligand. A brain MRI is negative for metastasis and blood work including LDH is normal. You schedule a visit to discuss treatment options. You sit with the patient and make the following recommendations:

    A. Surgical excision of the right chest wall mass and right lower lobectomy

    B. Single agent anti PD-1 treatment for 2 years

    C. Anti CTLA-4 antibody ipilimumab treatment at 3mg/kg every 3 weeks for four doses

    D. Ipilimumab at 3mg/kg plus nivolumab at 1mg/kg every 3 weeks for four doses followed by single agent nivolumab treatment for 2 years

5. A 43-year-old male presenting with symptoms of progressive weight loss of 10 pounds and right upper abdominal discomfort and lower back pain over preceding 3 months. His past history is significant for cutaneous melanoma of the upper back two and half year previously. The tumor was resected with negative margins and lymphoscintigraphy revealed positive sentinel lymph nodes in the axilla. Patient underwent completion lymphadenectomy and opted for close surveillance. Clinical examination reveal an anxious looking young male with discomfort in lower back and enlarged liver 4 cm below costal margin. An MRI of thoracic and lumbosacral spine showed evidence of metastatic tumor in second lumbar vertebra causing partial destruction of the vertebral body without evidence of cord compression. A peripheral blood test revealed normal liver and kidney functions but elevated LDH of 450 U/L (110-220). Whole body PET scan study revealed at least 7 multiple medium size (2 to 3 cm) metastasis in both the lungs, a single 2.5 cm enhancing mass in the right lobe of liver and an isolated metastasis in L2 vertebral body. Brain MRI with and without contrast showed no evidence of metastasis. A biopsy of the lung lesion confirmed metastatic melanoma and genetic study for BRAF mutational analysis reveal tumor to be BRAF wild type. The patient has a performance status of 1 and committed to his treatment. The patient underwent a radiofrequency ablation of the tumor in the L-2 vertebral body followed by external radiation therapy for pain relief.

   You sit down with the patient to discuss systemic treatment options and recommend following:

   A. Single agent anti PD-1 antibody

   B. Single agent anti CTLA-4 antibody

   C. Combination of anti PD-1 and anti CTLA-4 antibody

   D. High dose IL-2 treatment

6. A 68-year-old Caucasian male presents to his primary care provider with progressive pain in right lower chest, upper abdomen and shortness of breath. He has lost more than 25 pounds weight in the preceding 3 months and reports severe fatigue and loss of energy. Significant past medical history includes surgical excision of a cutaneous melanoma of the lower back 2 years previously. Clinical examination reveals a chronically ill looking male with pallor and discomfort due to right lower chest pain. A firm immobile mass measuring 4cm x 4cm is palpable in the right lower posterior chest wall. Pulse rate is 104/minute, regular and respiratory rate is

28/minute, oxygen saturation at 89% on room air (Performance status 3). Systemic examination reveal absent breath sounds in the right lower chest and findings consistent with moderate pleural effusion while liver is palpable at 3.5 cm below the right costal margins. A CAT scan of the chest/abdomen/pelvis reveal signs of right pleural effusion with bilateral lung nodules (at least 5 nodules counted) measuring between 1 to 2 cm in diameter and a solitary mass measuring 2.5 cm in the right lobe of liver. A brain MRI with and without gadolinium showed no evidence of brain metastasis while serum LDH level is 220 U/L (110-220). A genetic testing of his melanoma reveal BRAF mutation at V600E. The patient is provided supportive care and therapeutic pleural tap is performed for symptomatic relief confirms metastatic melanoma to the pleura on cytology. The most appropriate treatment recommendation is:

A. Combined ipilimumab plus nivolumab treatment

B. Anti BRAF treatment

C. Anti BRAF plus MEK therapy

D. Palliative care and hospice

E. Refer the patient to a clinical trial

7. A 64-year-old Caucasian male with significant history of sun exposure and heavy alcohol intake. He reported a nodule of the skin of the left side of the nose near the bridge that has progressively enlarged over 18 months. Evaluation by a dermatologist revealed a shiny pink nodule of the skin of the upper nose with central depression and rolled margins with marks of blood. A biopsy of the lesion was consistent with basal cell carcinoma. The patient did not follow up for surgical treatment planned by his dermatologist and the skin nodule has increased in size, ulcerated and started bleeding locally. Over the next year, the patient continued to report burning sensation over the left orbit that he covered with an eye shade as the tumor continued to grow into his left eye causing progressive loss of vision. Lately, the patient has been reporting episodes of intermittent bleeding from the left nostril leading to the emergency room visit. Clinical examination reveal a 64-year-old male with disfigured face and a large ulcerated tumor with everted margins involving left base of nose extending deep into the left side of the nose and into the left eyebrow and the left orbit with destruction of the left eye globe. There is no evidence of lymphadenopathy in the neck and imaging study of the orbit and soft tissue of the neck reveal tumor invading into the left orbit

and nasal cavity with destruction of the eye. A biopsy of the ulcer margin is consistent with basal cell carcinoma. Whole body CAT scan revealed no evidence of tumor in the chest or abdomen or pelvis. The patient is referred to an ENT surgeon who educated patient regarding nasal bleeds and temporary measures to control them. He also indicated the patient's not eligibility for surgical treatment based on local extent of the tumor. Patient is referred to you for medical treatment. You see the patient and recommend following:

A. External radiation therapy to the left side of nose to include tumor extension to the left orbit and eye

B. Systemic chemotherapy

C. Targeted therapy with hedgehog inhibitor agent

D. Palliative care and hospice

8. A 73-year-old woman from Florida presents with multiple erythematous swellings of the upper chest, back, and both arms that have progressively increased in size over last 3 months. Patient reports these lumps cause discomfort and burning sensation. Past history includes a small firm bluish purple nodule measuring about a centimeter in size surgically removed from her right upper chest wall that showed diagnosis of Merkel cell carcinoma. A lymphoscintigraphy procedure performed at the time of wide excision of the tumor, led to two right axillary sentinel lymph nodes positive for metastatic Merkel cell carcinoma. A right axillary lymph node dissection revealed 15 additional lymph nodes without metastasis. Patient completed external beam radiation to the site of cutaneous Merkel cell carcinoma and been on a close surveillance program. Patient has no comorbidities except for a well-controlled hypertension. Clinical examination reveals a 73-year-old woman looking chronically ill but not in acute distress. She has mild pallor and a performance status of 1. Skin examination reveal multiple erythematous subcutaneous nodules some showing skin breakdown and blood tinge fluid. Peripheral blood examination reveal hemoglobin of 10 gm%, hematocrit of 30 and LDH 300 U/L (110-220). A whole body PET scan showed multiple FDG avid tumors corresponding to the clinically palpable skin lumps. In addition a FDG avid lesion was found in the right lobe of liver measuring 3x 4 cm. Brain MRI showed no evidence of brain metastasis while liver lesion and subcutaneous lesion biopsies confirmed metastasis from Merkel cell carcinoma. The patient

accompanied by her daughter and husband request your opinion and wants to get better.

You sit down with the patient and the family and suggest following:

A. Systemic therapy with cisplatin plus etoposide

B. Palliative care and refer to hospice

C. Discuss the treatment to interrupt PD-1-PD-L1/2 axis in the tumor

D. Discuss the role of EBV virus in causation of this tumor

9. A 87-year-old male is referred to you by his dermatologist with a diagnosis of advanced squamous cell carcinoma. The patient is a lifetime nonsmoker and has significant history of sun exposure and previously resected squamous cell carcinoma of the skin of the scalp. Now he presents with lumps in the skin of the scalp, neck, and back in the preceding 3 months. Biopsy of the lesion reveal poorly differentiated squamous cell carcinoma. Blood examination shows mild azotemia and LDH is marginally elevated. Imaging studies reveal suspicious lung nodules biopsy of which confirmed squamous cell carcinoma. Patient is functional and has well controlled diabetes mellitus and hypertension. He has supportive wife and children who wants to try everything possible to help him get better:

You recommend following:

A. Systemic chemotherapy with 5-FU based agents

B. Single agent epidermal growth factor antagonist cetuximab given as a loading dose followed by weekly maintenance

C. Surgical consultations to resect subcutaneous tumors

D. Refer to a clinical trial with anti PD-1 agents

10. A 79-year-old woman with history of diabetes mellitus and congestive heart failure and adult onset rheumatoid arthritis involving joints of the upper extremities, presents to her primary care physician with a painless bluish nodule of the left leg adjacent to a previously resected cutaneous melanoma. A clinical examination reveal multiple bluish colored nodules each measuring 1 to 2 cm around the circumference of previously resected cutaneous melanoma. There is no evidence of lymph node enlargements

and systemic examination is normal. Surgical biopsy of one of the lesion is consistent with intra-cutaneous metastasis of melanoma and a genetic test to identify BRAF mutation showed BRAF to be wild type. A whole body PET study is negative for systemic organ metastasis and a brain MRI did not reveal metastasis to the brain. You sit down with the patient and discuss treatment options, as the tumor does not appear to be resectable. What are the treatment options for this patient?

A. External radiation therapy

B. Isolated limb infusion treatment

C. Combination of anti CTLA-4 and anti PD-1 agent

D. Intra lesional treatment with TVEK

ANSWERS TO REVIEW QUESTIONS

1. *ANSWER: A*

Rationale:

Based on a large AJCC melanoma-staging database on more than 27,000 patients with stage I and II melanoma is available for reliable assessment of prognosis and risk of recurrence. On a multivariate analysis, depth, ulceration, mitosis, and older age were independent prognostic factors associated with risk of recurrence. Presence or absence of regression or lympho-vascular invasion did not affect prognosis. In the absence of nodal metastasis, risk of recurrence was highest in stage IIB and IIC tumors compared to state IA/IB and IIA.

REFERENCES:

Balch CM et al. Prognostic factors analysis of 17,600 melanoma patients: validation of the American Joint Committee on Cancer melanoma staging system. *J Clin Oncol.* 2001;15:3622–3634.

Balch CM et al. Final version of 2009 AJCC melanoma staging and classification. *J Clin Oncol.* 2009;20:6199–6206. doi: 10.1200/JCO.2009.23.4799. Epub 2009 Nov 16.

2. *ANSWER: C*

Rationale:

The histological findings and stage of melanoma in this patient suggest high risk of recurrence between 60%–70% at 5 years and adverse outcome associated with it. Adjuvant treatment is recommended to prolong recurrence-free survival and overall survival. Two adjuvant treatment options are FDA approved that include HD IFN-alfa-2b and anti CTLA-4 antibody ipilimumab. HD IFN-alpha-2b treatment is given for one-year and confer relapse-free survival and overall survival. The side effects of HD IFN-alfa-2b include flu like symptoms, skin rashes, liver function abnormalities, and neuropsychiatric effects such as depression. Anti CTLA-4 anti-body treatment is recommended for 3 years and causes diverse symptoms of autoimmune diseases most common being diarrhea, colitis, skin rashes, autoimmune hepatitis, and endocrine hormone deficiency although any type of autoimmune side effects can occur leading to mortality of 1.1%. Of the two agents to choose from, anti CTLA-4 antibody treatment offer superior adjuvant benefit as noted by unequivocal relapse free and overall survival advantages. The patient in this scenario is a reasonable candidate for anti CTLA-4 antibody, as he wants the most effective treatment to prevent melanoma recurrence and prolong survival.

REFERENCES:

Kirkwood JM et al. High dose interferon alfa-2b significantly prolongs relapse-free and overall survival compared with the GM2-KLH/QS-21 vaccine in patients with resected stage IIB-III melanoma: results of intergroup trial E1654/S9512/C509801

Eggermont AM et al. Prolonged survival in stage III melanoma with ipilimumab adjuvant therapy. *N Engl J Med.* 2016 10; 375(19):1845–1855.

3. ANSWER: B

Rationale:

Cutaneous melanoma is inherited as a familial cancer in about 7% to 12% of patients, with autosomal dominant type of inheritance and high penetrance. Inherited melanoma is suspected in a patient with three or more primary cutaneous melanoma, or a family history of at least one invasive melanoma and two or more other diagnosis of melanoma and or pancreatic cancer among first- or second-degree relatives on the same side of the family. Germline mutation of the tumor suppressor gene cyclin dependent kinase 2A (CDKNK2A) is the most common and well-studied genetic abnormality that is associated with multiple atypical cutaneous melanocytic proliferations in a patient who is also at risk of developing pancreatic or brain cancers. Recent advances in molecular genetic technology has enabled detection of genetic abnormalities that share pathways with diverse other cancers in other organs leading to association of cutaneous melanoma with diverse internal malignancies. BAP-1 is one such gene, mutation of which is associated with cutaneous /ocular melanoma, mesothelioma, and renal cell carcinoma. Genetic testing might help to enhance understanding of the risk of new cutaneous melanoma as well as of other cancers in melanoma patients suspected to carry genetic mutations. A genetic testing should be preceded by appropriate counseling session by a genetic counselor so that results of the genetic testing could be appropriately interpreted. The most common genetic abnormality detected in about 40% of inherited melanoma is germinal mutation of CDKN2A gene while BAP-1 and POT-1 abnormalities account for about 10% of inherited cutaneous melanoma. This means that in almost half of patients suspected of familial melanoma, no known gene mutation may be detected as genetic abnormalities not previously known might be responsible. Genetic counselling will help understanding of risks of developing cutaneous melanoma and or internal malignancies so that close surveillance as well as appropriate life style modifications will lead to prevention and early diagnosis of cancer.

REFERENCES:

Ransohoff KJ et al. J Am Acad Dermatol. Familial skin cancer syndromes: increased melanoma risk. *Acad Dermatol.* 2016;74:423–434.

Soura E et al.. Hereditary melanoma: Update on syndromes and management: Emerging melanoma cancer complexes and genetic counseling. *J Am Acad Dermatol.* 2016;74(3):411–420.

4. ANSWER: B

Rationale:

There are two FDA-approved immune checkpoint inhibitors in three different regimens for use in patients diagnosed with metastatic melanoma. Ipilimumab is an anti CTLA-4 antibody that is approved as a single agent, pembrolizumab and nivolumab are two anti PD-1 agents approved as single agents for upto two years while combined anti CTLA-4 and anti PD-1 blockade is approved with ipilimumab and nivolumab administered every 3 weeks for four doses (induction) followed by single agent nivolumab administered every 2 weeks for 2 years (maintenance). While more than 80% responses following immune checkpoint inhibitor treatment are durable, autoimmune toxicity is a limiting factor and can be life threatening. Single agent anti PD-1 agent is effective in controlling metastatic melanoma in about 30% to 40% patients with favorable safety profile (grade 3/4 autoimmune toxicities of about 10% to 17%). Single agent anti CTLA-4 antibody result in about 20% to 25% of durable remissions but carry a higher grade 3/4 toxicity of about 20% to 27%. Combined anti CTLA-4 plus anti PD-1 combination is most effective with overall response rates of upto 60% but higher grade 3/4 autoimmune toxicities are seen in about 50% of patients. A large clinical trial comparing combination of ipilimumab and nivolumab in patients with stage IV or un-resectable stage III melanoma compared to single agent ipilimumab or nivolumab revealed comparable outcome with ipilimumab plus nivolumab or single agent nivolumab if patients had PD-1 ligand positive tumors and normal LDH and lower tumor bulk. Our patient who is 78-year-old male has PD-L1 positive tumor, low volume disease, and normal LDH and is likely to respond equally well to single agent anti PD-1 agent treatment compared to combined ipilimumab plus nivolumab. Other favorable factors of good outcome in our patient include oligo-metastases (3 or less organ sites) and good performance status. Single agent anti CTLA-4 agent is an option, but carries higher toxicity and inferior durable response rates. Surgical resection is an option in selected patients but carries higher risk of morbidity from surgical procedure, and a higher risk of recurrence following surgical treatment.

REFERENCES:

Postow MA, Chesney J et al. Nivolumab and Ipilimumab versus Ipilimumab in untreated melanoma. N Engl J Med. 372; 21.2015

Larkin J, Sileni-Chiarion R. et al. Combined Nivolumab and Ipilimumab or monotherapy in untreated melanoma. N Engl J Med. 373;1 2015

5. ANSWER: C

Rationale:

This is a relatively young male with stage IV melanoma and elevated LDH and committed to undergoing treatment. The likelihood of response to combined ipilimumab plus nivolumab is close to 60% with durable responses in more than 80% responding patients although risk of high grade 3/4 autoimmune side effect is high in the range of about 50%. Although elevated LDH levels confer adverse prognostic factor for single agent immune checkpoint inhibitor treatment, it does not affect outcome following combined immune checkpoint inhibitor treatment. Single agent anti CTLA-4 antibody or anti PD-1 antibody has lower efficacy and durable response in about 25% and 30% to 40% of patients with grade 3/4 autoimmune toxicities in 20% to 27% and 10% to 15% of patients respectively. High dose IL-2 treatment is not a superior option due to its higher toxicity from capillary leak syndrome and lower durable response rate of about 5% to 7% of patients. The tumor is negative for BRAF mutation hence patient is not eligible for targeted therapy.

REFERENCES:

Wolchok J et al. Nivolumab plus Ipilimumab in advanced melanoma. *N Engl J Med.* 2013; 69(2):122–133.

Postow MA et al. Nivolumab and Ipilimumab versus Ipilimumab in untreated melanoma. *N Engl J Med.* 2015;372:2006–2017.

6. ANSWER: C

Rationale:

The patient with stage IV melanoma is symptomatic from rapid tumor progression that is spreading to internal organs. A quick response is desirable for prompt relief of symptoms as supportive care is optimized. Although combined immune checkpoint inhibitor treatment is capable of rapid response, the patient's poor general condition and rapid progression of symptoms does not lend adequate window of time for reversal of symptoms with this strategy. Additionally, higher risks of developing serious autoimmune side effect following combined immune checkpoint inhibitor treatment and need to use of immune suppressive treatment to manage them could negatively affect patient's recovery and lead to adverse outcome. B-Raf is a serine/threonine kinase that occupies a central place in MAP kinase pathway regulating signals to the nucleus for gene expression important in maintaining tissue hemostasis. Activating mutations of BRAF gene result in uncontrolled downstream signals to the nucleus through MEK and ERK resulting in increased tumor cell proliferation, decreased differentiation and apoptosis. Vemurafenib and dabrafenib are two selective inhibitors of BRAF protein that have shown marked efficacy as single agents in patients with metastatic melanoma harboring BRAF mutation. However, acquired resistance to BRAF inhibitor agents lead to tumor recurrence and treatment failure. Addition of MEK inhibitor agent to BRAF inhibitor strengthens the MAP kinase pathway inhibition resulting in improved responses rates and progression-free survival (PFS) of 5.1 month versus 11.4 months and overall survival (OS) of 18.7 and 25.1 months, respectively. Recent analysis of data of patients receiving combined BRAF and MEK inhibitors over 3 years reveal flattening of the survival curve at around 3 years in about 30% patients that bear characteristics of low tumor burden (3 or less organ involvement), normal LDH and good performance status. Although our patient does not have favorable characteristics, a prompt tumor shrinkage and symptom improvement can help provide additional treatment options later. A clinical trial is a reasonable option but a poor performance status of this patient would likely make him ineligible for such an option.

REFERENCES:

Hauschild A et al. Dabrafenib in BRAF-mutated metastatic melanoma: a multicenter, open-label, phase 3 randomized controlled trial. *Lancet.* 2012;380:358–365.

Long GV, Stroyakovskiy D, Gogas H et al. Combined BRAF and MEK inhibition versus BRAF inhibition alone in melanoma. *N Engl J Med.* 2014;371:1877–1888.

7. ANSWER: C

Rationale:

This patient has a locally advanced basal cell carcinoma of skin of left side of the nose that extends into the left nasal cavity and orbit causing destruction of the globe of the left eye and intermittent bleeding from the nose. Imaging studies confirmed that the tumor is locally advanced without systemic metastasis. Although complete surgical excision is an option for cure of basal cell carcinoma, it is not a possibility in this patient whose tumor is unresectable. Basal cell carcinoma does not typically respond to systemic chemotherapy hence chemotherapy treatment is not indicated. Although first detected in a familial form of basal cell carcinoma, uncontrolled activity of hedgehog signaling pathway operates in approximately about 90% of sporadic forms of basal cell carcinoma due to an acquired mutation of at least one allele of PTCH1 gene.

Vismodegib is a first-in-class, small molecule inhibitor of smoothened (SMO) that is FDA approved at an oral dose of 150 mg daily for treatment of locally advanced or metastatic basal cell carcinoma. Response rates are described in 43% and 30% of patients with locally advanced and in metastatic setting with progression free survival of about 7.3 months. Common side effects include alopecia, dysgeusia (loss of taste), muscle spasms, fatigue and weight loss with serious side effects occurring in up-to 25% of patients. Sonidegib is second-in-class hedgehog inhibitor agent approved by the FDA at an oral dose of 200 mg/day for locally advanced or metastatic basal cell carcinoma. This patient who is not a candidate for surgical treatment would benefit from one of the two FDA approved agents and will need to be closely monitored for compliance and side effects associated with this agent.

REFERENCES:

Sekulic A et al. Efficacy and safety of Vismodegib in advanced basal-cell carcinoma. *N Engl J Med.* 2012;366(23):2171–2179.

Lear JT et al. Long-term efficacy and safety of Sonidegib in patients with locally advanced metastatic basal cell carcinoma: 30-month analysis of the randomized phase 2 BOLT study. *J Eur Acad Dermatol Venereol.* 2017; doi: 10.1111/jdv. 14542. [Epub ahead of print]

8. ANSWER: C

Rationale:

Merkel cell carcinoma is a very aggressive tumor caused by a Polyoma virus in more than 90% of cases. Patients with disseminated tumor have poor survival with traditional treatments that included multiple chemotherapeutic combinations. Although cisplatin plus etoposide combination result in high response rates in upto 50% to 60% of patients diagnosed with metastatic Merkel cell carcinoma, rapid tumor recurrences result in lack of survival benefit (median survival 8 to 10 months). Based on findings in tumor tissues of inflammatory footprints caused by tumor infiltrating lymphocytes as well as expression by tumor of PD-1L, PD-1/PDL-1 pathway has been studied as an important target for patients diagnosed with metastatic Merkel cell carcinoma. Avelumab is a first in class anti PD-1L antibody approved by the FDA in patients diagnosed with metastatic Merkel cell carcinoma administered intravenously every 2 weeks at 10 mg/kg dose. In a phase II study of patients diagnosed with metastatic Merkel cell carcinoma relapsed after previous chemotherapy, Avelumab, monoclonal antibody to PD-L1 was used at 10mg/Kg every 2 weeks. Results showed a response rate of 33% that included a complete response rate of 11.4% with more than 74% patients projected to have durable response at one year. The toxicities include autoimmune side effects such as diarrhea, skin rash, hepatitis and pneumonitis while infusional reactions were noted in about 0.2% patients.

REFERENCE:

Nghiem PT et al. PD-1 blockade with Pembrolizumab in advanced Merkel-cell carcinoma. *N Engl J Med.* 2016;374(26):2542–2552.

9. ANSWER: D

Rationale:

Although highly cured following surgical treatment, cutaneous squamous cell carcinoma rarely disseminate in advanced age patients believed to be due to weakened and dysfunctional immune function associated with aging. The prognosis is generally poor since tumor do not respond effectively to systemic chemotherapy agents or epidermal factor receptor antagonists while significant toxicities are limiting factors. Preliminary results of phase I clinical trials with anti PD-1 agents report encouraging durable responses in close to 50% patients. This 87 year old male has a performance status of 1 and appear to be eligible for clinical trial containing immune checkpoint inhibitor treatment.

REFERENCES:

Stevenson ML et al. Expression of Programmed Cell Death Ligand in Cutaneous Squamous Cell Carcinoma and Treatment of Locally Advanced Disease with Pembrolizumab. *JAMA Dermatol.* 2017 1:299-303. doi: 10.1001/jamadermatol.2016.5118.

Falchook GS et al. J Responses of metastatic basal cell and cutaneous squamous cell carcinomas to anti-PD1 monoclonal antibody REGN2810.*Immunother Cancer.* 2016; 15;4:70. doi: 10.1186/s40425-016-0176-3. eCollection 2016.

10. ANSWER: D

Rationale:

The patient has locally advanced disease in the lower extremity that is not surgically resectable (stage IV, M1a). Although systemic treatment with a single agent immune checkpoint inhibitor is a reasonable option, patient is concerned of autoimmune toxicities. The chance of severe autoimmune toxicity is much higher with combined immune checkpoint inhibitor treatment. Talimogene laherparepvec (T-VEC) is a first in class FDA-approved oncolytic virus for intra-tumoral injection of melanoma that contains a modified type I herpes simplex virus (HSV) designed to selectively enter and replicate in tumor cells causing tumor cell lysis and release of tumor epitope in the immediate tumor microenvironment. The expression by the herpes virus of GM-CSF gene promotes local inflammation and facilitates tumor presentation to the immune system as well as antimelanoma activity. In a phase III clinical trial of injecting T-VEC in directly in patient's tumors diagnosed with unresectable stage IIIB, IIIC, and IV M1a, clinical benefit was seen with most pronounced responses recorded in treatment naïve patients (response rate 26.4%, complete response rate 10.8%) with durable responses seen in 16.3% of patients compared to GM-CSF alone. The treatment is well tolerated and has minor side effects of flu like symptoms such as chills, fever, fatigue, nausea and injection site redness and pain. Phase I studies of T-VEC and anti PD-1 agent pembrolizumab show improved outcomes associated with T-VEC induced intra-tumoral CD8 T cell infiltration. External radiation therapy is less likely to be successful since melanoma is not very sensitive to radiation therapy. Isolated limb infusion is an alternative treatment that is more invasive and requires treatment center experienced to perform this procedure. Isolated lime infusion does confer local control of disease with no impact on overall survival.

REFERENCES:

Andtbacka RH et al. Talimogene Laherparepvec improves durable response rate in patients with advanced melanoma. *J Clin Oncol.* 2015;33:2780–2788.

Ribas A et al. Oncolytic Virotherapy Promotes Intratumoral T Cell Infiltration and Improves Anti-PD-1 *Immunotherapy.* Cell. 2017;170:1109–1119.e10. doi: 10.1016/j.cell.2017.08.027

Acute Leukemia 23

Aaron T. Gerds and Mikkael A. Sekeres

REVIEW QUESTIONS

1. A 32-year-old female presents with bruising, fatigue, and persistent fevers for 2 weeks. Her WBC is 2,700, hemoglobin is 6.4, and platelets count is 16. Her fibrinogen is <70 and PT is elevated at 22 (INR 2.2). What is the most appropriate next step in the management of this patient?

   A. Hydration and allopurinol

   B. Urgent bone marrow biopsy and aspiration

   C. Treatment with idarubicin or daunorubicin

   D. Initiation of ATRA

2. On reviewing a smear of her peripheral blood reveals blasts with numerous red to purple cytoplasmic granules that are darker and larger than normal neutrophil granules. Matchstick cells with numerous Auer rods were present as well. Flow cytometry revealed a blast cell population positive for CD117, 13/33, and MPO and negative for CD34 and HLA-DR. Which of the following cytogenetic abnormalities would confirm the diagnosis of APL?

   A. t(9;22)

   B. inv(16)

   C. t(15;16)

   D. t(8;14)

3. Cytogenetic testing and a bone marrow biopsy has confirmed the diagnosis of AML in this patient. What agent should be added to the ATRA as part of her treatment?

    A. Vincristine

    B. Arsenic trioxide

    C. Blinatumomab

    D. Corticosteroids

4. Eight days after starting treatment, her leukocyte count increases to 18,000,000. She also develops shortness of breath, swelling, and diffuse musculoskeletal pain. She is afebrile. Physical examination shows 2+ lower extremity edema. Auscultation of the lungs discloses bilateral basilar crackles. Initiation of which of the following is the most appropriate next step?

    A. Intravenous cryoprecipitate one unit over 15 minutes

    B. Amiodarone 50 mg/hr of continuous infusion

    C. Intravenous tocilizumab 4 mg/kg over one hour

    D. Intravenous dexamethasone 10 mg every 12 hours

5. A 62-year-old male was found to have pancytopenia on routine blood counts obtained by his primary care physician. A subsequent bone marrow biopsy confirms the diagnosis of acute myeloid leukemia (AML).

    He has a 45 pack-year history of smoking, and has been intermittently on steroids for diagnosis of asthma. 5 years ago, he was diagnosed with chronic lymphocytic leukemia and treated with bendamustine and rituximab. Exposure to which of the following is most likely related to the development of AML in this patient?

    A. Corticosteroids

    B. Cigarette smoke

    C. Alkylating agent

    D. Monoclonal antibody

6. A 51-year-old man is newly diagnosed with AML with cytogenetics revealing a translocation (8;21). He has no other significant comorbidities and has a good performance status. What would be the most appropriate course of therapy for this patient?

A. Induction chemotherapy followed by four cycles of low-dose cytarabine therapy

B. Induction chemotherapy followed by four cycles of high-dose cytarabine (HiDAC) therapy

C. Induction chemotherapy followed by autologous hematopoietic cell transplant

D. Induction chemotherapy followed by allogeneic hematopoietic cell transplant

7. A 59-year-old man is diagnosed with precursor B-cell ALL. He is found to be CD19 positive and CD20 negative. Cytogenetic analysis reveals t(9;22) resulting in a BCR-ABL fusion gene. What targeted therapy should be added to his chemotherapeutic plan?

   A. Rituximab

   B. Imatinib

   C. Alemtuzumab

   D. Ofatumumab

8. A 65-year-old woman presents to the emergency room with a 4-wek history of increasing fatigue and dyspnea on exertion. She also has a 2-week history of easy bruising. Her WBC is 45,600, hemoglobin is 6.4, and platelets count is 16. Review of her peripheral blood smear reveals 31% blasts.

   Initial management of acute leukemia in this patient includes which of the following?

   A. IV fluid hydration, allopurinol, and blood product transfusion

   B. Allopurinol, cyclophosphamide, and leukapheresis

   C. High-dose corticosteroids and allopurinol

   D. Infusional cytarabine, anthracycline, and allopurinol

9. The patient is found to have lethargy and elevated creatinine and lower extremity edema concerning for tumor lysis syndrome (TLS). Which of the following lab abnormalities would be consistent with TLS?

   A. Increased uric acid level

   B. Increased calcium level

C. Decreased phosphorous level

D. Decreased lactate dehydrogenase level

---

10. A 24-year-old man presents with a two-week history of fever, fatigue, and mild cervical lymphadenopathy. A peripheral blood sample was drawn, and he was found to have a white blood cell count of 16,000, absolute neutrophil count of 570, hemoglobin of 10.5, and a platelet count 76,000.

    Review of his peripheral blood and bone marrow aspirate reveals the presence of 54% blasts. Immunophenotyping of these cells by flow cytometry notes the expression of CD19, CD20 (subset), CD10, CD34, HLA-DR, sCD22, cCD22, CD38, and TdT and absence of surface and cytoplasmic IgM. Florescence in situ hybridization (FISH) identified a t(9;22) translocation.

    He was treated with a multidrug chemotherapy regimen and by day 28 achieves a complete remission. He does not have any living siblings. Which of the following is most appropriate treatment course after starting consolidation chemotherapy?

    A. At least 2 years of maintenance combination chemotherapy after completion of consolidation chemotherapy

    B. At least 2 years of maintenance rituximab after completion of consolidation chemotherapy

    C. Autologous hematopoietic cell transplantation after a single cycle of consolidation chemotherapy

    D. Allogeneic hematopoietic cell transplantation once an unrelated or alternative donor is identified

---

11. A 37-year-old female with relapsed acute lymphoblastic leukemia was given oral dexamethasone daily for the 2 days prior to hospital admission for blinatumomab. On day 3 of blinatumomab infusion, she developed fever, hypoxia requiring 4 LPM of oxygen via nasal cannula, diffuse pulmonary infiltrates on chest x-ray, hypotension, and is transferred from the regular medical floor to the intensive care unit. Blinatumomab is interrupted, IV fluids are given, and 5 hours later, his fever, hypoxia, and hypotension resolve. Which of the following is most appropriate time to restart blinatumomab?

    A. Restart blinatumomab now

    B. After premedication with tocilizumab

C. After premedication with dexamethasone

D. 24 hours after reaction began

---

12. A 32-year-old male presents with relapsed leukemia 17 months after completing a multidrug chemotherapy regimen. Immunophenotyping of the leukemic blast cells by flow cytometry notes the expression of CD2, cytoplasmic CD3, CD5, CD7, CD10 (subset), and CD38. What is the most appropriate agent to incorporate in the next line of treatment?

    A. Blinatumomab

    B. Rituximab

    C. Nelarabine

    D. Dasatinib

---

13. A 55-year-old man comes for evaluation of a one-month history of increasing fatigue and a two-week history of night sweats, fever, and lymphadenopathy. Analysis of the peripheral blood and bone marrow aspirate reveals the presence of 34% blasts positive for CD19, CD20, CD10, CD34, CD22, CD38, and TdT. Mutation analysis for BCR-ABL1 is negative. Addition of which of the following immunotherapies is most likely to improve overall survival in this patient?

    A. Blinatumomab

    B. Rituximab

    C. Brentuximab

    D. Alemtuzumab

---

14. A 55-year-old man comes for evaluation of a one-month history of increasing fatigue and a two-week history of night sweats, fever, and lymphadenopathy. Analysis of the peripheral blood and bone marrow aspirate reveals the presence of 34% blasts positive for CD19, CD20, CD10, CD34, CD22, CD38, and TdT. Mutation analysis for BCR-ABL1 is negative. Addition of which of the following immunotherapies is most likely to improve overall survival in this patient?

    A. Blinatumomab

    B. Rituximab

C. Brentuximab

D. Alemtuzumab

15. A 43-year-old man presents with a 3-week history of fatigue and abdominal pain. He is found to have splenomegaly on exam. Routine blood work reveals a white count of 68,000, hemoglobin of 8.9, and platelet count of 84. On a peripheral blood smear, 52% blasts, some with Auer rods, are identified. A subsequent bone marrow biopsy confirms the presence of AML. Metaphase cytogenetics reveal a normal male karyotype, but molecular testing reveals the presence of a FLT3-TKD mutation. Addition of which of the following immunotherapies is most likely to improve overall survival in this patient?

   A. Imatinib

   B. Ruxolitinib

   C. Dasatinib

   D. Midostaurin

ANSWERS TO REVIEW QUESTIONS

1. ANSWER: D

Rationale:

This patient has a very high suspicion of acute promyelocytic leukemia (APL) considering she is young, female, and appears to have disseminated intravascular coagulopathy (DIC). This is an oncologic emergency and ATRA therapy should be started as soon as APL is suspected. APL is a very curable disease, but unfortunately 10% of patients die early in the treatment course, typically from DIC and bleeding complications. Hydration and allopurinol are part of the initial therapy of acute leukemias, but are not the most important aspect for this patient. A bone marrow examination and cytogenetics will need to be performed, but ATRA therapy should be started regardless.

REFERENCE:

Abedin S, Altman JK. Acute promyelocytic leukemia: preventing early complications and late toxicities. *Hematology Am Soc Hematol Educ Prog.* 2016 Dec 2;2016(1):10–15.

2. ANSWER: C

Rationale:

The t(15;17) represents a translocation between the PML and RAR-alpha genes. The t(9;22) is typical for BCR-ABL, seen in chronic myeloid leukemia, while Inv 16 is associated with myelomonocytic leukemia. The t(8;14) involves the *myc* gene, seen in Burkitt's lymphoma.

REFERENCE:

Abedin S, Altman JK. Acute promyelocytic leukemia: preventing early complications and late toxicities. *Hematology Am Soc Hematol Educ Prog.* 2016 Dec 2;2016(1):10–15.

3. ANSWER: B

Rationale:

Arsenic trioxide (ATO) has been incorporated into up-front and postremission treatment strategies in APL, in which it has demonstrated a survival advantage over regimens excluding arsenic. The other agents are all used in regimens for ALL treatment.

REFERENCE:

Lo-Coco F, Cicconi L, Breccia M. Current standard treatment of adult acute promyelocytic leukaemia. *Br J Haematol.* 2016 Mar;172(6):841–854.

4. ANSWER: B

Rationale:

This patient has developed a potentially fatal complication of treatment, differentiation (retinoic acid) syndrome. It occurs in 25% of patients with APL during induction therapy with ATRA or arsenic trioxide. The mainstay of treatment is corticosteroids. Without treatment, mortality rates are high as 30%, principally from hypoxemic respiratory failure or from brain edema. With treatment, most patients improve within 12 hours and complete resolution of symptoms within 24 hours. Tocilizumab is used for severe cytokine release syndrome after blinatumomab or CAR T-cell therapy. Cryoprecipitate is used for patients with coagulopathies associated with APL. This patient does not have trial fibrillation; therefore, amiodarone would not be used.

REFERENCE:

Abedin S, Altman JK. Acute promyelocytic leukemia: preventing early complications and late toxicities. *Hematology Am Soc Hematol Educ Prog.* 2016 Dec 2;2016(1):10–15.

5. ANSWER: C

Rationale:

Alkylating agents can lead to AML development on average 5 to 7 years following exposure. Steroids are not associated with therapy-related AML. While cigarette smoking can increase the risk of AML slightly, it is not associated with t-AML. Monoclonal antibodies have no known association with AML.

REFERENCE:

Heuser M. Therapy-related myeloid neoplasms: does knowing the origin help to guide treatment? *Hematology Am Soc Hematol Educ Prog.* 2016 Dec 2;2016(1):24–32.

6. ANSWER: B

Rationale:

Patients with t(8;21) or inv(16) have a favorable prognosis and benefit most from HDAC consolidation. These patients do not seem to benefit from autologous or allogeneic transplant in first remission.

REFERENCE:

Lynch RC, Medeiros BC. Chemotherapy options for previously untreated acute myeloid leukemia. *Expert Opin Pharmacother.* 2015;16(14):2149–2162.

7. ANSWER: B

Rationale:

Approximately 25% to 30% of patients with ALL will have t(9;22). These patients are considered a very poor prognostic group. The addition of imatinib or second-generation tyrosine kinase inhibitor to standard ALL treatment regimens has been shown to be well tolerated with profound improvements in remission rates and survival. Rituximab and ofatumumab would not benefit this patient considering his disease does not express CD20. There are very limited data on the use of Alemtuzumab in patients will ALL.

REFERENCE:

Fielding AK, et al. UKALLXII/ECOG2993: addition of imatinib to a standard treatment regimen enhances long-term outcomes in Philadelphia positive acute lymphoblastic leukemia. *Blood.* 2014

Feb;123(6):843–850; Rousselot P, et al. Dasatinib and low-intensity chemotherapy in elderly patients with Philadelphia chromosome-positive ALL. *Blood*. 2016 Aug;128(6):774–782; Kim DY, et al. Nilotinib combined with multiagent chemotherapy for newly diagnosed Philadelphia-positive acute lymphoblastic leukemia. *Blood*. 2015 Aug;126(6):746–756.

8. ANSWER: A

Rationale:

IV fluid hydration, allopurinol, and blood product transfusion should be instituted upon presentation of a patient with either AML or ALL. Hydration can lessen the effects of leukostasis and tumor lysis syndrome, and allopurinol mitigates uric acid buildup from tumor lysis syndrome. Blood products are used to lessen bleeding risk or end-organ complications in patients with thrombocytopenia or anemia.

REFERENCE:

O'Donnell MR, et al. Acute myeloid leukemia, version 2.2013. *J Natl Compr Canc Netw*. 2013 Sep 1;11(9):1047–1055.

9. ANSWER: A

Rationale:

Tumor lysis syndrome is defined by elevated uric acid, decreased calcium, and increased phosphorous levels. Potassium can be either increased or decreased, and although not diagnostic LDH levels are commonly elevated indicating increased cellular turnover.

REFERENCE:

Coiffier B, et al. Guidelines for the management of pediatric and adult tumor lysis syndrome: an evidence-based review. *J Clin Oncol*. 2008; 26:2767.

10. ANSWER: D

Rationale:

This patient had newly diagnosed ALL. The presence of a *BCR-ABL* translocation indicates high-risk disease and is unlikely to be cured with chemotherapy alone, even with the addition of a tyrosine kinase inhibitor (i.e., imatinib). Therefore, in the setting of a complete remission, this patient should have HLA-typing completed and be considered for an allogeneic transplantation.

REFERENCE:

Marks DI, Alonso L, Radia R. Allogeneic hematopoietic cell transplantation in adult patients with acute lymphoblastic leukemia. *Hematol Oncol Clin North Am*. 2014 Dec;28(6):995–1009.

11. ANSWER: C

Rationale:

This patient had cytokine release syndrome. Patients are hospitalized around the time of infusion initiation to monitor for cytokine release syndrome and neurologic toxicity. Potential neurologic events include encephalopathy, convulsions, speech disorders, disturbances in consciousness, delirium, and coordination and balance issues. Other common toxicities include pyrexia, fatigue, headache, tremor, and leukopenia. Since the interruption was brief and the patient responded to symptomatic treatment of the cytokine release syndrome, it would be a grade 2 reaction. Therefore, repeating premedication with dexamethasone and restarting blinatumomab is the most appropriate next step. Tocilizumab is reserved for grade 3 or 4 cytokine release syndrome.

REFERENCE:

Topp MS., et al. Safety and activity of blinatumomab for adult patients with relapsed or refractory B-precursor acute lymphoblastic leukaemia: a multicentre, single-arm, phase 2 study. *Lancet Oncol.* 2015 Jan;16(1):57–66.

12. ANSWER: C

Rationale:

This patient has T-cell ALL by immunophenotyping. The leukemic blasts do not express CD19 or CD20, the targets for blinatumomab and rituximab. This patient's ALL does not harbor the *BCR-ABL* translocation, therefore dasatinib would be ineffective. Nelarabine, a prodrug converted in vivo to ara-GTP especially in T cells, has shown efficacy as a single agent relapsed T-cell ALL. Complete response rates of 20% to 35% have permitted some patients to go on to subsequent allogeneic hematopoietic cell transplantation.

REFERENCE:

Cohen MH, et al. Approval summary: nelarabine for the treatment of T-cell lymphoblastic leukemia/lymphoma. *Clin Cancer Res.* 2006;12(18):5329.

13. ANSWER: B

Rationale:

Rituximab, when added to chemotherapy for upfront treatment of B-cell ALL, improves overall survival in patients <60 years old. The patient's leukemia cells do not express CD30, the target for brentuximab. Blinatumomab and alemtuzumab have not been used in the first-line treatment of B-cell ALL.

REFERENCE:

Thomas DA et al. Chemoimmunotherapy with a modified hyper-CVAD and rituximab regimen improves outcome in de novo Philadelphia chromosome-negative precursor B-lineage acute lymphoblastic leukemia. *J Clin Oncol.* 2010;28(24):3880.

14. ANSWER: B

Rationale:

Rituximab, when added to chemotherapy for upfront treatment of B-cell ALL, improves overall survival in patients <60 years old. The patient's leukemia cells do not express CD30, the target for brentuximab. Blinatumomab and alemtuzumab have not be used in the first-line treatment of B-cell ALL.

REFERENCE:

Thomas DA et al. Chemoimmunotherapy with a modified hyper-CVAD and rituximab regimen improves outcome in de novo Philadelphia chromosome-negative precursor B-lineage acute lymphoblastic leukemia. *J Clin Oncol.* 2010;28(24):3880.

15. ANSWER: D

Rationale:

The FLT3 inhibitor, midostaurin, improves overall survival in patients <60 years old when added to anthracycline and infusional cytarabine (7+3) induction chemotherapy for upfront treatment of FLT3-mutated AML. This is irrespective of whether the leukemia cells harbor a FLT3-ITD or FLT3-TKD mutation, and variant allelic frequency of the mutation.

REFERENCE:

Pratz KW, Levis M., How I treat FLT3-mutated AML. *Blood.* 2017 Feb 2; 129(5): 565–571.

Chronic Lymphoid Leukemias **24**

Neel Trivedi and Chaitra Ujjani

REVIEW QUESTIONS

1. An 83-year-old gentleman presents to the emergency department at the direction of his primary care physician who noted abnormalities in his blood work on routine evaluation. He denies any fever, night sweats, infections, fatigue, or bleeding. His labs are notable for a hemoglobin of 10 g/dL, platelet count of $120 \times 10^3/\text{mm}^3$, and white blood cell count of $50 \times 10^3/\text{mm}^3$ with 60% lymphocytes. His chemistry profile is normal, and his peripheral smear is notable for several small mature lymphocytes and scattered smudge cells. You suspect a diagnosis of CLL. Which of the following characteristics are associated with a favorable prognosis?

    A. Expression of CD38

    B. Unmutated immunoglobulin variable region heavy chain

    C. NOTCH1 mutation

    D. Del 13q

2. A 55-year-old female with Rai stage I CLL whom you have been following with a watch and wait strategy for 2 years presents for follow-up with complaints of increasing fatigue over the past month. She has no other medical problems and her vital signs are normal. She denies bleeding and has no evidence of bruising or hematomas on examination. Her labs are notable for a hemoglobin of 7 g/dL, platelet count of $140 \times 10^3/\text{mm}^3$, and white blood cell count of $75 \times 10^3/\text{mm}^3$ with 50% lymphocytes. Her chemistry profile is normal except for an elevated indirect bilirubin and a

mild increase in the LDH. What is the most appropriate treatment for this patient at this time?

A. Transfusion of packed red blood cells

B. Fludarabine-based chemotherapy regimen

C. Corticosteroid therapy

D. Single-agent rituximab

3. A 77-year-old male nursing home resident with a history of moderate COPD, osteoarthritis, and diabetes mellitus 2 presents to your office with one month of fatigue, night sweats, and easy bruising. His spleen is palpable at 4 cm below the costal margin. A complete blood count shows a hemoglobin of 6.5 g/dL, platelet count of $60 \times 10^3/mm^3$, and white blood cell count of $144 \times 10^3/mm^3$ with 50% lymphocytes. Flow cytometry of the peripheral blood is consistent with CLL. He is lacking any cytogenetic abnormalities. Which of the following treatments would not be appropriate for this patient?

A. Fludarabine, cyclophosphamide, and rituximab

B. Ibrutinib

C. Bendamustine and rituximab

D. Chlorambucil and obinutuzumab

4. A 75-year-old man with a history of CLL presents for routine follow-up and is noted to have a new lymphocytosis of 95k from 11k three months prior and a new anemia with a hemoglobin of 9. He was previously treated with bendamustine and rituximab 5 years prior and achieved a complete remission. Given the relapse, fluorescence in situ hybridization (FISH) is ordered and you find that he has acquired del 17p. Which of the following is the best treatment for this patient?

A. Bendamustine and rituximab

B. Ofatumumab and chlorambucil

C. No treatment required, follow-up in 6 months

D. Venetoclax

5. A 55-year-old woman you successfully treated for CLL 1 year ago with fludarabine, cyclophosphamide, and rituximab returns to clinic after developing petechiae on her arms and legs. She also notes easy bruising for the past few weeks. A complete blood count shows a platelet count of 40×10^3/mm and a white blood cell count of 123×10^3/mm^3, consistent with relapsed disease. Her past medical history includes a mechanical heart valve, coronary artery disease, hypertension, and stroke. Her current medications include aspirin, warfarin, atorvastatin, metoprolol, and lisinopril. She is allergic to penicillins and sulfa drugs. On exam she has some splenomegaly but no palpable lymph nodes. Which of the following regimens is the most appropriate treatment for this patient's relapsed CLL?

   A. Fludarabine, cyclophosphamide, and rituximab

   B. Idelalisib and rituximab

   C. Ibrutinib

   D. Bendamustine and rituximab

ANSWERS TO REVIEW QUESTIONS

1. ANSWER: D. Del 13q is the most common cytogenetic abnormality in CLL, occurring in 50% of cases either alone or in combination with other genetic mutations. Patients who have del 13q as their only abnormality have a more favorable prognosis. Their disease follows a more indolent course and their survival is similar to age-matched controls. Mutation of NOTCH1, the expression of CD38 and unmutated IgVH are associated with a poorer prognosis. They are associated with a higher risk of relapse and inferior overall survival.

2. ANSWER: C. This patient most likely has AIHA, a known hematologic complication of CLL. Further evaluation may be notable for spherocytes on peripheral blood smear and a positive direct antiglobulin test, but neither is always present with AIHA. Other labs suggestive of hemolysis include an elevated indirect bilirubin, elevated LDH, and a low haptoglobin. Prednisone dosed at 1 mg/kg/day is the typical initial therapy for AIHA. Improvement in hemoglobin can be seen within a couple of weeks. Prednisone should be tapered off slowly once the hemoglobin and hemolysis labs normalize. This patient is hemodynamically stable with no history of cardiovascular disease, so a blood transfusion is not necessary at this time. Chemotherapy would only be indicated in this patient if corticosteroids were unsuccessful in controlling her AIHA. If corticosteroids were unsuccessful, fludarabine would not be the treatment of choice as it can potentiate AIHA. A bendamustine-based regimen would be more appropriate. Although rituximab can be used for AIHA, it is not typically used as a front-line option in part because of its cost relative to steroids.

3. ANSWER: A. This is an elderly patient with multiple comorbidities and poor performance status. He is symptomatic from CLL and requires treatment. While FCR has been shown to be an effective first-line therapy, it is poorly tolerated in elderly patients and/or those with significant comorbidities due to severe infections and cytopenias. Ibrutinib, BR, and Chl-Ob have been demonstrated to be well-tolerated in elderly patients.

4. ANSWER: D. This patient has relapsed CLL with a newly acquired mutation: del 17p. Patients with del 17p do not respond well to chemoimmunotherapy like BR and ofatumumab plus chlorambucil (choices A and B). A number of targeted therapies are approved for relapsed CLL and have shown to be effective for patients with del 17p including venetoclax (choice D), ibrutinib, and idelalisib. C is not correct because this patient is symptomatic and requires treatment.

5. ANSWER: B. This patient relapsed within one year of receiving FCR for her disease. She also has significant comorbidities including hypertension and a mechanical heart valve, which necessitates anticoagulation with warfarin. Ibrutinib and idelalisib are valuable options for patients with relapsed CLL who have failed chemoimmunotherapy. Ibrutinib is associated with hypertension and an increased risk of bleeding so the idelalisib and rituximab would be more appropriate (choice B).

Chronic Myeloid Leukemias 25

Samer A. Srour and Muzaffar H. Qazilbash

REVIEW QUESTIONS

1. A 37-year-old Hispanic gentleman presents to his physician with 25 lb weight loss, profound fatigue, and lower extremity edema. Initial laboratory studies showed a white blood cell count of 150 K/μL with normal hemoglobin and platelet count. Physical examination was notable for splenomegaly. He was started on hydroxyurea for cytoreduction. Bone marrow biopsy findings were consistent with chronic myeloid leukemia in chronic phase with no increased blasts. Cytogenetics confirmed Ph chromosome in 10/20 metaphases. BCR-ABL1 quantitative PCR was 32.12%. Patient was started on imatinib 400 mg PO daily. After 6 months of therapy, he had complete hematologic response and BCR-ABL1 by PCR decreased to 14.3%. Repeat bone marrow biopsy cytogenetics showed trisomy 8 in a Ph-negative clone in 10/20 metaphases and Ph chromosome in 10/20 metaphases. Mutation analysis revealed a new T315I mutation. What is the appropriate next step in management?

    A. Switch to dasatinib or nilotinib and repeat BCR-ABL1 quantitative PCR in 3 months.

    B. Switch to ponatinib, monitor with BCR-ABL1 quantitative PCR in 3 months, and repeat bone marrow biopsy at 9 months.

    C. Induction chemotherapy with or without second-generation tyrosine kinase inhibitor and check for potential donors in order to proceed to allogeneic stem cell transplant.

    D. Switch to ponatinib, continue monitoring with BCR-ABL1 quantitative PCR, and check for potential donors to proceed to allogeneic stem cell transplant.

2. A 65-year-old female patient with a diagnosis of chronic myeloid leukemia in chronic phase presents for her regular follow-up after 9 months of treatment with imatinib. She has achieved complete hematologic and cytogenetic response, and had major molecular response. However, she is poorly tolerating imatinib with refractory nausea and recurrent muscle cramps. Patient has a significant history of uncontrolled diabetes and severe peripheral artery disease. Which of the following is considered the best alternative treatment?

    A. Switch to a second generation tyrosine kinase inhibitor, and send HLA typing for patient and siblings, and refer for allogeneic stem cell transplant.

    B. Switch to Dasatinib 100 mg daily and continue BCR-ABL1 monitoring by PCR every 3 months.

    C. Switch to Nilotinib 300 mg twice a day and continue BCR-ABL1 monitoring by PCR every 3 months.

    D. Switch to Omacetaxine, sent for HLA typing for patient and siblings, and consider allogeneic stem cell transplant.

3. A 56-year-old male patient, previously healthy, presents with fatigue, early satiety, and weight loss. Initial workup showed elevated white blood cells at 42 K/µL, hemoglobin of 10 g/dL, and platelets of 110×10^9/L. Peripheral blood smear showed 70% neutrophils along with increased number of basophils (10%), eosinophils, myelocytes, metamyelocytes, and 3% blasts. Exam was unremarkable. Bone marrow biopsy showed 8% blasts and cytogenetics confirmed the presence of Philadelphia chromosome.

   What is an acceptable initial treatment for this patient?

    A. Imatinib, dasatinib, or nilotinib and monitor BCR-ABL1 by PCR every 3 months.

    B. Cytotoxic chemotherapy with or without dasatinib or nilotinib, and monitor BCR-ABL1 by PCR every 3 months.

    C. Bosutinib 500 mg PO daily and monitor BCR-ABL1 by PCR every 3 months.

    D. Ponatinib 30 mg daily and monitor BCR-ABL1 by PCR every 3 months.

4. A 53-year-old male patient who was previously healthy presents with fatigue, early satiety, and weight loss. Initial workup showed elevated white blood cells at 70 K/µL, hemoglobin of 10 g/dL, and platelets of 94 x 10^9/L. Peripheral blood smear showed 60% neutrophils along with increased number of basophils (22%), eosinophils, myelocytes, metamyelocytes, and 2% blasts. Exam was significant for splenomegaly. BCR-ABL1 fusion transcript was detected on peripheral blood fluorescence in situ hybridization. Bone marrow biopsy showed 11% blasts. What is the best treatment approach for this patient?

   A. Induction chemotherapy and HLA typing for patient and siblings.

   B. Imatinib, dasatinib, or nilotinib with or without cytotoxic chemotherapy and monitor BCR-ABL1 by PCR every 3 months.

   C. Dasatinib or nilotinib and consider referral for allogeneic stem cell transplant evaluation.

   D. Ponatinib 45 mg daily and monitor BCR-ABL1 by PCR every 3 months.

ANSWERS TO REVIEW QUESTIONS

1. ANSWER: D. The patient is considered a failure to first-line tyrosine kinase inhibitor (BCR-ABL1 by PCR >10%). In addition, he had no cytogenetic response, developed positive clonal evolution (a criterion for progression to accelerated phase), and has acquired T315I mutation. Cytogenetic clonal evolution and T315I portend for a poor prognosis, and therefore allogeneic stem cell transplantation should be considered. Due to his T315I mutation, ponatinib is the drug of choice. Neither dasatinib nor nilotinib is effective in patients with T315I mutation. Changing to ponatinib alone would not address his clonal evolution. Omacetaxine, a semisynthetic derivative of homoharringtonine, is an alternative option for patients with T215I mutation. Cytotoxic chemotherapy is considered in patients with advanced stage chronic myeloid leukemia, particularly those in blast phase.

2. ANSWER: B. Although the patient had an excellent response to first-line imatinib, he had significant toxicity. For patients who are intolerant to imatinib as first-line treatment, switching to any other approved tyrosine kinase inhibitor (TKI) in the first-line setting is indicated. Dasatinib is the preferred choice in this particular patient because nilotinib has significant cardiovascular adverse effects, including peripheral arterial occlusive disease (PAOD), and can cause hyperglycemia. Individual patient characteristics and drug safety profiles are important factors to select among the three FDA approved TKIs in the first-line setting (imatinib, dasatinib, and nilotinib). Omacetaxine, a semisynthetic derivative of homoharringtonine, is indicated for patients for failed or are intolerant to two or more TKIs and is an option for patients with T215I mutation.

3. ANSWER: A. The patient has chronic myeloid leukemia in chronic phase (blast cells in blood or marrow <10%, basophils in blood <20%, and platelets >100 × 10^9/L). Therefore, any of the three FDA-approved tyrosine kinase inhibitors (TKI) in the first-line setting (imatinib, dasatinib, and nilotinib) can be used. Individual patient characteristics, cost, and drug safety profiles are important factors to consider for drug selection. Bosutinib is indicated for second line treatment in patients who are resistant or intolerant to other first-generation or second-generation TKIs. Ponatinib is indicated for patients with T315I mutations and/or patients who are intolerant or failed other first-generation and second-generation TKIs.

4. ANSWER: C. The patient has chronic myeloid leukemia (CML) in accelerated phase; three criteria were met in this patient: blast cells in blood or marrow 10% to 19%, basophils in blood >20%, and platelets <100 × 10^9/L. Therefore, any of the second-generation tyrosine kinase inhibitors (TKI), dasatinib or nilotinib, can be used and referral for allogeneic stem cell transplantation is recommended. Allogeneic stem cell transplantation is indicated for selected patients with newly diagnosed accelerated phase CML based on response to TKI therapy and for all patients with disease progression from chronic phase to accelerated phase while on TKI therapy. Cytotoxic induction chemotherapy is indicated for majority of patients who present with lymphoid or myeloid blast phase CML. Ponatinib is indicated for patients with T315I mutations and/or patient who failed other first-generation or second-generation TKIs.

Chronic Myeloproliferative Neoplasms 26

Yogen Saunthararajah

REVIEW QUESTIONS

Mr. Jones is a 47-year-old active Caucasian male seen in the office of the internist Dr. Brown. His main complaint is increasing fatigue. He has noticed a decrease in his exercise tolerance, and a sense of fatigue that has been progressive in the 3 months preceding his visit to the clinic. He enjoys playing soccer, and usually participates in a "40 years and older" pick-up game every Saturday. For the past 2 months, he has not felt like playing.

Upon questioning, he states that he gets winded easily and feels fatigued after physical effort. It takes him longer to recover from effort than ever before. He denies any chest or abdominal pain and he has not had a change in his bowel habit or noticed any change in the color of his stool. His weight has not changed and his appetite remains good. He has not noticed blood in the toilet bowl after bowel movements. He has not experienced any recent colds, and he has not had recent cough, sore throat, fever, body ache, or headache. He denies night sweats, too. He has noticed some blood when rinsing after brushing his teeth, but, has noticed some bruises, although he wonders if these are from his soccer games. He has not had any bleeding from the nose.

He does not have any significant past medical history and initially he denied taking any medications. However, upon specific questioning regarding use of over-the-counter medications including pain medications, he mentions that he does use naproxen occasionally for pain and swelling in the knees after playing soccer. He has not used naproxen for more than 4 weeks.

He is a lawyer for a local law firm and has not had any unusual chemical exposures. He drinks alcohol only occasionally and in small amounts, and has not noticed swelling around the ankles, although his knees do swell after his soccer games, requiring use of postgame ice packs. He did travel to Thailand 5 years ago, had a good time, and was not unwell during or after the trip.

He has two siblings, one of whom was born before the patient, "was deformed at birth," and died as an infant. His other sibling, a brother aged 44, is alive and well without medical problems.

On examination, he is a fit-appearing Caucasian male. Although alert, he does appear fatigued and is pale without icterus. Bruises are noted on his lower extremities. There was no palpable lymphadenopathy. A spleen tip is palpated 12 cm below the left costal margin in the mid-clavicular line. There was no palpable hepatomegaly.

Labs

WBC	10.76	(4–11 K/μL)
RBC	1.82	(4.2–5.4 M/μL)
Hgb	7.3	(12–16 g/dL)
Hct	21	(37–47%)
MCV	105.2	(80–100 fL)
MCHC	34.9	(32–36%)
RDW-CV	12.4	(11.7–15%)
Platelets	70	(150–400 K/μL)
MPV	10.6	(7.3–11.1 fL)

1. What is the diagnosis, or what are the differential diagnoses, for Mr. Jones' condition?

    A. MDS

    B. MF

    C. Post-PV MF

    D. Post-ET MF

    E. All of the above

2. What additional investigations are indicated to establish a definitive diagnosis?

    A. Reticulocyte count and lactate dehydrogenase

    B. Evaluation for *JAK2* V617F mutation

    C. Bone marrow aspirate and biopsy for morphology and karyotype evaluation

    D. FISH studies to detect the *BCR-ABL* fusion

    E. All of the above

3. The *JAK2* V617 test was positive, and the bone marrow evaluation demonstrated an increase in reticulin fibrosis, and an increase in the myeloid: erythroid ratio, without an increase in megakaryocyte numbers. A 20q–chromosome abnormality was detected in 20 of 20 metaphases. Liver and renal function tests were normal. What are appropriate therapies for Mr. Jones?

   A. Allogeneic stem cell transplant

   B. *JAK2* inhibitor

   C. hydroxyurea

   D. Erythropoietin

   E. Iron supplements

ANSWERS TO REVIEW QUESTIONS

1. ANSWER: E. The myeloid neoplasms have overlapping clinical characteristics, because after all, many of the causative mutations can occur in the different categories of MPNs or MDS. Mr. Jones' demographic and constellation of symptoms, signs, and investigation observations thus far: shortness of breath, bruises, splenomegaly, macrocytic anemia, and thrombocytopenia are compatible with any of the above diagnoses. Other less likely differential diagnoses include portal hypertension from liver cirrhosis or portal vein thrombosis, since there were no suggestions of chronic liver disease risk factors, symptoms or signs in the history, and physical examination. Although he has had foreign travel to compel consideration of unusual protozoal illnesses such as malaria during the history and physical examination, this was sufficient to indicate that this diagnosis, or other protozoal illnesses, is highly unlikely. Determining the specific diagnosis, and Mr. Jones' risks for complications, will require further evaluation.

2. ANSWER: E. The reticulocyte count and lactate dehydrogenase are of course routine components in the evaluation of anemia, to better understand if the cause is from decreased production or increased destruction. Although the observations thus far do not place hemolytic anemia high on the differential diagnoses list, these parameters are nonetheless highly valuable baseline measures in the evaluation and management of myeloid malignancies, since they can be followed over time to confirm that the therapy is changing things in the right direction, with decreasing LDH and increasing functional marrow as represented by appropriate reticulocyte count levels for the degree of anemia. The JAK2 V617F mutation is part of the diagnostic criteria for the MPNs, because of its highly recurrent association with these conditions. Bone marrow aspirate for morphologic evaluation and karyotype analysis are invaluable in classifying an MPN and in evaluating risk, a very pertinent consideration in Mr. Jones who is a potential candidate for allogeneic stem cell transplant. Although the clinical picture suggests that chronic myeloid leukemia is a less likely MPN, the treatment implications of this diagnosis are profound, and there is a need to rule out this diagnosis. It can be legitimately argued, however, that the clinical picture of Mr. Jones does not compel urgent evaluation to rule out CML, and that instead of FISH analysis, Dr. Brown can wait for the results of standard metaphase karyotyping of the bone marrow.

3. ANSWER: A. The diagnostic evaluation suggests that the diagnosis is primary MF, although an MDS/MPN overlap neoplasm remains in the differential diagnosis. The clinical features and observations suggest that Mr. Jones is at least in an intermediate risk or even in a high-risk category (e.g., by the DIPSS plus risk classification system) of MF. Furthermore, he is relatively young. Thus, allogeneic stem cell transplant must be considered, and at a minimum, Mr. Jones and his sibling should be HLA typed. His predominant symptom complex relates to anemia, with a possibility also of platelet dysfunction in addition to the thrombocytopenia. Thus, pending evaluation for transplant, management of anemia is indicated, including transfusion if necessary, and consideration for androgens such as danazol. If Mr. Jones does not have a sibling match, and if unrelated donor transplant is not an option, then experimental therapies should be considered; these could include DNMT1-depleting drugs such as decitabine. Although Mr. Jones has splenomegaly, this is asymptomatic, and a JAK2 inhibitor is not indicated. For the same reasons, hydroxyurea is not indicated. Erythropoietin could be considered if erythropoietin levels are inappropriately low (e.g., <200 milliunits/mL). Although it is possible that they are, since levels were not checked, it seems unlikely given Mr. Jones' age and normal renal function tests. Iron supplements would only be indicated if Mr. Jones is iron deficient, again unlikely given the constellation of observations, the MCV, and Mr. Jones' sex. Of course, iron studies should be performed.

Multiple Myeloma 27

Arjun Lakshman and Shaji K. Kumar

REVIEW QUESTIONS

1. A 68-year-old lady is found to have IgA lambda M-spike of 3.1 g/dL on evaluation for lower back pain. Her hemoglobin is 12 g/dL, MCV 87 fL, and platelets $212 \times 10^9/\text{mm}^3$, and serum calcium and creatinine are normal. A skeletal survey reveals no lytic lesions. MRI pelvis and MRI lumbosacral spine are negative for bony deformities, but show a moderate disk bulge at L2 without neural impingement. Her bone marrow biopsy reveals 25% lambda restricted plasma cells. Congo red stain is negative. What is the most likely diagnosis?

   A. Monoclonal gammopathy of uncertain significance

   B. AL amyloidosis

   C. Smoldering multiple myeloma (SMM)

   D. Mutliple myeloma (MM)

2. In patients with newly diagnosed multiple myeloma receiving initial therapy with a combination of bortezomib, lenalidomide, and dexamethasone, addition of autologous stem cell transplant is associated with

   A. No additional benefit

   B. Improved progression-free survival

   C. Improved overall survival

   D. b and c

   E. Need for additional consolidation therapy post-transplant

3. In a meta-analysis of randomized trial of lenalidomide maintenance, all the following patient groups had improved survival with the use of lenalidomide maintenance except

   A. Initial therapy with lenalidomide prior to transplant

   B. Younger patients

   C. Patients with very good partial response or better after stem cell transplant

   D. Patients with high-risk FISH

4. In randomized trials, allogeneic stem cell transplant has been consistently shown to be superior to autologous stem cell transplant in which of the following patients?

   A. Patients with 17p deletion

   B. Younger patients <50 years of age

   C. Patients with high-risk translocations such as t(4;14), t(14;16)

   D. Patients with primary refractory disease

   E. None of the above

ANSWERS TO REVIEW QUESTIONS

1. ANSWER: C. This patient has an M-protein and has >10% plasma cells in the bone marrow in the absence of any end-organ damage. A useful acronym to remember is CRAB—hypercalcemia, renal failure, anemia, and bone lesions. MGUS patients also have no evidence of end-organ damage but have an M-spike <3 g/dL and <10% clonal plasma cells in the bone marrow. Negative congo red staining points against amyloid deposition. This patient does not have MM as she has no evidence of end-organ damage. The correct answer is SMM.

2. ANSWER: B. In the IFM DFCI 2009 study, patients with newly diagnosed multiple myeloma were randomized to receive three cycles of bortezomib, lenalidomide and dexamethasone (VRd) as induction, and ASCT with two more cycles of VRd after transplantation or five additional cycles of VRd. Patients in both arms received R maintenance. The ASCT arm showed better PFS and improvement in depth of response. But, the overall survival was similar in the two groups at 4 years.

3. ANSWER: D

4. ANSWER: E

Non-Hodgkin's Lymphoma 28

Christopher Melani and Mark Roschewski

REVIEW QUESTIONS

1. A 63-year-old previously healthy male is evaluated by his primary care physician for a "lump" in his right neck that was noted during shaving. Evaluation with a CT scan reveals diffuse lymphadenopathy in the neck, chest, abdomen, and pelvis up to 2.5 cm in size. No obvious extranodal masses are appreciated and a diagnosis of lymphoma is strongly suspected. Which of these tests will provide the greatest chance of obtaining a definitive diagnosis of lymphoma?

    A. Fine-needle aspirate of a cervical lymph node

    B. Core-needle biopsy of a cervical lymph node

    C. Excisional biopsy of a cervical lymph node

    D. Bone marrow biopsy and aspiration

2. A 46-year-old female presents to her local emergency room with a 1-month history of progressively worsening abdominal pain associated with a 10 lb. weight loss. CT scan of her abdomen and pelvis reveals bulky mesenteric, iliac, and inguinal lymphadenopathy up to 5 cm in size. Excisional lymph node biopsy of an inguinal lymph node reveals diffuse large B-cell lymphoma. Which of the following tests is **NOT** part of the standard work-up and staging of aggressive non-Hodgkin lymphoma?

    A. CT scan of the chest, abdomen, and pelvis

    B. Whole-body FDG-PET scan

    C. Bone marrow aspirate and biopsy

   D. HIV, HBV, and HCV testing

   E. Contrast-enhanced MRI brain

3. A 52-year-old male presents to his primary care physician with an enlarging left neck mass associated with unexplained fever and drenching night sweats for the past 3 weeks. Excisional lymph node biopsy reveals the diagnosis of diffuse large B-cell lymphoma and appropriate work-up and staging is performed. He is subsequently evaluated by a local oncologist and discusses the prognosis of his aggressive lymphoma. Which of the following factors is **NOT** required to calculate the International Prognostic Index (IPI) for this patient?

   A. Age

   B. ECOG performance status

   C. LDH level

   D. Hemoglobin

   E. Ann Arbor stage

4. Which of the following statements are true concerning chromosomal abnormalities in non-Hodgkin lymphoma?

   A. Burkitt lymphoma is associated with t(8;14), t(2;8), or t(8;22)

   B. Virtually all cases of mantle cell lymphoma harbor t(11;14), leading to overexpression of bcl-2

   C. Cyclin D1 is overexpressed in the majority of follicular lymphoma and is associated with t(14;18)

   D. Patients with anaplastic large cell lymphoma harboring t(2;5) have a worse prognosis than those without this translocation

5. A 70-year-old female with a history of hypertension and hyperlipidemia is evaluated in her local emergency room for a 1-day history of chest pain. As part of her work-up she undergoes a CT chest, which fails to reveal any acute pathology explaining her chest pain but does note bilateral axillary lymph nodes up to 2 cm in size. CT abdomen and pelvis reveals enlarged retroperitoneal and inguinal lymph nodes, which are all less than 3 cm in size and no evidence of splenomegaly. She is found to have a normal CBC

and denies any fevers, drenching night sweats, or weight loss. Excisional lymph node biopsy of one of the axillary lymph nodes reveals grade 1 to 2 follicular lymphoma. Which of the following is the most appropriate therapy for this patient?

    A. Observation ("watchful waiting")

    B. 6 cycles of bendamustine and rituximab

    C. 6 cycles of R-CHOP

    D. 4 weekly doses of rituximab

    E. High-dose chemotherapy with autologous stem cell transplantation

6. A 63-year-old male with a history of Waldenstrom macroglobulinemia presents to clinic to discuss treatment options. He initially presented with a 2-week history of headaches, blurred vision, and bruising consistent with hyperviscosity syndrome and received treatment with plasmapheresis and R-CHOP. He achieved a complete response following therapy but was found to have increasing IgM and worsening cytopenias with worsening symptoms of fatigue 5 years following initial treatment. Recurrent disease is confirmed on bone marrow biopsy and the decision is made to treat the patient with ibrutinib. Which of the following mutational profiles of the patient's lymphoma would be expected to result in the highest response rate to ibrutinib?

    A. MYD88 (WT) and CXCR4 (WT)

    B. MYD88 (L265P) and CXCR4 (WT)

    C. MYD88 (WT) and CXCR4 (WHIM)

    D. MYD88 (L265P) and CXCR4 (WHIM)

7. Which of the following statements is FALSE regarding the molecular biology of DLBCL?

    A. Patients with ABC-DLBCL have inferior PFS and OS compared to those with GCB-DLBCL

    B. The NF-κB pathway is constitutively activated in GCB-DLBCL

    C. PMBL has a molecular signature that is distinct from that of ABC- or GCB-DLBCL

D. PCNSL is typically of DLBCL histology

E. DLBCL cases that harbor both BCL-2 and MYC translocations constitute a highly aggressive subgroup that respond poorly to current therapies

8. A 55-year-old man presents to his primary care physician with progressive fatigue and night sweats. Physical examination reveals cervical and axillary lymphadenopathy, and laboratory analysis is notable for a hemoglobin of 11 g/dL, serum LDH 1.5 × ULN, and normal renal and hepatic function. He is referred for excisional biopsy of an enlarged left cervical lymph node, which reveals DLBCL. Subsequent oncologic staging workup includes a BM aspiration/biopsy, which reveals evidence of large malignant lymphocytes, and a PET/CT scan, which reveals hypermetabolic lymphadenopathy in the neck, axillae, hilum, and retroperitoneum, as well as multiple hypermetabolic lytic foci within nonweight-bearing bones. Serologic testing for chronic hepatitis and HIV are negative. MUGA scan demonstrates normal cardiac function. The patient has an ECOG performance status of 1, but does not wish to be referred for a clinical trial. Which of the following is the most appropriate approach to treating this patient?

   A. R-CHOP-21 for six cycles followed by posttherapy PET/CT scan and BM biopsy

   B. R-CHOP-14 with filgrastim for six cycles followed by posttherapy PET/CT scan and BM biopsy

   C. R-CHOP-21 for six cycles followed by posttherapy CT scan and BM biopsy

   D. R-CHOP-21 for four cycles if PET/CT after cycle 2 demonstrates complete response

   E. R-hyper-CVAD for eight cycles, followed by posttherapy CT scan and BM biopsy

9. A 50-year-old man with symptomatic stage III follicular lymphoma (histologic grade 2) is treated with six cycles of bendamustine and rituximab (BR) and obtains a complete remission. Three years later, he presents with worsening fatigue and frequent drenching night sweats. His examination reveals new anterior cervical and axillary lymphadenopathy and splenomegaly. Laboratory analysis reveals a hemoglobin of 9.5 g/dL, serum LDH

2 × the upper limit of normal, AST, and ALT 2× the upper limit of normal, and normal renal function. CT scan reveals multiple new enlarged cervical lymph nodes (2 cm maximal diameter), a 3 cm right axillary node, a 4 cm right external iliac node, splenomegaly (16 cm craniocaudal), and several enhancing foci within the liver (2 cm maximal diameter). Subsequent PET scan reveals moderate hypermetabolism (SUVs 5 to 10) within the cervical nodes and liver lesions, SUV of 14 within the right external iliac node, and SUV of 21 within the right axillary node. A surveillance CT scan performed 6 months ago revealed no abnormalities. What is the most appropriate next step in the management of this patient?

    A. Initiate salvage therapy for relapsed FL with R-CHOP

    B. Initiate salvage therapy for relapsed FL with ibritumomab tiutexan

    C. Initiate salvage therapy for relapsed FL with BR

    D. Obtain tissue biopsy of the right axillary lymph node

10. A 34-year-old woman presents to her primary care physician with progressive dyspnea on exertion and cough. Physical examination reveals mild facial plethora. Chest x-ray reveals mediastinal widening. Subsequent CT scan of the chest, abdomen, and pelvis is notable for a large mediastinal mass (13 cm in maximal diameter) compressing the SVC, and no other significant findings. Laboratory analysis reveals elevated LDH but is otherwise unremarkable. Tissue biopsy obtained via cervical mediastinoscopy reveals numerous large malignant lymphocytes in a sclerotic background that possess the following immunophenotype: CD20 strong+, CD23+, CD45+, CD79a+, Bcl6+, Mum1+, CD30 weak+, CD15−. What is the most likely diagnosis in this patient?

    A. Hodgkin lymphoma

    B. T-lymphoblastic lymphoma

    C. Primary mediastinal B-cell lymphoma

    D. Small Lymphocytic Lymphoma

    E. Mantle cell lymphoma

11. Epstein-Barr virus (EBV) has been implicated in the pathogenesis of multiple different subtypes of NHL in both immunocompetent and immunocompromised individuals.

    Which of these lymphoma subtypes is **NOT** frequently associated with EBV infection?

    A. PCNSL in immunocompetent individuals

    B. Endemic Burkitt lymphoma

    C. Plasmablastic lymphoma

    D. Primary effusional lymphoma (PEL)

    E. Extranodal NK/T-cell lymphoma, nasal type

    F. Post-transplant lymphoproliferative disorder (PTLD)

12. Marginal zone lymphoma (MZL) is a subtype of NHL that is known to be antigenically driven by both viral and bacterial pathogens. Which of these associations between the infectious pathogen and type of MZL is **INCORRECT**?

    A. *Helicobacter pylori*—gastric MALT lymphoma

    B. *Chlamydia psittaci*—ocular adnexal MALT lymphoma

    C. *Haemophilus influenza*—pulmonary MALT lymphoma

    D. *Campylobacter jejuni*—intestinal MALT lymphoma

    E. Hepatitis C virus (HCV)—splenic MZL

13. A 65-year-old male presents to his primary care physician complaining of worsening left lower quadrant abdominal pain over the past 2 weeks. Physical examination reveals splenomegaly with the spleen tip palpable 10 cm below the costal margin. Laboratory analysis reveals a hemoglobin of 9.0 g/dL and serum LDH 2 × the upper limit of normal. CT scan reveals splenomegaly (22 cm craniocaudal) without systemic lymphadenopathy. Bone marrow biopsy reveals a monoclonal B-cell population that is kappa restricted, expresses both IgM and IgD, and is CD20 positive but negative for CD5, CD10, CD23, CD103, and cyclin D1. HIV antibody, HBsAg, and HBcAb testing are negative but HBsAb, HCV antibody, and HCV PCR are positive. What is the most appropriate first step in the management of this patient?

    A. Observation

    B. Splenectomy

    C. Four doses of weekly rituximab monotherapy

    D. Six cycles of bendamustine and rituximab

    E. Hepatology consult for HCV antiviral treatment

14. A 56-year-old female has an excisional lymph node biopsy for evaluation of progressively enlarging left axillary lymphadenopathy. Pathologic examination of the lymph node reveals diffuse infiltration of the lymph node with large atypical lymphoid cells, which are positive for CD10, CD19, CD20, and Bcl-6 and negative for CD3, CD5, and MUM1. FISH analysis is negative for Myc, Bcl-2, or Bcl-6 rearrangements. Which of the following statements is **INCORRECT** regarding this patient's lymphoma?

    A. The immunophenotype is most consistent with GCB-DLBCL

    B. The outcome of this subtype of DLBCL is superior to its counterpart when treated with conventional chemoimmunotherapy

    C. This subtype of DLBCL frequently harbors mutations in the B-cell receptor (BCR) pathway that leads to chronic active BCR signaling

    D. Myc, Bcl-2, and Bcl-6 rearrangements are more common with this subtype of DLBCL

    E. Novel therapies, such as ibrutinib and lenalidomide, are typically associated with a lower response rate in this subtype of DLBCL

15. A 49-year-old male was evaluated in a local emergency room for a 1-month history of progressive fatigue as well as unexplained fevers and night sweats. Physical examination revealed palpable cervical and inguinal lymphadenopathy up to 2.5 cm in size. CT revealed cervical, mediastinal, retroperitoneal, and inguinal lymphadenopathy up to 4.7 cm in largest diameter in the mediastinum. Excisional lymph node biopsy of an inguinal lymph node revealed PTCL-NOS and the patient was treated with 6 cycles of CHOEP with complete response by PET. Three months following therapy, imaging revealed recurrent diffuse lymphadenopathy in the bilateral neck, axillae, mediastinum, retroperitoneum, pelvis, and inguinal regions. Repeat axillary lymph node biopsy confirmed relapsed disease and he received salvage treatment with ICE followed by high-dose chemotherapy with autologous stem cell rescue. Four months later the patient had recurrent lymphadenopathy on imaging associated with recurrent fatigue and night sweats. Cervical lymph node biopsy confirms

recurrent PTCL-NOS. Which of these novel agents is **NOT** currently approved for the treatment of relapsed/refractory PTCL?

   A. Romidepsin

   B. Belinostat

   C. Lenalidomide

   D. Pralatrexate

16. A 54-year-old female with a long-standing history of GERD with prior EGD showing Barrett's esophagus has been undergoing serial upper endoscopy as screening for the development of esophageal cancer. Her most recent EGD showed new nodularity in the gastric body and biopsy of this region revealed a monoclonal B-cell population that is positive for CD20 and negative for CD5, CD10, Bcl-2, and cyclin D1. *H. pylori* testing is positive and FISH analysis is positive for t(11;18). CT reveals several enlarged perigastic lymph nodes with low level FDG-uptake in both the stomach and perigastric lymph nodes on FDG-PET. Which of these treatments is **LEAST LIKELY** to result in a significant tumor response when used as monotherapy?

   A. Triple-antibiotic therapy

   B. Involved-site radiation therapy

   C. Rituximab

   D. Bendamustine and rituximab

17. An 85-year-old male with a history of mantle cell lymphoma presents to his oncologist's office for a routine follow-up appointment. He was initially diagnosed 5 years ago and received treatment with 6 cycles of bendamustine and rituximab after he was deemed ineligible for high-dose chemotherapy and autologous stem-cell transplant due to his advanced age. He achieved a complete remission following therapy by PET but relapsed 3 years later with enlarging diffuse lymphadenopathy in the neck, mediastinum, retroperitoneum, pelvis, and inguinal regions. After a 2-year period of "watchful waiting," steady progression in his pelvic and inguinal lymphadenopathy was observed, up to 8 cm in maximum diameter, resulting in recurrent left lower extremity swelling and recurrent

cellulitis. Which of these novel agents is **<u>NOT</u>** currently approved for the treatment of relapsed/refractory MCL?

A. Bortezomib

B. Lenalidomide

C. Ibrutinib

D. Idelalisib

ANSWERS TO REVIEW QUESTIONS

1. ANSWER: C. The gold standard for diagnosis of suspected lymphoma involves a properly evaluated and technically adequate excisional lymph node biopsy. Combination of core-needle biopsy and fine-needle aspiration has been utilized as an alternative method of diagnosis but fails to obtain a definitive diagnosis in approximately 20% to 25% of patients. There is a variability in bone marrow involvement at diagnosis between different types of lymphoma as well as issues with sampling error which make this method less likely to obtain a definitive diagnosis.

REFERENCE:

Amador-Ortiz C, Chen L, Hassan A, et al. Combined core needle biopsy and fine-needle aspiration with ancillary studies correlate highly with traditional techniques in the diagnosis of nodal-based lymphoma. *Am J Clinical Pathol.* 2011;135(4):516–524.

2. ANSWER: E. Accurate staging for aggressive non-Hodgkin lymphoma involves CT chest, abdomen, and pelvis, whole-body FDG-PET scan, bone marrow aspirate and biopsy, as well as lumbar puncture with CSF cytology and flow cytometry (in select cases). Additional tests that should be obtained prior to therapy and should be considered part of the workup but do not impact on disease stage include serology screens for HIV, hepatitis C, and hepatitis B. The International Harmonization Project revised response criteria for malignant lymphoma incorporates changes in nodal mass size on CT scan and FDG-avidity on FDG-PET into determining response to therapy. If bone marrow and/or CSF is positive at diagnosis it is important to reassess both these compartments following therapy to determine response. Contrast-enhanced MRI brain may be normal or show leptomeningeal enhancement if involved with lymphoma but is not part of the routine staging.

REFERENCE:

Cheson, B.D., et al., Revised response criteria for malignant lymphoma. *J Clin Oncol.* 2007;25(5):579–586.

3. ANSWER: D. The five clinical factors that comprise the IPI include age >60 years, ECOG performance status 2 or higher, LDH level greater than normal, two or more extranodal sites, and Ann Arbor stage III or IV disease. Hemoglobin <12g/dL is part of the Follicular Lymphoma International Prognostic Index (FLIPI) but is not one of the factors in the standard IPI score.

REFERENCES:

A predictive model for aggressive non-Hodgkin's lymphoma. The International Non-Hodgkin's Lymphoma Prognostic Factors Project. *N Engl J Med.* 1993;329(14):987–994.

Solal-Celigny P, Roy P, Colombat P, et al. Follicular lymphoma international prognostic index. *Blood.* 2004;104(5):1258–1265.

4. ANSWER: A. Although the majority of Burkitt lymphoma cases harbor t(8;14), other MYC-activating translocations can also occur in this disease.

The (11;14) translocation is present in virtually all cases of mantle cell lymphoma, but is associated with overexpression of cyclin D1. The (14;18) translocation is present in most cases of follicular lymphoma, but is associated with overexpression of bcl-2. The (2;5) translocation is associated with ALK-positive anaplastic large cell lymphoma, which has a better prognosis than its ALK-negative counterpart.

REFERENCES:

Campo, E., et al., The 2008 WHO classification of lymphoid neoplasms and beyond: evolving concepts and practical applications. *Blood*, 2011;117(19):5019–5032.

Swerdlow, S.H., et al., The 2016 revision of the World Health Organization classification of lymphoid neoplasms. *Blood*. 2016;127(20):2375–2390.

5. ANSWER: A. For patients with asymptomatic advanced-stage follicular lymphoma, chemotherapy has not been shown to improve overall survival compared to watchful waiting. This patient was diagnosed with FL incidentally during a workup for chest pain and has an overall low burden of disease, meeting none of the Groupe d'Etude des Lymphomes Folliculaire (GELF) criteria ($\geq$3 nodal sites, each with a diameter $\geq$3 cm; any nodal or extranodal tumor mass with a diameter $\geq$7 cm; B symptoms; splenomegaly; compression syndrome (ureteral, orbital, gastrointestinal) or pleural or peritoneal serous effusion; cytopenias (WBC <1.0 x 10^9/L and/or platelets <100 x 10^9/L); leukemia (>5 x 10^9/L malignant cells)). Treatment with BR, R-CHOP, and rituximab monotherapy are possible regimens used to treat patients with advanced symptomatic disease. High-dose chemotherapy with autologous stem cell transplantation is used for aggressive lymphomas generally in the relapsed/refractory setting and would not be indicated in this older female with asymptomatic indolent lymphoma and multiple comorbidities.

REFERENCES:

Ardeshna KM, Smith P, Norton A, et al. Long-term effect of a watch and wait policy versus immediate systemic treatment for asymptomatic advanced-stage non-Hodgkin lymphoma: a randomised controlled trial. *Lancet (London, England)*. 2003;362(9383):516–522.

Solal-Celigny P, Lepage E, Brousse N, et al. Doxorubicin-containing regimen with or without interferon alfa-2b for advanced follicular lymphomas: final analysis of survival and toxicity in the Groupe d'Etude des Lymphomes Folliculaires 86 Trial. *J Clin Oncol*. 1998;16(7):2332–2338.

6. ANSWER: B. Mutations in MYD88 and CXCR4 are highly prevalent in patients with WM and are associated with outcome in patients treated with ibrutinib. MYD88 (L265P) mutation results in increased BCR signaling through BTK and CXCR4 (WHIM) mutations confer resistance to ibrutinib. In the prospective study with ibrutinib in previously treated WM, the highest responses were seen in those patients who were MYD88 (L265P) mutated and CXCR4 (WT) with an ORR and major response rate of 100% and 91.2%, respectively.

REFERENCE:

Treon SP, Tripsas CK, Meid K, et al. Ibrutinib in previously treated Waldenstrom's macroglobulinemia. *N Engl J Med*. 2015;372(15):1430–1440.

7. ANSWER: B. The NF-κB pathway is constitutively activated in ABC-DLBCL, leading to upregulation of multiple antiapoptotic transcription factors. Targeting of NF-κB and its downstream regulators with novel agents such as ibrutinib and lenalidomide is currently a focus of intense research, and early studies are demonstrating promising results as monotherapy or in combination with cytotoxic chemotherapy for patients with ABC-DLBCL.

REFERENCES:

Wilson, W.H., et al. Targeting B cell receptor signaling with ibrutinib in diffuse large B cell lymphoma. *Nat Med.* 2015;21(8):922–926.

Nowakowski GS, LaPlant B, Macon WR, et al. Lenalidomide combined with R-CHOP overcomes negative prognostic impact of non-germinal center B-cell phenotype in newly diagnosed diffuse large B-Cell lymphoma: a phase II study. *J Clin Oncol: Official Journal of the American Society of Clinical Oncology.* 2015;33(3):251–257.

8. ANSWER: A. The patient has stage IV DLBCL with a high/intermediate IPI and requires immediate therapy with the current standard of care regimen, R-CHOP-21. R-CHOP-14 with growth factor support has not demonstrated any advantage over R-CHOP-21, and there is a trend toward increased toxicity with the former. R-hyper-CVAD is a dose-intensive regimen used in BL. Response assessment after completion of therapy using both metabolic (FDG-PET) and anatomic (CT) imaging is appropriate for DLBCL, as the achievement of PET-negative status without complete anatomic resolution of lymphadenopathy is now considered equivalent to anatomic complete response (CR). Imaging after two to four cycles of therapy is recommended to ensure chemoresponsive disease; however, evidence of good response on interim imaging should not be used to shorten the duration of therapy. Any patient with BM involvement at diagnosis must have documented clearance by repeat BM aspirate/biopsy prior to designation of CR.

REFERENCES:

Coiffier B, Lepage E, Briere J, et al. CHOP chemotherapy plus rituximab compared with CHOP alone in elderly patients with diffuse large-B-cell lymphoma. *N Engl J Med.* 2002;346(4):235–242.

Delarue R, Tilly H, Mounier N, et al. Dose-dense rituximab-CHOP compared with standard rituximab-CHOP in elderly patients with diffuse large B-cell lymphoma (the LNH03-6B study): a randomised phase 3 trial. *Lancet Oncol.* 2013;14(6):525–533.

9. ANSWER: D. There is a high suspicion for transformation of this patient's FL into an aggressive large cell lymphoma, given his rapidly progressive disease and the variably intense FDG uptake on PET. The approach to treating this patient may change considerably if transformation is identified, and consequently a biopsy of the most hypermetabolic and/or rapidly growing focus of disease (the site with the highest likelihood of transformation) is indicated prior to initiation of salvage therapy. Answers A, B, and C are all reasonable therapies for relapsed FL.

REFERENCES:

Karam, M., et al., Role of fluorine-18 fluoro-deoxyglucose positron emission tomography scan in the evaluation and follow-up of patients with low-grade lymphomas. *Cancer.* 2006;107(1):175–183.

Wondergem, M.J., et al., 18F-FDG or 3'-deoxy-3'-18F-fluorothymidine to detect transformation of follicular lymphoma. *J Nucl Med.* 2015;56(2):216–221.

10. ANSWER: C. This patient's clinical presentation and histologic findings are classic for PMBL. Classic Hodgkin lymphoma is characterized by the presence of Reed–Sternberg cells, and the malignant lymphocyte immunophenotype is typically CD30+, CD15+, and CD45–. T-lymphoblastic lymphoma is the nodal manifestation of T-ALL, and immunophenotype is consistent with T-cell origin (CD19/20–, CD2+, CD7+). SLL is the nodal/aleukemic manifestation of CLL, does not typically present as an isolated mediastinal mass, and consists of small malignant lymphocytes with dim CD20 expression. Mantle cell lymphoma is a variably aggressive lymphoma with a striking male predominance that typically presents with both nodal and extranodal (BM, peripheral blood, GI tract) involvement and is confirmed by the presence of t(11;14).

REFERENCE:

van Besien, K., M. Kelta, and P. Bahaguna, Primary mediastinal B-cell lymphoma: a review of pathology and management. *J Clin Oncol.* 2001;19(6):1855-1864.

11. ANSWER: A. EBV infection is associated with PCNSL in immunocompromised individuals, such as those with HIV infection, but is rare in immunocompetent patients with PCNSL. Plasmablastic lymphoma, endemic BL, extranodal NK/T-cell lymphoma, PEL and PTLD are all strongly associated with EBV infection. In many of these lymphomas, EBV is thought to drive lymphomagenesis by constitutively activating NF-κB and other cell signaling pathways, while in other lymphomas its pathogenic role remains unknown.

REFERENCE:

Krogh-Jensen, M., P. Johansen, and F. D'Amore, Primary central nervous system lymphomas in immunocompetent individuals: histology, Epstein-Barr virus genome, Ki-67 proliferation index, p53 and bcl-2 gene expression. *Leuk Lymphoma.* 1998;30(1–2):131–142.

12. ANSWER: C. *Chlamydia trachomatis* and *Chlamydia pneumonia*, not *Haemophilus influenza,* infections have been shown to be associated with pulmonary MALT lymphoma. *Helicobacter pylori, Chlamydia psittaci,* and *Campylobacter jejuni* infections have been associated with gastric, ocular adnexal, and intestinal MALT lymphoma, respectively. Remission can be achieved in a substantial proportion of patients with gastric MALT with triple-antibiotic therapy and oral adnexal MALT with doxycycline. Approximately one-third of cases of splenic MZL are associated with HCV infection and although rare, a proportion of cases of nodal MZL are associated with HCV.

REFERENCES:

Troppan, K., et al., Molecular Pathogenesis of MALT Lymphoma. *Gastroenterol Res Pract.* 2015;2015:102656.

Fischbach W, Goebeler-Kolve ME, Dragosics B, Greiner A, Stolte M. Long term outcome of patients with gastric marginal zone B cell lymphoma of mucosa associated lymphoid tissue (MALT) following exclusive Helicobacter pylori eradication therapy: experience from a large prospective series. *Gut.* 2004;53(1):34–37.

Ferreri AJ, Ponzoni M, Guidoboni M, et al. Regression of ocular adnexal lymphoma after Chlamydia psittaci-eradicating antibiotic therapy. *J Clinical Oncol: Official Journal of the American Society of Clinical Oncology.* 2005;23(22):5067–5073.

13. ANSWER: E. The clinical presentation along with bone marrow findings are most consistent with the diagnosis of splenic marginal zone lymphoma. Approximately one-third of cases of splenic MZL are associated with HCV and treatment with appropriate antiviral therapy alone can result in remission in a substantial proportion of these patients. For asymptomatic patients with splenic MZL not associated with HCV, observation alone is an appropriate treatment strategy. For symptomatic patients, splenectomy has been the historical standard of care; however, rituximab is increasing being used as an alternative or adjunct to surgical therapy. Treatment of advanced or relapsed/refractory disease generally follows that of follicular lymphoma with bendamustine and rituximab being an acceptable treatment regimen.

REFERENCES:

Arcaini L, Paulli M, Boveri E, et al. Splenic and nodal marginal zone lymphomas are indolent disorders at high hepatitis C virus seroprevalence with distinct presenting features but similar morphologic and phenotypic profiles. *Cancer.* 2004;100(1):107–115.

Tsimberidou AM, Catovsky D, Schlette E, et al. Outcomes in patients with splenic marginal zone lymphoma and marginal zone lymphoma treated with rituximab with or without chemotherapy or chemotherapy alone. *Cancer.* 2006;107:125–135.

14. ANSWER: C. The pathologic findings and immunophenotype is most consistent with GCB-DLBCL based on Hans classification, with positive CD10 and Bcl-6 and negative MUM1 by IHC. This subtype of DLBCL is more commonly associated with Myc, Bcl-2, and Bcl-6 rearrangements and has a superior outcome in terms of PFS and OS with conventional chemoimmunotherapy, compared to ABC-DLBCL. Mutations targeting the BCR pathway are more frequent in ABC-DLBCL, not GCB-DLBCL, which result in chronic active BCR signaling and increased responses are seen with novel targeted therapies, such as ibrutinib and lenalidomide.

REFERENCES:

Wilson, W.H., et al., Targeting B cell receptor signaling with ibrutinib in diffuse large B cell lymphoma. *Nat Med.* 2015;21(8):922–926.

Wilson, W.H., et al., The Bruton's Tyrosine Kinase (BTK) Inhibitor, Ibrutinib (PCI-32765), Has Preferential Activity in the ABC Subtype of Relapsed/Refractory De Novo Diffuse Large B-Cell Lymphoma (DLBCL): Interim Results of a Multicenter, Open-Label Phase 2 Study. *Blood.* 2012;120(21):686.

Nowakowski, G.S., et al., Lenalidomide combined with R-CHOP overcomes negative prognostic impact of non-germinal center B-cell phenotype in newly diagnosed diffuse large B-Cell lymphoma: a phase II study. *J Clin Oncol.* 2015. 33(3):251–257.

15. ANSWER: C. Lenalidomide is currently approved for MCL, multiple myeloma, and low to intermediate-1 risk MDS, but is not currently an approved treatment for PTCL-NOS. Romidepsin is approved based on a phase II trial showing an ORR of 25% and median DOR of 17 months. Belinostat was approved based on the phase II BELIEF study, based on an ORR of 25.8% and median DOR of 13.6 months. Pralatrexate was approved based on the PROPEL study, based on an ORR of 29% and median DOR of 10.1 months. All of these agents are acceptable salvage treatments for patients with PTCL-NOS but should be used as a bridge to more definite therapy, such as allogeneic transplantation.

REFERENCES:

Coiffier B, Pro B, Prince HM, et al. Results from a pivotal, open-label, phase II study of romidepsin in relapsed or refractory peripheral T-cell lymphoma after prior systemic therapy. *J Clin Oncol: Official Journal of the American Society of Clinical Oncology.* 2012;30(6):631–636.

O'Connor OA, Horwitz S, Masszi T, et al. Belinostat in patients with relapsed or refractory peripheral T-Cell lymphoma: Results of the Pivotal Phase II BELIEF (CLN-19) Study. *J Clin Oncol: Official Journal of the American Society of Clinical Oncology.* 2015;33(23):2492–2499.

O'Connor OA, Pro B, Pinter-Brown L, et al. Pralatrexate in patients with relapsed or refractory peripheral T-cell lymphoma: results from the pivotal PROPEL study. *J Clin Oncol: Official Journal of the American Society of Clinical Oncology.* 2011;29(9):1182–1189.

16. ANSWER: A. The t(11;18) translocation is predictive of a lack of response for gastric MALT lymphoma to *Helicobacter pylori* eradication with triple-antibiotic therapy. Symptomatic patients who require treatment and possess this translocation should be considered for alternative treatment modalities including ISRT, rituximab monotherapy, or combination chemotherapy.

REFERENCE:

Liu, H., et al., T(11;18) is a marker for all stage gastric MALT lymphomas that will not respond to H. pylori eradication. *Gastroenterology,* 2002;122(5):128–694.

17. ANSWER: D. Idelalisib is not currently approved for the treatment of MCL and is approved in combination with rituximab for relapsed CLL and also as monotherapy for patients with relapsed FL and SLL in patients who have received at least two prior therapies. Bortezomib resulted in an ORR of 33% with median DOR of 9.2 months as monotherapy in patients with relapsed/refractory MCL and is approved in patients who have received at least one prior therapy. Lenalidomide monotherapy was compared to investigator's choice in the randomized phase II SPRINT study and demonstrated a significant improvement in PFS in patients ineligible for intensive chemotherapy or stem-cell transplantation and is approved after at least two prior therapies, at least one including bortezomib. Ibrutinib showed an ORR of 68% with median DOR of 17.5 months in relapsed/refractory MCL and is approved after at least 1 prior therapy.

REFERENCES:

Fisher RI, Bernstein SH, Kahl BS, et al. Multicenter phase II study of bortezomib in patients with relapsed or refractory mantle cell lymphoma. *J Clin Oncol: Official Journal of the American Society of Clinical Oncology.* 2006;24(30):4867–4874.

Trneny M, Lamy T, Walewski J, et al. Lenalidomide versus investigator's choice in relapsed or refractory mantle cell lymphoma (MCL-002; SPRINT): a phase 2, randomised, multicentre trial. *Lancet Oncol.* 2016;17(3):319–331.

Wang ML, Rule S, Martin P, et al. Targeting BTK with ibrutinib in relapsed or refractory mantle-cell lymphoma. *N Engl J Med.* 2013;369(6):507–516.

Hodgkin Lymphoma 29

Robert Dean and Matt Kalaycio

REVIEW QUESTIONS

1. A 19-year-old heterosexual, single African American male presented with a 2-month history of right supraclavicular lymph node enlargement. He denied weight loss, night sweats, or unexplained fevers. Physical examination showed a 2 cm firm lymph node in the right supraclavicular fossa and a 3 cm lymph node in the right axilla. An excisional biopsy of the right axillary node was consistent with nodular sclerosis CHL. A PET/CT scan showed hypermetabolic activity confined to nonbulky right supraclavicular and right axillary nodal areas. His CBCs, differential, and chemistries were within normal limits. ESR was 22. Echocardiogram showed a left ventricular ejection fraction of 65% and pulmonary function tests showed normal spirometric parameters. What is the next best step in this patient's management before starting treatment?

    A. Unilateral bone marrow aspiration and biopsy

    B. Bilateral bone marrow aspiration and biopsy

    C. Sperm banking

    D. MRI brain with and without contrast

    E. Infuse-A-port insertion

2. What is the best therapy option for the 19-year-old African American man in question 1?

    A. Four cycles of ABVD followed by 30 Gy of involved field radiation therapy

    B. Two cycles of ABVD followed by 20 Gy of involved field radiation therapy

C. Six cycles of chemotherapy with R-CHOP

D. Subtotal nodal radiation therapy

E. Four cycles of dose-escalated BEACOPP followed by 30 Gy of involved field radiation therapy

3. A 45-year-old schoolteacher with stage IIIA mixed cellularity CHL is undergoing first-line chemotherapy with ABVD. She is tolerating chemotherapy well. A PET/CT scan performed after two cycles showed complete remission. She presents now to start cycle 4 of chemotherapy with ABVD. She reports no nausea, vomiting, or fevers with the previous cycle. Her blood work today showed normal hepatic and renal function. Blood counts showed an absolute neutrophil count (ANC) of 880/μL and platelet count of 145/μL. What is the best next step in management?

A. Delay chemotherapy until ANC >1,000/μL

B. Delay chemotherapy until ANC >1,000/μL and add growth factor support to the next cycle of chemotherapy

C. Continue ABVD without delay and add growth factor support

D. Continue ABVD without delay and without growth factor support

E. Continue ABVD with 25% dose reduction in doxorubicin and bleomycin

4. A 55-year-old man with advanced-stage nodular sclerosis CHL presented with new-onset right axillary lymph node enlargement. He was treated with six cycles of ABVD 3 years ago. An excisional biopsy of the right axillary node confirmed relapsed disease. A PET/CT scan showed widespread hypermetabolic lymphadenopathy above and below the diaphragm. Bone marrow biopsy was negative. He goes on to achieve a second complete remission after three cycles of salvage chemotherapy with ICE. He has four siblings. You now recommend

A. High-dose therapy and autologous hematopoietic cell transplantation

B. Matched sibling allogeneic hematopoietic cell transplantation

C. Six cycles of ICE followed by watchful waiting

D. Six cycles of ICE followed by brentuximab vedotin maintenance therapy

ANSWERS TO REVIEW QUESTIONS

1. ANSWER: C. In young HL patients, measures to ensure fertility preservation before starting chemotherapy are of paramount importance. While infertility due to ABVD chemotherapy is uncommon, sperm banking (which is relatively inexpensive and readily available) in a male patient before starting treatment is important for two reasons: (1) To document normal sperm count and motility at baseline, since suboptimal sperm count and quality is not uncommon in HL patients even before initiating chemotherapy. (2) Sperm banking is often not feasible in patients who have refractory disease after ABVD chemotherapy before starting salvage regimens associated with high probability of causing infertility. Bone marrow aspiration biopsy is not required in patients with stage IA or IIA disease, and bilateral bone marrow biopsies are not needed in HL. Infuse-A-port is often inserted before starting chemotherapy, but ABVD-like regimens can be safely administered using peripheral intravenous access only.

2. ANSWER: B. The patient in this question has favorable risk, early-stage (IIA) HL, according to the German Hodgkin Study Group (GHSG) criteria. The HD10 trial by GHSG showed that in patients with favorable early-stage HL, two cycles of ABVD followed by 20 Gy of involved field radiation was not inferior to more aggressive options. Option A is appropriate for patients with *unfavorable* nonbulky early-stage HL. R-CHOP (C) is not an option of HL (at least in the front-line setting). Subtotal radiation therapy is inferior of chemotherapy combined with involved field radiation therapy and is not recommended.

3. ANSWER: D. HL is a highly curable hematologic malignancy; however, delays in administering chemotherapy on time (A and B) or reducing dose intensity (E) can negatively impact the probability of long-term disease control and are not recommended. Administration of growth factors (e.g., filgrastim) with ABVD has been shown to be associated with increased pulmonary toxicity and is not routinely recommended (B and C). ABVD can be safely administered to HL patients with growth factor support and regardless of ANC at the day of chemotherapy.

4. ANSWER: A. The patient in this question shows evidence of chemosensitive disease after second-line therapy with ICE regimen. High-dose therapy and autologous transplantation are curative for relapsed, chemosensitive patients with HL and remains the standard of care of this patient population (A). Patients with relapsed HL should be referred to a transplant center for transplant planning soon after a relapse is confirmed (ideally before starting salvage chemotherapy regimens). Chemotherapy alone (C) in this setting is inferior to chemotherapy followed by autologous transplantation. Similarly allogeneic transplantation (B) is generally not indicated in first relapse, outside the setting of a clinical trial. There is no role of brentuximab vedotin maintenance after chemotherapy (D).

Hematopoietic Cell Transplantation 30

Abraham S. Kanate, Michael Craig, and Mehdi Hamadani

REVIEW QUESTIONS

1. Which of the following is the most correct statement about true hematopoietic stem cells (HSC)?

    A. HSC have self-renewal capacity and remain in an "active" proliferative state at all times making them susceptible to toxins and chemotherapy.

    B. HSC can differentiate to form only myeloid specific cells (e.g., granulocyte, erythrocyte, platelets) but not lymphoid cells.

    C. True HSC have the capability of reconstituting the entire hematopoietic system and are characterized by their unlimited self-renewal capacity, pluripotency (ability to differentiate), quiescence and extensive proliferative capacity.

    D. HSC are only found in the bone marrow space and thus obtaining them for a transplant requires multiple aspirations from the bone marrow under general anesthesia (harvest).

2. A 55-year-old man is referred for bone marrow transplant evaluation. 2-weeks ago the man presented with mild fatigue and (L) upper quadrant discomfort. Initial evaluation showed splenomegaly, 3-cm below the left costal margin. WBC count was 154,000/mcL with maturing myeloid series at various stages of differentiation along with mild basophilia (3%) and eosinophilia (2%) and no myeloblasts (0%). Hemoglobin was 14.6 and platelet count 536,000/mcL. A bone marrow aspirate and biopsy performed 2 days ago showed chronic phase—chronic myeloid leukemia with

fluorescent in-situ hybridization confirming the presence of Philadelphia chromosome; t(9;22). What is the most appropriate approach at present?

A. Obtain HLA typing of the patient and his siblings to proceed to allogeneic HCT without delay

B. Start therapy with interferon-alpha, but obtain HLA typing of patient and sibling to plan an allogeneic HCT in 3 to 6 months

C. Start evaluating the patient for high-dose chemotherapy and autologous HCT

D. Plan to initiate *bcr-abl* tyrosine kinase inhibitor (TKI) at present as there is no role for an allo-HCT at this time.

3. A 36-year-old Caucasian female with no siblings was diagnosed with acute myeloid leukemia (AML) with normal cytogenetics. She received standard "3 + 7" induction chemotherapy and entered complete remission and completed four cycles of consolidation therapy. Six months later she presents with peripheral blasts and bone marrow evaluation confirms relapse. Apart from admitting the patient for re-induction chemotherapy and supportive care, what other step should be initiated at this time?

A. Consider high dose therapy and autologous hematopoietic cell transplantation (HCT)

B. HLA type the patient and run a preliminary search for unrelated donor allogeneic HCT

C. HLA type the patient, but defer allogeneic HCT for next relapse

D. Do nothing, allogeneic HCT is not a treatment option for this patient

4. A 53-year of female was diagnosed with IgA kappa multiple myeloma when she presented with anemia (Hemoglobin = 7.6 gm/dL) and multiple lytic bone lesions in the appendicular and axial skeleton and noted to have 5.4 gm/dL of IgA kappa monoclonal protein and 30% atypical plasma cells in the bone marrow aspirate/biopsy. She was initiated of triple drug therapy with bortezomib, lenalidomide and dexamethasone (VRD) as well as bisphosphonate therapy. After 2 cycles of therapy the patient has achieved a very good partial remission and has been referred for transplant evaluation. Which of the following statements made by the transplant physician is most accurate?

A. "High-dose melphalan followed by autologous HCT is a curative treatment for myeloma and should be pursued immediately"

B. "Although not a curative treatment, high dose melphalan followed by autologous HCT has shown to improve survival in myeloma and should be considered as one of the treatment options in eligible patients"

C. "There is no role for autologous HCT in myeloma and the current recommendation is to continue VRD therapy for 6 cycles followed by observation"

D. "Obtain HLA typing of the patient to consider allogeneic HCT in first remission

5. A 55-year-old male with relapsed Hodgkin lymphoma underwent high dose therapy with BEAM (carmustine + etoposide + cytarabine + melphalan) followed by autologous peripheral blood progenitor cell infusion. Hematopoietic recovery occurred by day +14 and he was discharged from the transplant center by day +25. He reports to your clinic on day +48 with 3 days onset of progressive dyspnea and dry cough. His current medications include trimethoprim-sulfamethoxazole and acyclovir. On examination his pulse is 110, BP 108/70, respiratory rate 34 and pulse-oximetry reads 88% on room air. Chest X-ray shows non-specific interstitial markings. What should be the next step in his management?

A. Initiate the patient on intravenous azithromycin and ceftriaxone

B. Stop trimethoprim-sulfamethoxazole and start the patient on inhaled pentamidine

C. Start IV ganciclovir and immunoglobulin

D. Obtain pulmonary function test and start the patient on steroid therapy

6. You are evaluating the 40-year old HLA-matched brother of a patient with acute myeloid leukemia (AML) with complex cytogenetics in CR1. The potential donor is in good health, has no medical complaints and is not on any medications except a history of basal cell carcinoma that was resected 3 years ago. When counselling the patient regarding peripheral blood progenitor cell collection which of the following statements is accurate?

A. The history of basal cell carcinoma rules him out as a donor for allogeneic hematopoietic cell transplantation.

B. The procedure consists of giving a single dose cyclophosphamide followed by growth factors for mobilization and progenitor cell collection by apheresis

C. The procedure is well tolerated with the most common side effect being self-limiting bone pain and a very rare risk of splenic rupture

D. The history of AML in his sibling (recipient), increases significantly the risk of future AML in the brother and so he cannot serve as a donor

7. A 50-year-old female with history of chronic myeloid leukemia underwent mismatched unrelated donor (7/8 match) peripheral blood progenitor cell allogeneic hematopoietic cell transplantation 16 days ago after cyclophosphamide and busulfan conditioning. She had myeloid engraftment on day +12. She complains of diffuse abdominal pain that is more prominent in the right upper quadrant. Her stool output is documented as 150 mL of liquid stool over the last 24 hours. Volume status shows that she is 3 litres positive with a weight gain of 2.5 Kg compared to the day before. Blood work shows; hyperbilirubinemia (3 mg/dL), stable hemogram, creatinine 1.1 and normal peripheral smear. What is the most likely diagnosis?

A. Sinusoidal obstruction syndrome (SOS)

B. Acute graft-versus-host-disease (GVHD)

C. Hepato-splenic candidiasis

D. Thrombotic microangiopathy

8. A diagnosis of sinusoidal obstruction syndrome (veno-occlussive disease) is established in the patient in Question #7. She is managed conservatively for 2 days when on rounds it is reported that her creatinine is 2.1 and she has significant dyspnea and hypoxia requiring oxygen support. She continues to have tender hepatomegaly, worsening hyperbilirubinemia (4.5 mg/dL) and weight gain. Apart from aggressive supportive management what other approved therapeutic option may be available for this patient.

A. Anticoagulation with low dose heparin

B. Plasmapheresis

C. Caspofungin

D. Defibrotide

---

9. A 36-year female underwent myeloablative matched unrelated donor, allo-HCT for a history of acute lymphoblastic leukemia with peripheral blood progenitor cells as graft source. She had prompt engraftment noted on day +14 and was discharged to the outpatient setting. Today is day +26 and she presents with >50% body surface area erythematous rash, jaundice along with >1.5 liter/day diarrhea. Lab evaluation show serum bilirubin at 7 mg/dL. She is currently on tacrolimus 2.5 mg PO twice daily as well as appropriate antimicrobial prophylaxis. What is the most appropriate management at this time?

   A. Schedule for colonoscopy and biopsy next week to identify the cause of diarrhea, but continue the current therapy.

   B. Obtain diagnostic skin biopsy of the affected area and start patient on prednisone 1 mg/kg BID, as well as continue tacrolimus to maintain therapeutic levels.

   C. Stop tacrolimus as it has been ineffective and start mycophenolate mofetil instead.

   D. Plan to obtain liver biopsy and initiate defibrotide for sinusoidal obstruction syndrome.

---

10. A 42-year-old male with history if IgG kappa multiple myeloma with normal cytogenetics by fluorescent in situ hybridization and karyotype underwent high dose melphalan and autologous hematopoietic cell transplantation. On day +95 a complete myeloma panel including bone marrow evaluation reveals that the patient has achieved very good partial remission (VGPR). The patient inquires of post-transplant treatment for multiple myeloma. What would be the most appropriate next step?

   A. Discuss role of allogeneic hematopoietic cell transplantation as a consolidative strategy

   B. Consider lenalidomide maintenance therapy

   C. Consider consolidation triple drug therapy with velcade, lenalidomide, and dexamethasone (VRd)

   D. There is no available data to recommend any further therapy

ANSWERS TO REVIEW QUESTIONS

1. ANSWER: C. CRITIQUE: True HSC are characterized by their unlimited self-renewal capacity, pluripotency (ability to differentiate), quiescence (stays inactive thus evading toxins and damage), and extensive proliferative capacity. They are capable of reconstituting the entire hematopoietic system (myeloid and lymphoid) at the single cell level. About 1 in 100 HSC are found in the peripheral blood, a property that is exploited when chemokines such as G-CSF are used to mobilize the stem cells to the periphery which can then be collected for transplantation.

2. ANSWER: D. CRITIQUE: Chronic myeloid leukemia used to be one of the most common indications for allogeneic HCT in the pre-*bcr-abl*-TKI era. With the advent of oral tyrosine kinase inhibitors (e.g.: imatinib, dasatinib, nilotinib) that block the phosphate binding site of *bcr-abl*, the fusion protein formed as a result of reciprocal translocation, t(9;22) also called Philadelphia chromosome, (a) immediate allo-HCT and (b) interferon use is not considered the initial standard of care. Allogeneic-HCT may still be considered in cases of intolerance to multiple TKIs, or progression of disease despite optimal use of these drugs usually due to resistance. There is no role for (c) autologous transplantation in CML.

3. ANSWER: B. CRITIQUE: This patient with normal cytogenetics AML (intermediate-risk) is treated upfront with induction and consolidation therapy followed by close observation in CR1. At the time of first relapse, apart from re-induction chemotherapy, every attempt must be made to HLA type the patient at the earliest and find a suitable donor for an allogeneic HCT in CR2. Since she does not have a sibling donor, a National Marrow Donor Program search must be initiated to locate a suitable donor. Time is vital as it takes 3 to 6 months to obtain an allograft from an unrelated donor. She has a 70% chance of finding a HLA-matched donor. Choice (a) is not a therapeutic option for this patient, autologous HCT is sometimes considered as consolidation therapy in CR1, ideally in a clinical trial setting; (c) and (d) are wrong as allogeneic HCT should be considered in first relapse or CR2 and deferring it will considerably worsen her prognosis.

4. ANSWER: B. CRITIQUE: Randomized phase III trials have clearly shown that high dose melphalan followed by autologous HCT, although not considered a curative therapy does improve progression free survival and overall survival when compared to patients not undergoing auto-HCT. When a patient is started on induction therapy that includes an immunomodulatory drug such as lenalidomide, it is optimal to consider mobilization and stem cell collection after 4 to 6 cycles as continued use of these drugs may damage stem cells thus potentially impairing mobilization and collection. Allogeneic HCT in myeloma is best considered experimental and is usually not considered as standard of care in the initial treatment plan.

5. ANSWER: D. CRITIQUE: Use of carmustine (BCNU) as part of high dose therapy can cause delayed interstitial pneumonitis and present with typical findings as described in the question. The correct management includes obtaining pulmonary function test including diffusion lung capacity of carbon monoxide and the use of steroids (d). BCNU can cause pulmonary fibrosis which may take years to manifest. The described symptoms, lack of productive cough, and negative chest x-ray points against bacterial pneumonia and hence choice (a) is not the best answer. The compliant use of trimethoprim-sulfamethoxazole effectively protects the patient against *Pneumocystis* pneumonia and hence switching to inhaled pentamidine (b) is not indicated. Cytomegalovirus pneumonia typically complicates allogeneic hematopoietic cell transplantation and so choice (e) is incorrect.

6. ANSWER: C. CRITIQUE: Evaluation of the potential donor (sibling and unrelated) is an important part of pretransplant workup. Only serious or life-threatening illness that endangers the donor or history of malignancy within the past 5 years (except nonmelanoma skin cancers) are considered absolute contraindications (a). While there is a theoretical risk for AML with the use of growth factors, this has not been observed in healthy donors and family history does not pose an increased risk either (d). Sub-ablative chemotherapy (e.g., cyclophosphamide) prior to growth factor mobilized progenitor cell collection is only considered for autotransplant. Growth factor mobilized progenitor cell collection is very well tolerated barring minor bone pain, a rare risk of spontaneous splenic rupture and no long-term effects (c).

7. ANSWER: A. CRITIQUE: The triad of findings (hyperbilirubinemia, right upper quadrant pain and weight gain/ascites) in the first 3 weeks after myeloablative allogeneic hematopoietic cell transplantation should strongly raise the suspicion of SOS. Pre-existing liver disease, conditioning regimens containing combination of cyclophosphamide with busulfan and higher dose total body irradiation, prior exposure to gemtuzumab ozogamicin are all risk factors for developing SOS. With the advent of intravenous busulfan with levels and restricting the radiation dose to 12 to 13 Gy has dramatically decreased the incidence. Acute GVHD must be considered in the differential and sometimes liver biopsy is required. In this case choice (b) is wrong as the clinical features fit SOS. Hepato-splenic candidiasis, once common is very effectively prevented with azole prophylaxis and thrombotic microangiopathy is unlikely with normal peripheral smear (c and d).

8. ANSWER: D. CRITIQUE: In 2016, the Food and Drug Administration (FDA) approved defibrotide for the management of SOS/VOD with associated renal or pulmonary dysfunction. Defibrotide is administered 6.25 mg/kg every 6 hours given as a 2-hour intravenous infusion, for a minimum of 21 days or continue treatment until resolution. The drug is an oligonucleotide mixture with profibrinolytic properties and its exact mechanism of action has not been fully described. Defibrotide was evaluated in two prospective and one expanded access single arm clinical trials which showed improved day +100 survival rates compared to historical controls.

9. ANSWER: B. CRITIQUE: Clinically the patient has acute GVHD of the skin, gastrointestinal tract and liver. While biopsy may be obtained to confirm diagnosis, therapy should not be delayed until results are available (a). The standard initial treatment is to start 2 mg/kg/day of prednisone usually in divided doses. This patient may benefit from inpatient hospitalization and iv steroid use along with iv hydration and repletion of electrolyte abnormalities etc. Tacrolimus (at optimal levels) and prophylactic antimicrobials should be continued. If the patient shows poor response to initial steroid therapy, mycophenolate (c) may be considered in addition. The above case is not consistent with sinusoidal obstruction syndrome and hence (d) defibrotide is the incorrect choice.

10. ANSWER: B. CRITIQUE: Based on the weight of current evidence the most appropriate next step in this patient would be to consider lenalidomide orally as a maintenance therapy. Large randomized trials have showed progression free survival advantage but were limited by the fact that they were not powered to detect overall survival differences. A recent meta-analysis including the patients enrolled in 3 large trials (n=1208) confirmed the progression-free survival advantage and demonstrated significant median overall survival advantage in the lenalidomide maintenance (not reached) compared to placebo arm (86 months). No current data exists that justifies the use of allogeneic transplantation in this setting in myeloma. The role of a second autotransplant (tandem auto) and post-transplant consolidation with VRd are more debatable and may be considered in high risk patients. Recently, reported randomized phase III trial did not however, show any benefit with tandem auto-HCT or post-transplant VRd consolidation compared to single auto transplantation. Hence, in this standard risk patient who has achieved a VGPR after auto-transplant, maintenance lenalidomide should be considered the most appropriate next best step.

Carcinoma of Unknown Primary **31**

F. Anthony Greco

REVIEW QUESTIONS

1. Which of the following statements is incorrect?

   A. CUP is a clinical pathologic syndrome and these patients have a predictable similar biologic behavior.

   B. In autopsy series, the majority (about 75%) of CUP patients have their small anatomical primary sites identified.

   C. The incidence of CUP is not precisely known since many patients are arbitrarily assigned a specific primary site/cancer type based on the physician's clinical opinion or the pathology report.

   D. The cause of the CUP clinical pathologic syndrome is unknown.

2. A 50-year-old woman is referred following a core-needle biopsy diagnosis of adenocarcinoma involving a mass in her right axilla. Physical examination revealed a 3x2 cm right axillary mass. Mammography and breast MRI were normal and CT scans of her chest, abdomen, and pelvis showed only a right axillary lesion. The axillary mass was surgically resected. Further pathology revealed only a CK7 positive immunostain on the biopsy specimen with multiple negative other stains including ER, PR, and HER2/neu. A molecular cancer classifier was obtained on the biopsy specimen and was reported as unclassifiable/inconclusive. Which of the following is the best course of action?

   A. Right axillary node dissection followed by close follow-up.

   B. Radiation therapy to the right axillary.

C. Empiric chemotherapy with gemcitabine and cisplatin.

D. Neoadjuvant chemotherapy with a breast cancer chemotherapy regimen followed by primary radiation therapy to the right axilla and breast.

3. A 70-year-old woman with abdominal pain was found to have several liver lesions and a right adrenal mass seen on CT scan. No other lesions were found by CT scanning of her chest, abdomen, and pelvis. A core-needle liver biopsy showed adenocarcinoma and the following immunostains were negative: CK7, CK20, TTF-1, and CDX2. The pathologist felt this was most likely arising from the upper gastrointestinal tract. Esophagogastroduodenoscopy and colonoscopy were unremarkable. What is your next recommendation?

   A. Begin treatment with empiric chemotherapy for CUP with paclitaxel and carboplatin.

   B. Obtain several serum tumor markers including CEA, CA19-9, and CA125.

   C. Order a molecular cancer classifier assay on the biopsy specimen.

   D. Begin liver directed therapy with radioactive microspheres.

4. A 56-year-old woman presents with back pain and is found to have a lytic lesion of the L-3 vertebral body and several liver lesions seen on CT scan of the chest, abdomen, and pelvis. A biopsy of a liver lesion revealed adenocarcinoma and immunostaining was not specific. A molecular cancer classifier assay was performed on the biopsy specimen and showed a 96% probability of lung adenocarcinoma. What is the most appropriate next test to order?

   A. Mammogram

   B. Genetic testing of the biopsy specimen for EGFR mutational status, ALK/ROS1 rearrangements, and PDL-1 staining.

   C. Bronchoscopy

   D. PET scan

5. A 40-year-old homosexual gentleman presented with a 3x3 cm inguinal mass. A biopsy showed squamous cell carcinoma. A p16 stain was positive in the cancer cells. Physical examination is normal except for this large right inguinal mass. A CT scan of his chest, abdomen, and pelvis showed the inguinal mass and an enlarged right iliac node measuring 2 × 3 cm. He refuses surgery. What treatment is indicated?

   A. Empiric chemotherapy with paclitaxel and carboplatin

   B. Empiric chemotherapy with gemcitabine and cisplatin

   C. Radiotherapy to the inguinal area, iliac, and retroperitoneal nodal areas

   D. Chemoradiation with 5-FU, mitomycin C and radiotherapy to include the anal canal, right inguinal, and iliac areas

ANSWERS TO REVIEW QUESTIONS

1. ANSWER: A

Rationale:

CUP is a heterogeneous group of different metastatic cancers, which share in common very small clinically occult anatomical primary sites, but are biologically different from one another, usually behaving similarly to their counterparts with known recognizable primary cancers. Autopsy series have documented that most CUP patients have a small identifiable primary site. The incidence of CUP is difficult to precisely determine, since many patients with CUP are assigned a specific cancer type and therefore are not included in tumor registries as CUP. The mechanisms at play causing CUP remain an enigma.

REFERENCES:

a. Greco FA, Hainsworth JD. Cancer of unknown primary site. In: DeVita VT Jr., Lawrence TS, Rosenberg SA, eds. *Cancer: Principles and Practice of Oncology.* 10th ed. Philadelphia, PA: Wolters Kluwer Publishers; 2015:1720–1737.

b. Pentheroudakis G, Golfinopoulos V, Pavlidis N. Switching benchmarks in cancer of unknown primary from autopsy to microarray. *Eur J Cancer.* 2007;43:2026–2036.

c. Greco FA. Cancer of unknown primary site: still an entity, a biological mystery and a metastatic model. *Nat Rev Cancer.* 2014;14:3–4.

2. ANSWER: D

Rationale:

Women with CUP who have an axillary adenocarcinoma usually have an occult breast cancer on the ipsilateral side and if no other metastasis are identified represent a putative clinical stage II breast cancer. In this patient, her cancer is triple negative and immunostains and molecular cancer classifier were unable to substantiate the diagnosis of breast cancer. However, she falls within a favorable subset of CUP and her prognosis when treated like stage II breast cancer is similar to known stage II breast cancer.

REFERENCES:

a. Pentheroudakis G,Lazaridis G, Pavlidis N. Axillary nodal metastasis from carcinoma of unknown primary (CUPAx): a systematic review of published evidence. *Breast Cancer Res Treat.* 2010;119:1–11.

b. Greco FA, Hainsworth JD. Cancer of unknown primary site. In: DeVita VT jr., Lawerence TS, Rosenberg SA, eds. *Cancer: Principles and Practice of Oncology.* 10th ed. Philadelphia, PA: Wolters Kluwer Publishers; 2015:1720–1737.

3. ANSWER: C

Rationale:

The patient has CUP and the cancer type is unknown based on clinical standard pathologic features, although the pathologist suspected an upper gastrointestinal origin. A molecular cancer classifier assay may diagnose the cancer type and is about 90% accurate. There are several possible occult primary sites, many of which are treatable with specific treatments (for example breast, lung, and renal carcinomas to name a few), which could benefit this patient and precise therapy depends on a specific diagnosis. A molecular cancer classifier assay complements standard pathology and in many patients diagnoses the specific cancer type.

REFERENCES:

a. Greco FA. Improved diagnosis, therapy and outcomes for patients with CUP. *Nat Rev Clin Oncol.* 2017;14:5–6.

b. Hainsworth JD, Greco FA. Gene expression profiling in patients with carcinoma of unknown primary site; from translational research to standard of care. *Virchows Arch.* 2014;464:393–402.

c. Greco FA, Lennington WJ, Spigel DR, Hainsworth JD. Molecular profiling diagnosis in unknown primary cancer: accuracy and ability to complement standard pathology. *J Natl Cancer Inst.* 2013;105:782–790.

4. ANSWER: B

Rationale:

The patient has CUP, but the molecular assay reveals a gene expression pattern consistent with lung adenocarcinoma at a very high probability. The next most important step is to determine if the cancer cells contain a target which can be treated with relatively effective targeted drugs such as EGFR inhibitors or ALK/ROS1 inhibitors, or immunotherapy with an immune checkpoint inhibitor.

REFERENCES:

a. Hainsworth JD, Greco FA. Lung adenocarcinoma with anaplastic lymphoma kinase (ALK) rearrangement presenting as carcinoma of unknown primary site: recognition and treatment implications. Drugs Real World Outcomes. 2016;3:115–120.

b. Greco FA. Improved diagnosis, therapy and outcomes for patients with CUP. *Nat Rev Clin Oncol.* 2017;14:5–6.

5. ANSWER: D

Rationale:

In his setting, the most likely diagnosis is an occult anal squamous primary with metastasis to the inguinal and iliac nodes. The positive p16 stain of the cancer cells highly suggest that this is an HPV associated anal carcinoma. Therapy with 5-FU, mitomycin C and radiotherapy is potentially curative in his setting.

REFERENCE:

a. Glynne-Jones R, Adams R, Lopes A, Meadows H. Clinical endpoints in trials of chemoradiation for patients with anal cancer. *Lancet Oncol.* 2017;18:218–227.

Central Nervous System Tumors **32**

Emanuela Molinari and Mark R. Gilbert

REVIEW QUESTIONS

1. **Testing point:** Recall knowledge. **Task:** Pathophysiology/basic science
   Stem: What is the main innovation brought by 2016 WHO classification CNS tumors, and why it is so important?

   Key and Distractors:

   A. It adds new entities and increases the numbers of tumors recognized, which is important as provide a diagnosis for all tumor patients

   B. It uses molecular parameters combined to histology features to define tumor entities that are important for understanding tumor etiology, predicting clinical course and response to treatment and prognosticate outcomes

   C. It changes parameters of staging and grading based on histological features redefining clinical phenotypes based on conventional histology

   D. There is no innovation but a regular update on previous 2007 classification

2. **Testing point:** Recall knowledge. **Task:** Differential diagnosis
   Stem: Although not diagnostic and specific, which brain tumors frequently presents with calcifications at neuroimaging?

Key and Distractors:

A. Lymphoma

B. Medulloblastoma

C. Meningiomas and oligodendroglioma

D. Almost all astrocytomas

3. **Testing point**: Judgement. **Task**: Management decision

   Stem: A 68-year-old patient presents to medical attention for new onset of headache and memory problems. He is otherwise fit and well with controlled hypertension on medical treatment. Neuroimaging reveals a single lesion on right fronto-temporal lobe with irregular enhancing margins and surrounded by vasogenic edema but no midline shift. Partial tumor resection was well tolerated and pathology confirmed the suspicion of Glioblastoma, MGMT promoter methylated. What is the best adjunctive treatment in this scenario?

Key and Distractors:

A. No adjunctive treatment as the prognosis is too poor for the elderly to embark in treatment with likely toxicity related side effects

B. Conventional radiotherapy of 60 Gy (in 30 fractions over a period of 6 weeks) in combination with temozolomide as there is no need for late effects concerns given the age of the patient

C. Only whole brain radiotherapy at high dose as patient methylation status does prognosticate poor response to chemotherapy

D. Short course of radiotherapy at the total dose of 40 Gy in 15 fractions over 3 weeks with concurrent and adjuvant temozolomide, as this combination provides the longer progression-free survival and overall survival coupled with better tolerability in elderly patients

4. **Testing point**: Synthesis. **Task**: Clinical features

   Stem: A 45-year-old lady presents with 4-month history of nonspecific headache with tension type features and fatigue to the neurologist. Her neurological examination is unremarkable. She does have a past history of breast cancer, which was treated the previous year and she is under surveillance with no evidence of recurrence. A head MRI reveals a single right frontal lobe lesion with apparent infiltrative margin surrounded by some edema. As the differential diagnosis includes brain metastasis and primary brain tumor, it is a solitary, the patient is scheduled for surgery that will also allow pathology confirmation. Before going to the operating room, the best management would include:

Key and Distractors:

A. Blood tests analysis including coagulation status as per standard routine prior to surgery

B. Heparin prophylaxis as she may have a malignant glioma and this could increase the risk of thromboembolism

C. Prophylactic antiepileptic regime as whether she has primary or secondary brain tumor, she has 25% risk of developing seizure at diagnosis and further 20% risk through the illness course

D. Steroids treatment in case she develops mass effects due to surgery

5. **Testing point**: Judgement. **Task**: Management Decision

   Stem: A 28-year-old man seeks a second opinion regarding an imaging finding. He was diagnosed with oligodendroglioma grade II, IDH1 mutated on the left frontal lobe that presented with focal seizure nine years ago. He was initially monitored with neuroimaging and then treated two years after with temozolomide. After two years from end of treatment he developed seizure recurrence and neuroimaging showed changes in keeping with tumor progression. He underwent surgery, which revealed progression to anaplastic oligodendroglioma and he was treated with a combination of proton beam RT and chemotherapy, which he completed three years ago. He has been well and asymptomatic since, but the two most recent imaging at 3-month interval shows mild changes, which are mostly characterized by increased signal in FLAIR sequences on periventricular area and with linear pattern and without enhancement. Spectroscopy does not reveal 2 hydroxyglutarate (2HG) peak. What would be a most likely diagnosis and appropriate management?

Key and Distractors:

A. Biopsy is warranted to have diagnostic confirmation before proceeding with any decision

B. Radiation therapy should be initiated as soon as possible as his tumor has already proved to have evolved to a more aggressive grade

C. Active imaging monitoring as the imaging and clinical data support treatment related effects more than disease recurrence or progression

D. Enrolling in available clinical trials as he clearly failed standard treatments in the past

6. **Testing point**: Judgement. **Task**: Treatment

   Stem: A 35-year-old woman presents with a history of posterior fossa ependymoma grade II diagnosed four years ago. She underwent surgery with total resection on imaging followed by radiotherapy at tumor site. The patient does not have genetic disease association. Recently she has complained of back pain which affects her ability to walk distances and lower limbs paresthesia. Neuroimaging of the brain show stability and no recurrence of the disease, and neuroimaging of the spine reveals punctiform new lesion in the thoracic area and more evident lesion in lumbar area at L3 plus sugar coating appearance of the thoraco-lumbar spine at post contrast imaging. What would you offer as next step?

Key and Distractors:

A. Palliative care as when ependymoma disseminates, there is no cure and no effective treatment

B. Radiation therapy, optimally with proton beam to the whole spine and follow up to decide if further adjunctive treatment is needed

C. Therapy should be aimed to control the disease at this point, with conventional targeted radiotherapy at the lumbar site that shows more prominent lesion producing symptoms

D. Surgery on the lumbar area followed by chemotherapy, likely temozolomide, as the tumor recurred after radiation

7. **Testing point**: Judgement. **Task**: Management decision

   Stem: 24 year old woman presents in A&E with first seizure event. At head CT a lesion is found in the left occipital lobe with some hemorrhage and calcifications noted. After evaluating her for stroke factors and detailing the lesion with head MRI, it is felt she has a probable low-grade tumor. The lesion seems infiltrating but does not cross the midline and is less than 6 cm in maximum diameter. She does not have neurological deficits and her visual field is full in both eyes. First imaging scan at three months shows stable appearance. What would be the best approach?

Key and Distractors:

A. Start her on antiepileptic medication with new AED class, active monitoring the imaging with longitudinal follow-up to detect any clinical or neuroimaging changes that would warrant intervention

B. Biopsy the lesion to get a diagnosis and start early treatment even if it is likely she will have new visual deficits from surgery as this approach will give her a survival advantage

C. Targeted radiation therapy to the occipital lesion as the lesion will grow and therapy is more effective with less toxicity when tumor size is less

D. Combination of targeted radiotherapy and temozolomide as chances are it is a oligodendroglioma and it is possible its genetic profile may respond to the combined treatment

8. **Testing point:** Knowledge. **Task**: Natural history/epidemiology

   Stem: A 3-year-old patient presents with a 4-week history of morning vomiting and clumsiness. Examination reveals a mild VI cranial nerve palsy and swelling of optic discs. Head MRI is performed and reveals a midline posterior fossa mass enhancing post contrast and causing moderate hydrocephalus. Spinal MRI does not reveal metastases. Surgical resection achieves total gross resection at post surgery imaging and pathology confirms medulloblastoma diagnosis detailing tumor profiling as SHH subgroup with p53 wildtype. Adjunctive chemoradiotherapy is the next treatment step. What would you say to the parents to inform the decision process?

Key and Distractors:

A. Preparing the parents for the worst as brain tumor in childhood have poorer outcomes than in adult population

B. The child's medulloblastoma subtype with appropriate treatment may have 5-year survival of around 80%. However, given the age of the child, detailed discussion of long-term side effects on neurocognitive development should take place with the parents

C. Reassuring the parents that the child is out of risk as surgery cures the child's subtype of medulloblastoma

D. No prognostication can be done until the child has reached 5 years of age as the pathologist has not given the histology definition and genetic profiling is not a prognosticating factor

9. **Testing point**: Synthesis. **Task**: Clinical features

Stem: A 32-year-old lady presents with previous diagnosis of right frontal glioblastoma multiforme IDH mutated, MGMT methylated. She underwent surgery with maximal subtotal resection, followed by radiation therapy and temozolomide. The follow-up MRI after 3 months of radiation treatment shows increased area of T1 post contrast enhancing and increased signal at T2 FLAIR (upper row images, from left to right). Her neurological examination is stable and she feels fatigued but overall better in herself. The neuro-oncologist decided to go ahead with temozolomide treatment (lower row images show same sequences at follow-up scan after 3 months interval from previous one). What would you conclude as being the most likely scenario?

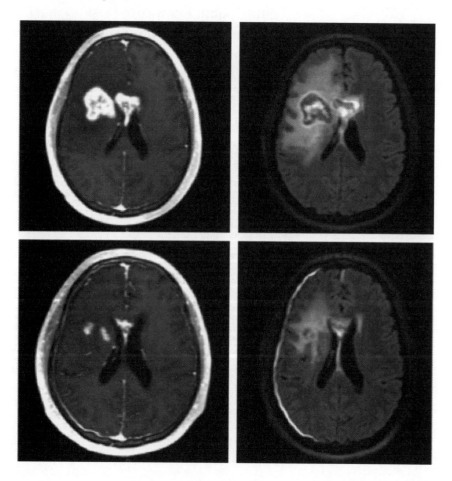

Upper row at 3 months after radiation treatment and lower row at 3 months follow up while on adjunctive temozolomide. On the left T1 sequences post contrast and on the right T2 FLAIR.

Key and Distractors:

A. It is a classical example of surgery induced changes

B. It is a good example of pseudo-progression

C. Fluctuations during treatment are the norm, so you should always wait the end of the adjunctive treatment and related number of scans before reaching a conclusion regarding treatment efficacy

D. She is an extraordinary case and you could not draw any conclusion

10. **Testing point:** Recall knowledge. **Task:** Clinical features, natural history/ epidemiology

   Stem: A 38-year-old lady was found to have breast nodule during pregnancy and she was diagnosed with breast cancer. After delivery she underwent surgical removal plus chemotherapy with good systemic response. However, she developed headache and brain MRI revealed one small asymptomatic lesion in the right frontal lobe in keeping with brain metastases. Pathology from breast surgery revealed HRE2-positive tumor. What would be the next treatment plan?

Key and Distractors:

A. Prognosis is too poor and palliative care would optimize the quality of life for the remaining life expectancy

B. Whole brain radiotherapy coupled with a chemotherapy agent that cross BBB as brain metastases takes the lead in the management plan over systemic disease, being the main prognostic factor of survival

C. It is likely that brain metastases have the same genomic profile of the tumor of origin so there is no need to address specifically the brain metastases apart from steroids if edema is present

D. Stereotactic radiosurgery of brain metastases associated with continuing chemotherapy agent targeted to the original tumor that has been controlled

ANSWERS TO REVIEW QUESTIONS

1. ANSWER: B

Rationale:

The 2016 WHO classification for CNS tumors augments previous classifications that were based on histological features and it incorporates molecular parameters into the classification, helping defining tumor by clinical phenotype and adding information that are useful in clinical practice for prognostication, response to treatment, and clinical course.

REFERENCE:

Louis D, Perry A, Reifenberger G, et al. The 2016 World Health Organization Classification of Tumors of the Central Nervous System: a summary. *Acta Neuropathol.* 2016;131:803.

2. ANSWER: C

Rationale:

Integrating information from different investigations is helpful in increasing diagnostic accuracy. Intracranial tumors present with a variety of features at neuroimaging. Calcifications are commonly seen in slow growing tumors, as meningioma and oligodendroglioma, and other tumors as craniopharyngioma, pineal parenchyma tumors, ependymoma, dermoid cysts, and much less frequently in astrocytomas.

REFERENCE:

Kiroğlu Y, çalli C, Karabulut N, et al. Intracranial calcifications on CT. *Diagn Interv Radiol.* 2010;16:263–269.

3. ANSWER: D

Rationale:

Although the prognosis for glioblastoma worsen with age, advanced age alone should not necessarily preclude treatment options. As elderly brain is more susceptible to radiation toxicity due to less physiological reserve, it became of great relevance a recent study by Perry et al. showing that surgical resection followed by short course of radiotherapy in association with chemotherapy improved outcomes (progression-free survival and overall survival) in elderly patients, and the greater benefits was seen in the subgroup of patients with MGMT methylated status.

REFERENCES:

Perry JR, Lapierre N, O'Callaghan CJ, et al. Short-course radiation plus Temozolomide in elderly patients with glioblastoma. *N Engl J Med.* 2017;376(11):1027–1037.

Wick W, Platten M, Meisner C, et al. Temozolomide chemotherapy alone versus radiotherapy alone for malignant astrocytoma in the elderly: the NOA-08 randomised, phase 3 trial. *Lancet Neurol.* 2012;13(7):707–715.

4. ANSWER: A

Rationale:

The patient does not have localizing or focal neurology signs and does not have had any seizure activity. There is no evidence based data that would support antiepileptic prophylaxis in patients who do not present with seizures. She is ambulant and she does not have a past history of thromboembolism and she is not taking chemotherapy agents that increase the risk of venous thromboembolism, that would support heparin prophylaxis and she does not have significant peritumor edema and mass effects to justify steroids.

REFERENCES:

Bergen DC. Prophylactic antiepileptic drugs in patients with brain tumors. *Epilepsy Curr.* 2005;5(5):182–183.

Mikkelsen T, Paleologos NA, Robinson PD, et al. The role of prophylactic anticonvulsants in the management of brain metastases: a systemic review and evidence-based clinical practice guideline. *J Neuro Oncol.* 2010;96(1):97–102.

O'Donnell M, Weits JI. Thromboprophylaxis in surgical patients. *Can J Surg.* 2003;46(2):129–135.

5. ANSWER: C

Rationale:

Neuroimaging appearances couple with lack of clinical symptoms and signs further support treatment related effects. The imaging findings do point towards proton beam radiation treatment effect in his diagnosis, and spectroscopy gives more weight towards treatment effect. Management would be continuing active monitoring with serial neuroimaging. Starting treatment now would not be appropriate and have the risk of not being able to discern treatment failure given the underlying process of the imaging appearance. Biopsy has low chances of sampling the small area of mild change with the above characteristics.

REFERENCE:

Hygino da Cruz HLC, Rodriguez I, Domingues RC, et al. Pseudoprogression and pseudoresponse: imaging challenges in the assessment of posttreatment glioma. *Am J Neuroradiol.* 2011; 32(11):1978–1985.

6. ANSWER: B

Rationale:

There are no standard guidelines in adult ependymomas and tailored management should be addressed in individual cases. Treatment of recurrent ependymoma remains a challenge and it does not have a good outcome generally. The above scenario reveals a leptomeningeal drop metastasis in the lumbar area, possibly in the thoracic area as well, and involvement of the whole spine. Initial tumor seemed to have responded well to radiation. Although tumor is likely to progress acquiring more aggressive features over time, it may still be radiosensitive. In adult patients, it is important to preserve the bone marrow and proton beam radiation does offer this advantage in addition to be better tolerated. Chemotherapy is not very effective and carries risks of bone marrow toxicity that limit further options without providing clear benefits, so that it can be pursued as last option.

REFERENCE:

Wu J, Armstrong T, Gilbert M. Biology and management of ependymomas. *Neuro Oncol.* 2016;18(7):902–913.

7. ANSWER: A

Rationale:

The above patient is young and has no current neurological and visual deficit. It is likely she has a slowly growing tumor, possibly a oligodendroglioma given the imaging appearances with calcification and seizure onset is a positive predictive factor of outcome. She experiences a seizure and should be started on antiepileptic medication, preferably with new AEDs that does not interact with chemotherapy agents that may be needed. There are no current evidence-based data suggesting that early intervention versus active observation and intervention at changes does impact on overall survival. It is generally better to get a molecular diagnosis to more accurately diagnose the tumor and decide the optimal treatment. Nonetheless, for lesions suggesting slowly growing low-grade gliomas, the management is controversial and should be individualized. Patient's view is important and informed decision has to be based on current evidence-based data. For young patients, with well controlled epilepsy and no neurological or visual deficits, the risks on impacting the quality of life with surgery-related deficits and risks do not outweigh the possible benefits of earlier intervention.

REFERENCE:

Schaff LR, Lassman AB. Indications for Treatment: Is observation or chemotherapy alone a reasonable approach in the management of low-grade gliomas? *Semin in Radiat Oncol.* 2015;25(3):203–209.

8. ANSWER: B

Rationale:

The 2016 WHO classification combining histological and molecular profiling of medulloblastomas stratifies patients risks and outcomes. SHH subtype in children aged below four with p53 wildtype have a reasonable good prognosis with appropriate treatment but despite 5 years old survival of almost 80%, neurotoxic sequelae due to chemo/radio-therapies strongly impact the neurocognitive development of such young children.

REFERENCES:

Pietsch T, Haberler C. Update on the integrated histopathological and genetic classification of medulloblastoma – a practical diagnostic guideline. *Clin Neuropathol.* 2016;35(6):344–352.

Brodin PN, Munck Af Rosenschöld P, Aznar CA, et al. Radiobiological risk estimates of adverse events and secondary cancer for proton and photon radiation therapy of pediatric medulloblastoma. *Acta Oncol.* 2011;50(6):808–816.

Askins MA, Bartlett DM. Preventing Neurocognitive Late Effects in childhood cancer survivors. *J Child Neurol.* 2008;23(10):1160–1171.

9. ANSWER: B

Rationale:

The combination of type of tumor and time from chemoradiation treatment, coupled with the lack of clinical symptoms progression raised the suspicion of pseudo-progression and the neuroimaging improvement at follow-up scan did confirm this. MGMT methylation in GBM often correlates with imaging finding of pseudo-progression after radio-chemotherapy in the first three months. Pseudo-progression reflects an increased inflammatory response and it is linked to better outcome, so it would be a miss to interrupt prematurely a treatment that works.

REFERENCES:

Brandes AA, Franceschi E, Tosoni A, et al. MGMT promoter metylation status can predict the incidence and outcome of pseudoprogression after concomitant radiochemotherapy in newly diagnosed glioblastoma patients. *J Clin Oncol.* 2008;26(13):2192–2197.

Fabi A, Russillo M, Metro G, et al. Pseudoprogression and MGMT status in Glioblastoma patients: implications in clinical practice. *Anticancer Res.* 2009;29(7):2607–2610.

10. ANSWER: D

Rationale:

The patient's breast tumor belongs to a subtype with reasonably good prognosis and systemic disease has responded to treatment. Addressing the systemic disease leads the treatment as it is dominant in survival prognostication and overall response to treatment. Brain is considered a sanctuary site but recent studies showed that treatment response in brain metastases depends more on choosing an agent effective in controlling the primary tumor than specifically crossing the BBB, so with controlled systemic disease and single asymptomatic brain lesion, there would be no indication to change the chemotherapy agent. The lesion is in a reasonably good location for safe resection. Surgery would provide tissue for pathology that also confirms genetic profiling of the brain metastases. As tumor may change with time and disease progression, pathology may provide information useful at later stage. It is important to consider long-term side effects in such categories as young patients with good systemic disease control and prognosis, therefore avoiding whole brain radiation treatment when appropriate as in single (or less than 4) brain lesion.

REFERENCE:

Leone JP, Leone BA. Breast cancer brain metastases: the last frontier. *Exp Hematol Oncol.* 2015;4:33.

Endocrine Tumors **33**

Jaydira Del Rivero and Ann W. Gramza

REVIEW QUESTIONS

1. A 36-year-old woman is found to have a 3-cm thyroid mass, enlarged neck lymph nodes, and multiple subcentimeter bilateral pulmonary nodules. Subsequent biopsies of both a lung nodule and the thyroid mass revealed PTC. What is the appropriate next step in this patient's management?

    A. Diagnostic radioactive iodine whole-body scan to evaluate sites of disease

    B. Total thyroidectomy and lymphadenectomy

    C. Radioactive iodine treatment

    D. Doxorubicin-based combination chemotherapy

    E. Clinical trial with a kinase inhibitor

2. A 62-year-old woman with a long history of metastatic papillary thyroid cancer with pulmonary nodules that had been relatively stable over the prior 3 years presented to clinic for evaluation. She underwent a total thyroidectomy and lymph node dissection at the time almost 13 years ago. She subsequently received ^{131}I-radioactive iodine ablative treatment on three separate occasions. Her most recent radioactive iodine (RAI) scan performed a month ago was negative for uptake. FDG-PET with cross-sectional imaging revealed a dramatic increase in the activity, number, and size of innumerable pulmonary metastases. Which of the following is the most appropriate systemic management choice for this patient?

    A. Chemotherapy with paclitaxel

    B. Radioactive iodine

C. Lenvatinib

D. Pazopanib

---

3. A 23-year-old male with a history of MEN2A and MTC presents for follow-up. He was originally diagnosed 5 years ago when a thyroid mass was noted incidentally following a car accident. He subsequently underwent a total thyroidectomy with central and right neck dissections. Today, his review of systems is negative. On physical examination, his neck is notable for well-healed surgical scars and no palpable nodules or lymph nodes. The rest of the examination is unremarkable. Laboratory studies reveal normal serum chemistries, CBC, and TSH. His calcitonin from today is 93 and has been stable since his thyroidectomy. Which of the following is the most appropriate next step in his management?

    A. Radioactive iodine whole-body scan and treatment with radioactive iodine if the scan is positive for disease.

    B. Contrast-enhanced CT or MRI of the neck, chest, and abdomen with liver protocol for initial staging followed by treatment with vandetanib 300 mg daily. Repeat calcitonin in 2 to 3 months.

    C. Contrast-enhanced CT or MRI of the neck, chest, and abdomen with liver protocol for staging. If imaging is negative, repeat serum calcitonin in 6 months.

    D. Treat his neck with external beam radiotherapy.

    E. Increase his levothyroxine dose to suppress TSH to <0.1. Repeat his calcitonin and TSH levels in 6 weeks.

---

4. A 50-year-old woman with a history of metastatic medullary carcinoma of the thyroid presented for routine follow-up. She was originally diagnosed with medullary thyroid cancer about 10 years ago and was treated initially with total thyroidectomy. Soon after diagnosis she was found to have asymptomatic nodules that remained relatively stable, so she was followed with active surveillance. Recently, she received external-beam radiation therapy to palliate pain related to a new bone lesion and was also found at that time to have enlargement of bilateral pulmonary nodules. Tumor marker levels including calcitonin and carcinoembryonic antigen have also doubled in the last 6 months. Which of the following is the most appropriate treatment option for this patient?

    A. Lenvatenib

    B. Radioactive iodine

C. Doxorubicin and cisplatin

D. Vandetanib

Measurement	4 Years Ago	3 Years Ago	2 Years Ago	Last Year
Urinary epinephrine, μg/24 h (nmol/d)	58 (316)	68 (371)	49 (267)	56 (305)
Urinary norepinephrine, μg/24 h (nmol/d)	264 (1561)	221 (1307)	235 (1390)	251 (1484)
Urinary metanephrine, μg/24 h (nmol/d)	587 (2976)	610 (3093)	602 (3052)	615 (3118)
Urinary normetanephrine, μg/24 h (nmol/d)	1146 (6257)	1235 (6743)	1180 (6443)	1220 (6661)

5. A 58-year-old woman presents to your clinic after relocating from another state. She has a history of pheochromocytoma, and unilateral adrenalectomy was performed 5 years ago. One year later, she presented with recurrent disease that required further debulking surgery; she did not receive any adjuvant therapy. To today's appointment, she has brought a list of investigations performed at her previous endocrine center since her last operation:

Three years ago, ^{123}I *meta*-iodobenzylguanidine (MIBG) scintigraphy and single-photon emission CT revealed no MIBG-avid lesions. Two years ago, fluorodeoxyglucose (FDG) positron emission tomography (PET)–CT documented multiple small "hotspots" in the ribs, thoracic spine, and lungs consistent with metastatic pheochromocytoma. She feels well, with no symptoms suggestive of catecholamine excess. She is taking doxazosin, 4 mg daily, and her blood pressure is 138/79 mm Hg (supine). Height is 64 in (162.6 cm), and weight is 135 lb (61.4 kg) (BMI = 23.2 kg/m²). You organize updated investigations, the findings of which are shown here:

Urinary epinephrine = 51 μg/24 h (278.2 nmol/d)

Urinary norepinephrine = 248 μg/24 h (1466.7 nmol/d)

Urinary metanephrine = 561 μg/24 h (2844.3 nmol/d)

Urinary normetanephrine = 1116 μg/24 h (6093.4 nmol/d)

FDG-PET/CT shows multiple small "hotspots" as previously reported with no significant interval change. Which one of the following is the most appropriate next step in this patient's management?

A. Surveillance only

B. Off–label sunitinib

C. MIBG

D. CVD

E. Radiolabeled octreotide

6. Which gene causing PHEO/PGL should be tested first in a patient with metastatic disease?

   A. VHL

   B. SDHB

   C. SDHA

   D. SDHC

   E. RET

7. A 45-year-old man is referred for evaluation of incidentally discovered bilateral adrenal masses. CT of the chest and abdomen was performed during routine follow-up of treated esophageal adenocarcinoma. The esophageal malignancy was diagnosed 7 years ago. It was resected after neoadjuvant treatment with radiation and chemotherapy. His appetite is normal and body weight is stable. He has no dysphagia or back pain. He is taking no medications. There is no history of hypertension or palpitations. On physical examination, his height is 67 in. (170.2 cm) and weight is 153 lb (69.5 kg) (BMI = 24 kg/m²). Blood pressure is 145/75 mm Hg, and pulse rate is 84 beats/min. Laboratory evaluation with a basic metabolic panel and random plasma cortisol was normal. He does not appear cushingoid (no striae or edema). Findings from heart and lung examinations are normal. CT scan shown below. Which of the following is the best next step in this patient's care?

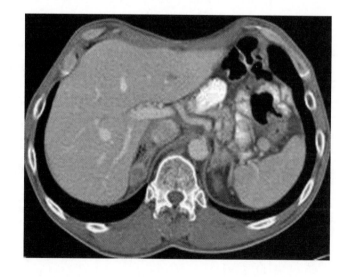

A. Perform and FDG-PET scan

B. Perform a CT-guided FBA of the adrenal

C. Measure 24-hour urinary metanephrines and catecholamines

D. No additional testing now, follow up CT in 3 to 6 months

8. A 55-year-old male presents with severe abdominal pain and diarrhea. Evaluation by EGD reveals a 1 cm duodenal ulcer, and biopsies are negative for *Helicobacter pylori*. A serum gastrin level is elevated at 1,300 pg/mL. What is the next appropriate step in his evaluation?

A. Octreotide scan

B. Secretin stimulation test

C. EUS

D. CT scan of the abdomen

E. ^{131}I-MIBG scan

9. A 65-year-old patient undergoes a CT scan of her chest for suspected pulmonary embolism (PE). No evidence of PE is found, but incidentally, the CT scan shows multiple large intrahepatic lesions suspicious for metastatic disease. Further workup includes a dedicated CT scan of abdomen and pelvis, which confirms the presence of about eight heterogeneously enhancing lesions in the liver measuring up to 5 cm. In addition, a 3-cm mass is found in the body of the pancreas without evidence of peripancreatic lymphadenopathy. An ultrasound-guided biopsy of the liver metastases reveals a well-differentiated neuroendocrine tumor with a Ki67 proliferation index of less than 1%. Upon clinical presentation, the patient did not report any tumor-related symptoms. Which of the following is the best next step in the treatment of this patient?

A. Start systemic therapy with everolimus

B. Start systemic therapy with sunitinib

C. Consider debulking resection of the liver metastases

D. Do not start any tumor-directed therapy and repeat imaging within the next 3 to 6 months

10. A 50-year-old female with a history of ACC presents for consultation regarding further management. She underwent resection 1 year ago, and now presents with left flank pain, weight gain, weakness, and uncontrolled hypertension. She is found to have a 7.5 cm mass in the left renal fossa and multiple lesions consistent with metastatic disease. A CT-guided biopsy confirms ACC recurrence. She is judged unresectable. Of the treatment options listed, which should be started immediately?

   A. Streptozocin

   B. Combination chemotherapy with cisplatin, doxorubicin, and etoposide

   C. Sunitinib

   D. Mitotane

   E. Hydrocortisone

ANSWERS TO REVIEW QUESTIONS

1. ANSWER: B. The purpose of this question is to understand the management of patients with previously untreated metastatic PTC. Unlike most malignancies, resection of the primary tumor and lymph nodes should be performed in all patients with metastatic disease. This is because these patients are still potentially curable with subsequent radioactive iodine treatment. Complete responses are seen in approximately 45% of patients. This is particularly the case for young patients with multiple pulmonary metastases. A preoperative diagnostic radioactive iodine scan would not be useful for two reasons: all of the iodine would concentrate in the thyroid, and the patient has had a recent CT scan with IV contrast. Iodinated contrast will interfere with the diagnostic scan by increasing the circulating iodine. For this reason (and because radioactive iodine is intended for remnant ablation and metastases, not primary tumors), treatment with radioactive iodine is not an appropriate first step in this patient's management. Doxorubicin-based chemotherapy and clinical trials with kinase inhibitors are reserved for patients with radioactive iodine refractory disease.

2. ANSWER: C. The FDA approved lenvatinib for the treatment of locally recurrence or progressively metastatic differentiated thyroid cancer that does not respond to RAI. Lenvatinib is an inhibitor of the vascular endothelial growth factor receptor 2 (VEGFR2). Doxorubicin and cisplatin have some activity but its use is supported by low-quality evidence. Pazopanib has been studied but it is not approved yet for radioiodine refractory papillary thyroid cancer.

3. ANSWER: C. The purpose of this question is to recognize the appropriate time to initiate therapy with a kinase inhibitor in advanced MTC. Vandetanib and cabozantinib are tyrosine kinase inhibitors that are approved for the treatment of symptomatic or progressive MTC in patients with unresectable locally advanced or metastatic disease. Both were approved based on improvement in progression-free survival compared to placebo, but demonstrated no improvement in overall survival. Therefore, given the treatment-related risks, use in patients with indolent, asymptomatic, or slowly progressing disease is typically not recommended. Answer B is incorrect because we do not know the results of his imaging. Asymptomatic patients with elevated calcitonin and negative imaging should not receive vandetanib. If disease is present, there are several options to be considered depending on the disease burden and location. They include surgical resection if feasible, localized therapy such as radiofrequency ablation or chemoembolization, vandetanib, or cabozantinib therapy. Answers A and E are incorrect because MTC is derived from parafollicular or C cells. This cell type does not incorporate iodine or have TSH receptors. Therefore, TSH suppression and radioactive iodine are not effective therapies. Answer D is incorrect because while external beam radiation is sometimes used, it is not done empirically without imaging to assess for resectable disease. Further, MTC is not particularly radiosensitive. Answer C is the best answer. If his imaging is negative, his calcitonin should be repeated in 3 to 6 months. If it is stable, no further imaging is indicated. If it continues to rise, it rapidly increases, or he develops new symptoms, further imaging should be done.

4. ANSWER: D. Vandetanib, an oral inhibitor of VEGFR, RET, and epidermal growth factor receptor (EGFR) has been approved in April 2011 by the U.S. Food and Drug Administration (FDA) for the treatment of advanced (metastatic or unresectable locally advanced) medullary thyroid cancer based on an international randomized phase III trial. Median progression-free survival was improved in patients randomly assigned to vandetanib versus placebo (hazard ratio 0.45, 95% CI, 0.30 to 0.69). The overall response rate was 45%. Objective responses were durable on the basis of the median duration of response not being reached at 24 months of follow-up. Cabozantinib is another oral TKI recently approved for its clinical activity in patients with MTC. A double-blind, phase III trial comparing cabozantinib with placebo demonstrated an estimated median PFS of 11.2 months for cabozantinib versus 4.0 months for placebo. Prolonged PFS with cabozantinib was observed across all subgroups including by age, prior TKI treatment, and RET mutation status (hereditary or sporadic). Lenvatinib is approved for the treatment of radioiodine refractory differentiated thyroid cancer.

5. ANSWER: A. The purpose of this question is to recognize the appropriate time to start systemic therapy. This patient is asymptomatic from his disease and with no evidence of disease progression on repeated scans. CVD therapy is not indicated in every patient with metastatic PHEO/PGL, but should be considered in the management of patients with symptoms, with rapidly progressive disease and where tumor shrinkage might be beneficial. Targeted radiotherapy using 131-I MIBG is an option in systemic treatment for patients with progressive disease and positive MIBG scan. Radiolabelled somatostatin analogues are being investigated. There is limited data with sunitinib but limited activity has been reported. Less than 40% of patients with metastatic PHEO respond (usually partial rather than complete response) to currently used therapeutic modalities such as MIBG or chemotherapy.

6. ANSWER: B. Mutations in the succinate dehydrogenase subunit B (*SDHB*) have been linked to more aggressive tumor behavior and patients with germline SDHB mutations are more likely to present with metastatic disease than are patients with the sporadic form of PHEOs/PGL. The rate of metastasis of *SDHB*-related PHEO/PGL has been reported to be between 34% and 71%, with a 5-year survival rate of 36% after the diagnosis of metastasis. Other *SDH* mutations have approximate metastatic rates as follows: *SDHA*, 0-14%; *SDHC*, rarely malignant; *SDHD*, <5%; RET, rarely malignant; VHL, <5%.

7. ANSWER: C. This 45-year-old man has bilateral, 1.5-cm vascular and heterogeneous adrenal masses. In the contrast-enhanced CT image, the right adrenal mass appears to arise from the posterior aspect of the lateral adrenal limb; the mass in the left adrenal gland appears to occupy the body of the adrenal and has expanded it in a triangular shape. The possibility of metastatic disease to the adrenal glands should be at the top of the list of diagnostic possibilities. Metastases are the cause of adrenal incidentalomas in approximately one-half of patients who have a history of malignant disease, but account for only 0.7% to 2.5% of all adrenal incidentaloma cases. Tumors that commonly metastasize to the adrenal glands include carcinomas of the lung, kidney, colon, breast, esophagus, pancreas, liver, and stomach. Metastases to the adrenal glands are frequently bilateral. The primary malignancy is usually already recognized when an adrenal incidentaloma is discovered; metastatic cancer to the adrenal without a known primary is extremely rare. Image-guided FNA biopsy is useful to distinguish adrenal from nonadrenal tissues (e.g., metastases or infection) and is relatively safe; Because performing FNAB on a pheochromocytoma may result in hemorrhage and hypertensive crisis, biochemical testing should always be performed to exclude the possibility of this catecholamine-secreting tumor before the procedure. Although the patient does not have symptoms suggestive of a pheochromocytoma, lack of symptoms does not exclude this tumor and evaluation should be performed. Although the imaging is not suggestive of a pheochromocytoma, measurement of 24-hour urine catecholamines should still be done. Alternatively, plasma fractionated metanephrines can be measured. Additional imaging studies can be performed to evaluate adrenal incidentalomas, but they are not always necessary. Imaging with FDG may be useful in patients with a history of malignancy or in those with inconclusive adrenal CT imaging, but it is not the best next step in this vignette. In patients in whom hormonal dysfunction has been excluded and imaging characteristics yield low pretest probability for malignancy (size <4 cm, unilateral location, homogeneous density, low Hounsfield units), repeated imaging to assess for interval growth is reasonable. However, this patient has not yet had a complete hormonal evaluation and does not have low-risk imaging characteristics.

8. ANSWER: B. The purpose of this question is to understand the clinical presentation and diagnosis of Zollinger–Ellison syndrome and gastrinoma. This patient's clinical symptoms are suggestive of Zollinger–Ellison syndrome, the condition associated with a gastrinoma that is characterized by refractory peptic ulcer disease, diarrhea, and gastric hyperacidity. Patients who are suspected of gastrinoma with an elevated gastrin level should undergo a secretin stimulation test as the next step in diagnosis. Secretin stimulates secretion of gastrin from gastrinomas, but not from normal G cells. As a result, gastrin levels will rise after secretin infusion in patients with gastrinomas. A positive secretin stimulation test is generally considered a rise in gastrin of ≥200 pg/mL. After the diagnosis of gastrinoma is made, it must be localized using imaging. EUS, octreotide scan (somatostatin receptor scintigraphy), CT, and MRI are all useful imaging modalities to localize gastrinomas. ^{131}I-MIBG is structurally similar to norepinephrine and is typically used to diagnose pheochromocytomas.

9. ANSWER: D. In asymptomatic well-differentiated nonfunctional neuroendocrine tumor, the fact that it was found incidentally makes watchful waiting the best option for this patient. Everolimus and sunitinib have been shown to be effective in the treatment of advanced pancreatic neuroendocrine tumors; however, it is used when there is evidence of rapid disease progression. Debulking procedures can play a role in functional neuroendocrine tumors in order to reduce the hormone-excess causing symptoms.

10. ANSWER: D. The purpose of this question is to understand the role of mitotane for the treatment of ACC. Mitotane is an adrenocortolytic therapy with objective tumor responses seen in approximately one-third of patients with metastatic disease. Its primary benefit (achieved in approximately 75% of cases) is the reduction of symptoms related to the ectopic hormone production of these tumors. This patient has associated Cushing syndrome with weight gain, weakness, and hypertension and is therefore particularly in need of an adrenocortolytic therapy. Both streptozocin and the combination of cisplatin, doxorubicin, and etoposide (EDP) are often used with mitotane. These two regimens, in combination with mitotane, were studied head to head in a clinical trial as first-line therapy for patients with locally advanced or metastatic disease that is not amenable to surgery. EDP with mitotane was superior to streptozocin and mitotane with regard to overall response rate and progression-free survival; however, there was no overall survival advantage.

Hematopoietic Growth Factors 34

Philip M. Arlen and Andreas Niethammer

REVIEW QUESTIONS

1. Which of the following benefits of ESA has been consistently demonstrated in RCTs and meta-analyses as compared to the others?

    A. Reduced requirement for blood transfusion

    B. Decrease in symptoms related to anemia

    C. Decreased mortality in cancer patients

    D. Decreased cardiac complications related to anemia

    E. Improved quality of life

2. Who among the following is the best candidate for ESA if the goal is to reduce the need for blood transfusions?

    A. A 55-year-old female with stage II breast cancer on adjuvant chemotherapy with asymptomatic hemoglobin of 10 g/dL.

    B. A 60-year-old female with metastatic breast cancer on palliative chemotherapy with symptomatic anemia of hemoglobin 8 g/dL.

    C. A 55-year-old male with metastatic prostate cancer on palliative chemotherapy with asymptomatic anemia of hemoglobin 9 g/dL.

    D. A 50-year-old female with stage III breast cancer on adjuvant chemotherapy with asymptomatic hemoglobin level of 10.5 g/dL.

    E. None of the above.

3. Which of the following clinical cases LEAST justifies the use of G-CSF?

   A. A 50-year-old male on 12th cycle of FOLFIRI with bevacizumab for metastatic colon cancer presents with febrile neutropenia with ANC 220. He has no other complaints.

   B. A 49-year-old female with stage II triple negative breast cancer is coming to receive cycle three of dose dense AC-T. Prior cycle without G-CSF support was complicated by prolonged febrile neutropenia.

   C. A 40-year-old female with cervical cancer with history of extensive pelvic radiation presents with fever and ANC of 90. Otherwise, the patient has no complaints.

   D. A 69-year-old male with metastatic nonsmall cell lung cancer presents on cycle three of cisplatin and vinorelbine presents with febrile neutropenia and increased productive cough and shortness of breath.

   E. A 69-year-old male presenting to start induction chemotherapy with TPF for unresectable hypopharyngeal carcinoma.

4. Which of the following is the TRUE statement about the evidence concerning colony-stimulating factors?

   A. A dose-dense chemotherapy regimen supported by pegfilgrastim showed superior clinical benefit, compared with the regimen supported by filgrastim in elderly patients with aggressive lymphoma.

   B. Cochrane meta-analysis of lymphoma clinical trials showed that CSF as a primary prophylaxis reduced the risk of neutropenia, febrile neutropenia and infection, but no benefit in overall survival.

   C. Meta-analysis clinical trials of G-CSF for chemotherapy-induced febrile neutropenia showed that CSFs reduced the hospital stay, shorter time to neutrophil recovery and infection related mortality

   D. ASCO 2006 updated guideline recommends that the use of CSFs when the risk of febrile neutropenia is approximately 40%.

   E. Meta-analysis of randomized controlled trials that evaluated addition of CSFs during and following chemotherapy in patients with AML, showed that CSF decreases the occurrence of bacteremia and invasive fungal infection but no difference in all-call mortality.

ANSWERS TO REVIEW QUESTIONS

1. ANSWER: A

Explanation:

Decrease in transfusion rates is the only benefit of ESAs consistently demonstrated in RCTs and meta-analyses. Consistent evidence does not exist for the rest of the attributes provided in the choices (especially at higher hemoglobin levels). Strikingly, in the case of choice C, at least one meta-analysis of 53 pooled RCTs showed that the use of ESAs is signifcantly associated with shorter survival.

REFERENCE:

Seidenfeld J, Piper M, Bohlius J, et al. Comparative effectiveness of epoetin and darbepoetin for managing anemia in patients undergoing cancer treatment: Comparative Effectiveness Review No. 3.

2. ANSWER: C

Explanation:

As per the current guidelines and FDA label, the ESAs are best recommended for cancer-induced anemia to decrease the need of blood transfusions when the hemoglobin levels fall below 10 g/dL. Between 10 and 12 g/dL there is a lack of consistent evidence to say that ESAs would decrease transfusion requirement. There is also an emerging body of evidence that shows that ESAs are associated with significantly increased mortality. For the patient in choice B, the symptomatic anemia may warrant a blood transfusion instead for quick relief. Although there still lacks a consensus data on the use of ESA based on the intent of chemotherapy regimen, FDA labelling does restrict the use to those being treated with palliative intent.

REFERENCE:

Rizzo JD, Brouwers M, Hurley P, et al. American Society of Hematology/American Society of Clinical Oncology clinical practice guideline update on the use of epoetin and darbepoetin in adult patients with cancer. *Blood.* 2010;116:4045–4059.

3. ANSWER A:

Explanation:

Routine adjunctive use of CSF for febrile neutropenia is not recommended unless patient has risk factors for infection-associated complication, including age >65, expected prolonged neutropenia (>10 days), profound neutropenia (<100/mcl), sepsis syndrome, hospitalization, pneumonia, invasive fungal infection, or uncontrolled primary disease.

Explanation B:

The use of G-CSF may be justified as **a secondary prophylaxis.** Citron et al. showed that dose-dense regimen supported by G-CSF has superior clinical outcome. ASCO guideline recommends administering CSF to patients who had dose-limiting neutropenic event that could otherwise impact planned dose of chemotherapy from a prior cycle of chemotherapy when no CSFs were given.

Explanation C:

The use of G-CSF may be justified as a treatment of febrile neutropenia. She has febrile neutropenia with ANC that is profoundly low (<100/mcl). Profound neutropenia is one of the high-risk features.

Explanation D:

The use of G-CSF may be justified as a treatment of febrile neutropenia. Patient has febrile neutropenia and at least two high-risk features—age above 65 and likely a postobstructive pneumonia.

Explanation E:

The use of G-CSF may be justified as primary prophylaxis. TPF regimen is myelosuppressive and goal of induction therapy is curative. Patient has one high-risk feature (age above 65).

4. ANSWER: B

Explanation:

Cochrane meta-analysis reported by Bohlius J et al. concluded that CSF when used as a prophylaxis in patients with malignant lymphoma undergoing conventional chemotherapy, reduce the risk of neutropenia, febrile neutropenia, and infection (2). No evidence exists to suggest that either G-CSF or GM-CSF provides a significant advantage in terms of complete tumor response, freedom from treatment failure, or overall survival.

Explanation A:

No data exists that compared pegfilgrastim and filgrastim in this disease setting. Citron et al. reported that dose-dense regimen supported by G-CSF had superior clinical outcome compared with conventional chemotherapy in node positive breast cancer patients (1).

Explanation C:

The meta-analysis by Clark et al. showed that the overall mortality was not influenced significantly by the use of CSF (odds ratio [OR] = 0.68; 95% CI, 0.43 to 1.08; P = .1).(3) A marginally significant result was obtained for the use of CSF in reducing infection-related mortality (OR = 0.51; 95% CI, 0.26 to 1.00; P = .05). Patients treated with CSFs had a shorter length of hospitalization (hazard ratio [HR] = 0.63; 95% CI, 0.49 to 0.82; P = .0006) and a shorter time to neutrophil recovery (HR = 0.32; 95% CI, 0.23 to 0.46; P < .00001).

Explanation D:

CSFs are recommended for use with first- and subsequent-cycle chemotherapy to prevent febrile neutropenia (FN) when risk of FN is >20% (4).

Explanation E:

Gurion R et al. reported that the addition of CSFs to chemotherapy yielded no difference in all-cause mortality at 30 days and at the end of follow-up (RR 0.97; 95% CI, 0.80 to 1.18 and RR 1.01; 95% CI, 0.98 to 1.05, respectively) or in overall survival (HR 1.00; 95% 0.93 to 1.08).(5) There was no difference in complete remission rates (RR 1.03; 95% CI, 0.99 to 1.07), relapse rates (RR 0.97; 95% CI, 0.89 to 1.05) and disease-free survival (HR 1.00; 95% CI 0.90 to 1.13). CSFs did not decrease the occurrence of bacteremias (RR 0.96; 95% CI, 0.82 to 1.12), nor the occurrence of invasive fungal infections (RR 1.40; 95% CI, 0.90 to 2.19). CSFs marginally increased adverse events requiring discontinuation of CSFs as compared to the control arm (RR 1.33; 95% CI, 1.00 to 1.56).

REFERENCES:

1. Citron ML, Berry DA, Cirrincione C, et al. Randomized trial of dose-dense versus conventionally scheduled and sequential versus concurrent combination chemotherapy as postoperative adjuvant treatment of node-positive primary breast cancer: first report of Intergroup Trial C9741/ Cancer and Leukemia Group B Trial 9741. *J Clin Oncol.* 2003;21(8):1431–1439.

2. Bohlius J, Herbst C, Reiser M, Schwarzer G, Engert A. Granulopoiesis-stimulating factors to prevent adverse effects in the treatment of malignant lymphoma. *Cochrane Database Syst Rev.* 2008(4):CD003189.

3. Clark OA, Lyman GH, Castro AA, Clark LG, Djulbegovic B. Colony-stimulating factors for chemotherapy-induced febrile neutropenia: a meta-analysis of randomized controlled trials. *J Clin Oncol.* 2005;23(18):4198–4214.

4. Smith TJ, Khatcheressian J, Lyman GH, et al. 2006 update of recommendations for the use of white blood cell growth factors: an evidence-based clinical practice guideline. *J Clin Oncol.* 2006;24(19):3187–3205.

5. Gurion R, Belnik-Plitman Y, Gafter-Gvili A, et al. Colony-stimulating factors for prevention and treatment of infectious complications in patients with acute myelogenous leukemia. *Cochrane Database Syst Rev.* 2012;6:CD008238.

Infectious Complications in Oncology

35

Lekha Mikkilineni and Juan C. Gea-Banacloche

REVIEW QUESTIONS

1. A 26-year-old woman with relapse AML is undergoing consolidation with HiDAC (high-dose cytarabine). On day 10 of her chemotherapy she develops her first episode of fever (38.6°C), despite having been on prophylaxis with levofloxacin, fluconazole and acyclovir. The patient is hemodynamically stable. The physical examination reveals oropharyngeal erythema and shallow ulcers. There is *no* erythema or tenderness around her right Hickman catheter exit site or tunnel. The rest of physical examination is unremarkable. The ANC is 0.07 (70/µL). Which of the following is the best choice regarding treatment?

    A. Obtain blood cultures and start oral antibiotics.

    B. Obtain blood cultures and start IV cefepime.

    C. Obtain blood cultures and start vancomycin and cefepime.

    D. Obtain blood cultures and start vancomycin + meropenem + amikacin.

    E. Obtain blood cultures and observe for 1 hour to be sure that the fever is real.

2. The patient was started on cefepime but the fever persisted and after 48 hours her blood pressure dropped from 130/80 to 90/65, and her heart rate was 130. Blood cultures came positive for coagulase-negative *Staphylococcus* (one out of six bottles). Reviewing the records from previous hospitalizations showed that the patient was colonized with

vancomycin-resistant enterococcus (VRE) and that she had had a UTI 3 months prior caused by an ESBL-producing *Klebsiella pneumoniae*. What is the best approach at this time?

A. Add empirical antifungal treatment with amphotericin B.

B. Add an antibiotic with VRE coverage to enterococcus (e.g., linezolid) and remove the catheter.

C. Add vancomycin to the cefepime, and do not remove the catheter.

D. Add vancomycin to the cefepime, and remove the catheter.

E. Change antibiotics to meropenem and daptomycin and add caspofungin.

---

3. Cultures were positive for ESBL-producing *K. pneumoniae*. The patient's blood pressure and heart rate recovered with the new antibiotic regimen and fluid resuscitation, but the fever never went away for more than 24 hours. Five days later the patient continues to be febrile and neutropenic. The blood pressure is stable. What do you think is the best strategy at this point?

A. Maintain same antimicrobial agents until the ANC more than 0.5, unless there is further hemodynamic instability.

B. Stop daptomycin because VRE was never found in the blood and continue with meropenem.

C. Get a CT scan of the chest looking for signs of fungal infection.

D. Get a CT scan of the chest and sinuses to look for signs of fungal infection and start amphotericin B.

E. Discontinue the meropenem to test for β-lactam-induced drug fever.

---

4. A 58-year-old man patient with diffuse large B cell lymphoma (DLBCL) is about to be treated with R-CHOP (CHOP chemotherapy + rituximab). His hepatitis B serology shows HBsAb⁻ and HBcAb⁺. His liver enzymes are normal. He is not aware of having had hepatitis, and has never received blood products. What of these options is the best management?

A. Start entecavir 0.5 mg daily a week before starting chemotherapy and continue it until 3 months after completing treatment.

B. Monitor HB DNA weekly after starting chemotherapy.

C. Start lamivudine 100 mg daily a week before starting chemotherapy and continue it until 3 months after completing treatment.

D. The serology is most consistent with a falsely positive anticore antibody (HBcAb): no monitoring or preemptive treatment is indicated.

E. Obtain a HB DNA viral load now. If no HB DNA is detected no intervention is necessary.

5. A 56-year-old woman received an allogeneic bone marrow transplant 9 days ago. She was neutropenic even before transplant, so her total duration of neutropenia was 35 days. She developed a new fever (38.9° C) while receiving prophylaxis with ceftazidime, fluconazole, and acyclovir. She denied any symptoms, her blood pressure was 130/70 mmHg, heart rate 97 bpm, O_2 Sat 98% on room air. Her physical exam was unrevealing, but a CT of the chest showed four new dense, well circumscribed nodules on the lingula and left upper lobe, one of them exhibiting the halo sign. What is the best of the following management recommendations?

A. Discontinue fluconazole and start caspofungin

B. Discontinue fluconazole and start voriconazole

C. Discontinue fluconazole and start liposomal amphotericin B

D. Discontinue fluconazole and start posaconazole

E. Discontinue fluconazole, start liposomal amphotericin B and caspofungin, schedule a bronchoscopy for bronchoalveolar lavage and substitute meropenem and levofloxacin for ceftazidime.

6. A 40-year-old woman with high-risk Ph+ ALL in remission (after 4 cycles of R-hyper-CVAD and 2 of clofarabine + etoposide + cyclophosphamide) was admitted for allogeneic hematopoietic stem cell transplant (allo-HCT). She was receiving anti-infective prophylaxis with voriconazole 200 mg PO bid, azithromycin 250 mg PO daily, and acyclovir 800 mg PO bid. While in the hospital, she developed worsening cough and shortness of breath over several days. On physical exam, she is sitting comfortably with normal vital signs and O_2Sat 98% while on nasal cannula with O2 at 2 l/min. The only finding on the physical exam are diffuse fine crackles on both lungs. Her chest CT showed multifocal ground-glass opacities. A nasopharyngeal swab was positive for rhinovirus/enterovirus. Her

sputum grew light *Aspergillus niger*, 1 colony of *Penicillium* and 1 colony of *Fusarium*. Her CBC showed Hb 7.7, ANC 450/μL, Platelets 16,000 (stable after her chemotherapy). Chemistries are normal. A fungitell assay is positive (220 ng/mL, normal < 80). What of the following is the best option?

A. Obtain a voriconazole level and increase the voriconazole to 300 mg IV

B. Obtain an ABG, schedule a BAL as soon as possible and start IV TMP/SMX

C. Start piperacillin-tazobactam and vancomycin for healthcare-associated pneumonia

D. Start piperacillin-tazobactam and vancomycin for healthcare-associated pneumonia and add liposomal amphotericin B

E. Add caspofungin

7. A 31-year-old woman received an allo-HCT for her Ph+ ALL a year ago, and has been in molecular remission for the last 9 months. Unfortunately, she developed chronic extensive GVHD and is on 1 mg/kg/prednisone, tacrolimus and mycophenolate mofetil (MMF). Her anti-infective prophylaxes include voriconazole, acyclovir, and TMP/SMX. Two days after being admitted to the hospital electively to adjust her GVHD treatment, she developed right-sided pleuritic chest pain. Her CT showed multiple nodules, some of them cavitated. A Gram-stain of her BAL showed long, branching, beaded Gram-positive rods. Cultures are pending. What is the best option?

A. Start levofloxacin for community-acquired pneumonia

B. Start vancomycin and piperacillin-tazobactam and levofloxacin for healthcare-associated pneumonia

C. Start vancomycin and piperacillin-tazobactam and levofloxacin for healthcare-associated pneumonia and add amphotericin B lipid formulation

D. Start vancomycin only

E. Start meropenem, TMP/SMX, and amikacin and schedule a brain MRI with gadolinium

8. A 42-year-old woman with GATA-2 immunodeficiency and myelodysplastic syndrome underwent a matched, unrelated donor (MUD) allo-HCT. On Day 17 her routine CMV PCR became positive (4.32 Log10 UI/ml) and IV

ganciclovir 5 mg/kg/12h was started. Surprisingly, both she and her donor were CMV negative by serology. After 2 weeks of treatment the CMV viral load was 4.92 Log10 UI/mL. What is the appropriate management?

A. Continue the current treatment

B. Increase ganciclovir to 7.5 mg/kg IV q 12h

C. Switch to valganciclovir 900 mg PO bid

D. Switch to foscarnet 90 mg/kg/12h and send the CMV DNA for genotypic resistance testing

E. Switch to combination treatment ganciclovir 2.5 mg/kg/12h and foscarnet 45 mg/kg/12h and send the CMV DNA for genotypic resistance testing

9. A 42-year-old Ethiopian woman underwent cord blood allo-HCT for her Ph+ ALL. Her early course was complicated by engraftment syndrome that required steroids, aspergillosis of the lung, several urinary tract infections (Enterococcus and Klebsiella), Campylobacter jejuni colitis, Staphylococcus epidermidis CLABS and GVHD on treatment with prednisone 0.5 mg/kg/d and tacrolimus. She is on prophylaxis with voriconazole, acyclovir, and inhaled pentamidine. She is admitted with a two-day history of fever and aphasia. Her toxoplasma IgG was +. The MRI showed three lesions: left frontal lobe, left parietal lobe, and inferior aspect of the left frontal lobe with mass effect. All three are hyperintense on T2 and hypointense on T1. The CT of the chest showed a residual cavitary lesion. The laboratory studies are unrevealing except for HHV6 in blood, which was positive at 1500 copies/mL. What of these options is best regarding diagnosis and management?

A. Obtain a brain biopsy and treat accordingly

B. Start amphotericin B for aspergillosis and pyrimethamine + sulfadiazine for toxoplasmosis and repeat the MR in two weeks

C. Obtain a lumbar puncture and send cytology, flow cytometry, HHV6, toxoplasma PCR and aspergillus antigen in the CSF and treat according to the results

D. Start ganciclovir for HHV6 encephalitis

10. A 23-year-old man who just received induction chemotherapy for AML (FLAG) comes to the Day Hospital because he was 38.7 at home and he knows he is neutropenic. His only symptom is headache. On physical

exam, he is pale and diaphoretic. Temperature 40.8°C; blood pressure 124/71; heart rate 124bpm; respiratory rate 16rpm, O_2 sat 98% on room air. No focal findings. Chemistries are normal. CBC: WBC 0.12, H/H 8.5/23.5, Platelets 11000. Chest X ray is normal. You send blood cultures and start ceftazidime. One hour later, after 1000 cc of NS and his first dose of antibiotics his vital signs are repeated with blood pressure 40.2°C; blood pressure 115/59; heart rate 143 bpm; respiratory rate 28rpm; O_2 sat 98% on room air. What do you give?

A. Ceftazidime

B. Ceftazidime + amikacin

C. Ceftazidime + vancomycin

D. Piperacillin-tazobactam

E. Meropenem + vancomycin + amikacin

ANSWERS TO REVIEW QUESTIONS

1. ANSWER: C. **Obtain blood cultures and start vancomycin and cefepime.**
This patient has several risk factors for bacteremia caused by Streptococcus mitis (prophylaxis with levofloxacin, high-dose cytarabine, and severe mucositis), which may be associated with severe sepsis and ARDS. Expert opinion supports adding vancomycin to the initial regimen in this setting, although it has not proven to be beneficial. Treatment with meropenem would be an acceptable choice, as few isolates of S. mitis are resistant to meropenem.

This is high-risk neutropenic fever (prolonged, profound neutropenia) so oral antibiotics should not be used (Option A is wrong). The addition of aminoglycosides (Option D) is not appropriate in the absence of hemodynamic instability or suspected antibiotic resistance, as it has been associated with increased toxicity and not superior overall outcome than monotherapy. Finally, a temperature of 38.6° C constitutes fever and treatment should be started without delay.

2. ANSWER: E. **Change antibiotics to meropenem and daptomycin IV and add an echinocandin as empirical antifungal**
The important concept on this question is that when the patient worsens clinically (hypotension and tachycardia) the antibiotic regimen must be changed immediately to cover potentially resistant pathogens. The history of colonization with VRE and infection with a cephalosporin-resistant K. pneumoniae mandate empirical treatment of both organisms.

Changing or adding an antifungal agent with activity against Candida is appropriate but it should not be the sole intervention, as hypotension is more common with bacterial infections and fungal infection is unlikely after only two days of fever (Option A is wrong). An antibiotic with activity against VRE should be added, but there is no indication to remove the catheter since there is no evidence it is the source of the fever. A single culture bottle with coagulase-negative *Staphylococcus* suggests contamination during the blood culture draw (a colonized or infected catheter would result in multiple positive blood cultures), so Option B is wrong. Options C and D do not address the problem (hypotension during cefepime treatment) and are not acceptable.

3. ANSWER: D. **Get a CT scan of the chest and sinuses to look for signs of fungal infection and start amphotericin B.**
This question is about persistent fever during neutropenia. Persistent fever in the absence of new microbiological or clinical findings is not an indication to change the antibacterial regimen, but it is a clue that there may be a hidden fungal infection and, at a minimum, efforts to find it should be undertaken, so Options A and B are inadequate. Some authorities recommend withholding antifungal therapy in persistent fever unless there are other data suggesting fungal infection, but even if one chooses this approach just a CT of the chest is not sufficient diagnostic workup, so Option C is also insufficient. Option E is wrong: stopping antibiotics during persistent fever in neutropenic patients was associated with septic shock and death in early trials in the 1980s.

4. ANSWER: A. Start entecavir 0.5 mg daily a week before starting chemotherapy and continue it until 3 months after completing treatment. The answer to this question is based on a randomized controlled trial (Huang H. et al. *JAMA*. 2014;312: 2521–2530) that proved entecavir superior to lamivudine (Option C is wrong). Even patients with undetectable HBV DNA were at risk of Hepatitis B reactivation, so d and e are wrong. As reactivation of HBV can result in fulminant liver failure and death, b is not recommended by the current guidelines.

5. ANSWER: E. Discontinue fluconazole, start liposomal amphotericin B and caspofungin, schedule a bronchoscopy for bronchoalveolar lavage and substitute meropenem and levofloxacin for ceftazidime. The best approach in this setting is not known so our recommendation of Option E is strictly "expert opinion." Given the prolonged neutropenia the patient is at high risk for mold infection (most commonly aspergillus) and has a typical presentation with fever, no systemic toxicity, and four pulmonary nodules described as "dense and well circumscribed," one of them with a characteristic (if not pathognomonic) halo sign. Options A through D are insufficient because they do not include any diagnostic intervention. Furthermore one may argue both with the antifungal choice (Options A and B would not treat mucormycosis, which is a less likely but possible cause of this clinical picture) and the fact that none of them modifies the antibacterial coverage, which in clinical practice would most likely be changed.

6. ANSWER: B. Obtain an ABG, schedule a BAL as soon as possible and start IV TMP/SMX. This patient with severe compromise of her T cell immunity after her chemotherapy, shortness of breath, diffuse crackles, and multifocal ground glass opacities is likely to have Pneumocystis jirovecii pneumonia (PJP or PCP), and Option B is the only that addresses this concern (hence the best option). The fungitell assay is typically positive in PCP. In many cases in clinical practice other antibiotics may be started for possible hospital-acquired pneumonia (Options C and D) but the possibility of PCP must be addressed. Invasive mold infection is not a real concern in this case: despite the findings in the sputum culture, the patient does not have profound neutropenia (making Fusarium highly unlikely) and the CT does not support mold infection. Furthermore, Aspergillus niger and Penicillium almost never cause disease.

7. ANSWER: E. Start meropenem, TMP/SMX, and amikacin and schedule a brain MRI with gadolinium. This patient had Nocardia infection (as revealed by the Gram stain of the sputum and subsequent modified AFB stain). The point of this question is to remind the reader of nocardiosis, which may happen in immunocompromised patients (particularly transplant recipients and those taking corticosteroids) and is NOT prevented by TMP/SMX at the doses usually given to prevent PCP. Susceptibility to antibiotics may be predicted once the species is identified, but to be certain one is covering it and until final identification and suscepti-bilities are available the combination of meropenem, TMP/SMX, and amikacin is appropriate (linezolid could be substituted for amikacin). Nocardia is not a nosocomial infection and typically presents subacutely, so it is safe to assume the patient brought it with her to the hospital. There is risk of disseminated infection (preferentially to the brain) so an MRI with gadolinium to look for abscess is indicated.

8. ANSWER: A. Continue the current treatment.

CMV infection when both recipient and donor are CMV negative by serology is distinctively uncommon (2% to 4%) when leukodepleted blood products are used. The point of the question, however, is that controlling CMV may take time (probably longer in the setting of what must be considered primary infection) and that a persistently high virus level that is not increasing is not an indication for either changing treatment of ordering genotypic testing (Options D and E are wrong). Ganciclovir and foscarnet are considered equally effective against CMV, the choice is based on the risk of toxicity (bone mar-row suppression with ganciclovir, nephrotoxicity with foscarnet), so Option D is wrong. The combination of both at reduced doses was attempted on a trial and shown to be less effective and more toxic (Option E is wrong). There is no reason to increase the ganciclovir dose or to switch to valganciclovir, which is just the prodrug of ganciclovir (Options B and C are wrong).

9. ANSWER: C. Obtain a lumbar puncture and send HHV6, toxoplasma PCR, and aspergillus antigen in the CSF and treat according to the results

There is no evidence-based answer for this question, but c is probably the best answer. The main considerations in this case are toxoplasmosis (due to the IgG+ recipient, cord transplant, and lack of systemic prophylaxis by using inhaled pentamidine instead of TMP/SMX), aspergillosis (due to the history, but unlikely while the patient is receiving voriconazole) and leukemia. Option B, commonly used in AIDS patients, has no role in this setting. One cannot argue with a brain biopsy (Option A) except because it carries higher morbid-ity than a lumbar puncture, which may be diagnostic. If the CSF is not diag-nostic, a biopsy is indicated. HHV6 does not present with aphasia or lesions with mass effect, and treatment would not be indicated in the absence of a positive PCR in the CSF (Option D is wrong).

10. ANSWER: E. Meropenem + vancomycin + amikacin

This is a very straightforward question: the patient shows signs of sep-sis, so expanded antibacterial and antifungal coverage are mandatory. More important (but not mentioned in the options) is transfer to the ICU for aggres-sive fluid resuscitation and pressors.

Oncologic Emergencies and Paraneoplastic Syndromes 36

Meena Sadaps and James P. Stevenson

REVIEW QUESTIONS

1. Which of the following statements regarding SVC syndrome is INCORRECT?

   A. Common symptoms include dyspnea and facial swelling

   B. SVCS is a clinical diagnosis

   C. Tissue diagnosis should precede further treatment in nonemergent cases

   D. Complete occlusion of the SVC is a contraindication to stent placement

   E. Indwelling venous catheters do not have to be removed if SVCS is detected early

2. Which of the following measures can be used to reduce intracranial pressure?

   A. Elevation of the head of the bed above 30 degrees

   B. Osmotic diuresis

   C. Dexamethasone

   D. Mechanical hyperventilation

   E. All of the above

3. A 60-year-old male with multiple myeloma presents with back pain and lower extremity weakness of two days duration. The back pain is described as being of maximum intensity upon awakening in the morning. What is the most sensitive imaging modality to make the diagnosis?

   A. CT myelography

   B. CT spine

   C. MRI with contrast

   D. Lumbar puncture

   E. X-ray of spine

4. What common metabolic abnormality can be seen in patients with elevated ICP?

   A. Hypokalemia

   B. Hyperkalemia

   C. Hyponatremia

   D. Hypernatremia

   E. Hypocalcemia

5. A 48-year-old female with Burkitt lymphoma who has recently been started on a multiagent immunochemotherapy regimen presents after labwork incidentally noted uric acid of 7 mg/dl, calcium of 6 mg/dl, and phosphorus of 6.7 mg/dl. Patient is asymptomatic. What is the recommended treatment for the patient's hypocalcemia?

   A. Calcium gluconate 1g, administered slowly

   B. Calcium acetate 667 mg TID

   C. Sodium polystyrene sulfonate 15 g

   D. Allopurinol 300 mg

   E. Dialysis

6. Which electrolyte abnormality is NOT seen in tumor lysis syndrome?

   A. Hypokalemia

   B. Hyperuricemia

   C. Hyperphosphatemia

D. Hypocalcemia

E. Elevated lactate dehydrogenase (LDH)

7. Ectopic ADH production is most commonly associated with which of the following malignancies:

    A. Head and neck squamous cell carcinoma

    B. Nonsmall cell lung cancer

    C. Breast cancer

    D. Small cell lung cancer

    E. Non-Hodgkin's lymphoma

8. A 46-year-old female with breast cancer presents with hypercalcemia that has been resistant to bisphosphonate therapy. What is the next step in management?

    A. Plicamycin

    B. Calcitonin

    C. Hospice/Comfort Care

    D. Gallium nitrate

    E. Denosumab

9. A 30-year-old female with angiosarcoma of the breast presents to the emergency department with a temperature of 102° F and neutrophil count that reads "too few to count." She has no other past medical history and review of systems is otherwise negative. Blood and urine cultures are drawn and CXR is normal. What is the next step in management?

    A. Discharge home with 7 day course of ciprofloxacin and augmentin and close outpatient follow-up

    B. Discharge home with no antibiotics and close outpatient follow-up

    C. Admit to the hospital for IV zosyn until cultures result

    D. Admit to the hospital for IV vancomycin and zosyn until cultures result

    E. Admit to the hospital for IV zosyn and PO fluconazole until cultures result

10. What scoring system is used to stratify patients with febrile neutropenia as either low risk or high risk?

    A. Cairo and Bishop classification

    B. MASCC index

    C. Gleason grading system

    D. Nottingham score

    E. Karnofsky score

ANSWERS TO REVIEW QUESTIONS

1. ANSWER: D. Complete occlusion of the SVC is NOT a contraindication for stent placement.

2. ANSWER: E. All of the aforementioned interventions may be used to help decrease ICP.

3. ANSWER: C. MRI with contrast of the spine is the most sensitive diagnostic imaging study for malignant cord compression.

4. ANSWER: C. Patients with elevated ICP are commonly noted to have hyponatremia in the setting of SIADH.

5. ANSWER: B. The hypocalcemia should resolve after treating the underlying hyperphosphatemia with phosphate binders. Furthermore, the patient is asymptomatic from the hypocalcemia, further confirming that targeted treatment is not necessary at this time.

6. ANSWER: A. Patients with tumor lysis syndrome are noted to have hyperkalemia due to the release of intracellular potassium with cell lysis.

7. ANSWER: D. Ectopic ADH production is most commonly seen with small cell lung cancer.

8. ANSWER: E. Denosumab is used in the treatment for bisphosphonate-refractory malignant hypercalcemia.

9. ANSWER: A. This patient can be treated as an outpatient with oral antibiotics given her MASCC risk index score is greater than 21, placing her at low risk of complications.

10. ANSWER: B. The MASCC risk index score is used to stratify febrile neutropenic patients as either low risk or high risk. This then helps to determine further management.

Psychopharmacologic Management in Oncology 37

Donald L. Rosenstein, Maryland Pao, Sheryl B. Fleisch, and Daniel E. Elswick

REVIEW QUESTIONS

1. Which of the following antidepressants would be the safest choice for a patient with breast cancer taking tamoxifen?

    A. Citalopram

    B. Venlafaxine

    C. Paroxetine

    D. Fluoxetine

2. A 67-year-old male is receiving interferon-α for metastatic melanoma. He develops pneumonia and is admitted to the inpatient oncology service. He begins treatment with IV antibiotics and shows improvement over 2 days of admission. He becomes confused on the third day of admission with agitation, difficulty sleeping, and fluctuating level of consciousness. He is afebrile and hemodynamically stable. What should be done next?

    A. Start a low dose of alprazolam as needed for sleep and agitation.

    B. Schedule low-dose haloperidol just prior to bedtime.

    C. Change the patient's antibiotic regimen.

    D. Review the patient's medication list and systematically look for medical causes of the confusion.

3. Which of the following is true regarding initiation of psychopharmacology for cancer patients?

   A. There are established guidelines from the NCCN that outline decision making for treating mood and anxiety disorders and other forms of psychological distress.

   B. Only a psychiatrist should start psychoactive medications.

   C. Only a psychiatrist with psycho-oncology training should start medications.

   D. There are no clear guidelines for treating mood and anxiety disorders.

4. A 78-year-old male with advanced pancreatic cancer has been struggling with his diagnosis and treatment. He has had severe abdominal pain, which has been difficult to control and has essentially stopped eating over the past few weeks. He feels burdensome to his wife and daughter and becomes more detached from those around him. His family is concerned because he has made several statements that he does not feel he deserves to live anymore and his cancer is a "punishment for his life sins." What would be most important in assessing the patient's risk for self-harm?

   A. His current functional status

   B. Any past history of self-harm

   C. His current medications

   D. His financial status

5. Which of the following agents would be a reasonable first choice for Interferon-alpha associated depression?

   A. Propranolol

   B. Haloperidol

   C. Paroxetine

   D. Alprazolam

ANSWERS TO REVIEW QUESTIONS

1. ANSWER: B. Tamoxifen is broken down to its active metabolite, endoxifen, by cytochrome P-450 2D6. Many antidepressants have an inhibitory effect on 2D6 substrates and therefore could potentially inhibit the conversion to endoxifen. Venlafaxine (Effexor) has minimal inhibitory effect at 2D6 and would be the best antidepressant choice in this patient. Paroxetine or fluoxetine would be a poor choice as they are potent inhibitors at 2D6.

2. ANSWER: D. Delirium is an acute disturbance of consciousness with reduced ability to focus, sustain, or shift attention. Patients may demonstrate an array of symptoms including changes in cognition, memory deficits, disorientation, speech/language disturbances, delusions, and perceptual abnormalities. A medical workup is required as delirium, by definition, has an underlying medical or neurologic cause. Haloperidol would be a reasonable choice for management of agitation in a patient without contraindications such as QTc prolongation or other cardiovascular risk factors. BZDs such as lorazepam should generally be reserved for delirium related to alcohol or BZD withdrawal. The Academy of Psychosomatic Medicine has an online monograph on evidence-based management of delirium available at: http://www.apm.org/library/monographs/delirium/APM-EACLPP_DeliriumMonograph.pdf.

3. ANSWER: A. There are established National Comprehensive Cancer Network Guidelines that are helpful for establishing a strategy for identifying and treating distress among cancer patients including depression and anxiety. These guidelines are updated frequently and are available through the NCCN website.

4. ANSWER: B. The patient's age and gender are major contributors to risk factors for self-harm. The strongest predictor of self-harm is a prior history of self-harm. The other issues listed such as his financial status or his medications could potentially contribute to self-harm but are not as predictive as prior history. Recent data suggest a correlation to receiving a diagnosis of cancer and suicide, with highest risk of suicide in the first 4 weeks of cancer diagnosis. Highest rates of suicide in cancer patients are seen in advanced esophageal, pancreatic, liver, and lung cancer.

5. ANSWER: C. Paroxetine is a selective serotonin reuptake inhibitor (SSRI) which is commonly used for major depressive disorder and anxiety disorders and other associated psychiatric conditions. Paroxetine (and other SSRIs) has shown benefit in ameliorating the psychiatric symptoms associated with Interferon-alpha. Haloperidol is an antipsychotic that is used for delirium and psychosis and alprazolam (a benzodiazepine) is indicated for anxiety disorders. Propranolol is a beta-blocker that has shown some benefit for anxiety in addition to hypertension.

Management of Emesis 38

David R. Kohler

REVIEW QUESTIONS

The following questions reference evidence-based consensus guidelines published by the American Society of Clinical Oncology (ASCO)[1,2], the Multinational Association of Supportive Care in Cancer (MASCC) and the European Society of Medical Oncology (ESMO)[3], and the National Comprehensive Cancer Network® (NCCN)[4] for preventing and treating emetic symptoms in patients who receive antineoplastic medical and radiation therapies.

1. A 57-year-old female with breast cancer returns to the outpatient clinic to receive her first cycle of adjuvant chemotherapy with docetaxel 75 mg/m^2, doxorubicin 50 mg/m^2, and cyclophosphamide 50 mg/m^2. All three drugs are administered intravenously on the first day of a 3-week cycle. Which of the following regimens is most consistent with antiemetic primary prophylaxis recommended by MASCC/ESMO, ASCO, and NCCN guidelines?

    A. A single dose of dolasetron 100 mg PO + dexamethasone 20 mg PO + fosaprepitant 150 mg IV prior to chemotherapy.

    B. Any serotonin (5-HT$_3$)-receptor antagonist + dexamethasone 20 mg PO prior to chemotherapy + a 3-day regimen of aprepitant (125 mg PO on day 1 before chemotherapy, then 80 mg/day PO days 2 and 3).

    C. Palonosetron 0.25 mg IV + fosaprepitant 115 mg IV + dexamethasone 12 mg IV on day 1, followed by dexamethasone 8 mg/day PO on days 2 and 3.

    D. Granisetron 2 mg PO + dexamethasone 12 mg PO + fosaprepitant 150 mg IV prior to chemotherapy, followed by dexamethasone 8 mg/day PO for one dose on day 2, then dexamethasone 8 mg twice daily on days 3 and 4.

E. Ondansetron 24 mg IV + rolapitant 180 mg PO prior to chemotherapy.

---

2. At presentation in clinic, the same patient's height and weight are measured. Her height is 170.2 cm (67 inches); current weight is 110 kg (243 lb.).

    A pretreatment analysis of serum chemistries revealed the following (results outside of normal ranges identified by up and down arrows):

Na	↓ 130 mmol/L	Albumin	↓ 2.2 mg/dL
K	3.2 mmol/L	Ca	↓ 1.95 mmol/L
Cl	↓ 93 mmol/L	Mg	↓ 0.58 mmol/L
Total CO$_2$	27 mmol/L	P	3.4 mg/dL
BUN	11 mg/dL	Alkaline phosphatase	92 U/L
creatinine	↓ 0.52 mg/dL	ALT	22 U/L
glucose	↑ 226 mg/dL	AST	↑ 43 U/L
		Total bilirubin	0.4 mg/dL
		Total protein	6.6 g/dL

Her medical history includes the following:

1. Type 2 diabetes managed with extended-release metformin 2000 mg daily

2. Hypertension controlled with losartan 100 mg + hydrochlorothiazide 12.5 mg/day

3. A 2-year history of depression for which she takes controlled-release paroxetine 50 mg daily

What factors should the patient's health care providers take into consideration in selecting antiemetic agents?

A. Dexamethasone should be excluded from her antiemetic regimen to prevent exacerbating hyperglycemia.

B. A potential for pharmacokinetic drug interactions between paroxetine and both 5-HT$_3$-receptor antagonists (dolasetron, ondansetron, palonosetron) and rolapitant.

C. Recommendations for empiric antiemetic doses (not based on body weight) should be doubled to compensate for obesity.

D. A potential for adverse pharmacokinetic and pharmacodynamic drug interactions between 5-HT$_3$-receptor antagonists (dolasetron, granisetron, ondansetron, palonosetron) and paroxetine.

E. Choices B and D.

3. In addition to the emetogenicity of antineoplastic treatment, what patient-specific factors place the patient at increased risk for sub-optimal emetic control?

    A. Co-morbid pathologies associated with diabetes

    B. Female sex

    C. Depressive disorder

    D. History of motion sickness

    E. Difficulty with emesis during pregnancy

    F. Chronic constipation

4. A 20-year-old male with a recent diagnosis of nonseminomatous germ cell tumor presents for his first course of BEP chemotherapy (bleomycin 30 Units/dose IV for 3 doses on days 1, 8, and 15 + etoposide 100 mg/m^2 per day IV for 5 consecutive days, on days 1 to 5 + cisplatin 20 mg/m^2 per day IV for 5 consecutive days, on days 1 to 5). What anti-emetic regimen would you choose for primary prophylaxis?

    A. Aprepitant 125 mg PO on day 1 before chemotherapy, then 80 mg/day PO on days 2 to 5 with granisetron 2 mg/day PO + dexamethasone 20 mg/day PO both given before chemotherapy for 5 days on days 1 to 5.

    B. Any 5-HT$_3$ receptor antagonist daily before chemotherapy for 5 days + fosaprepitant 150 mg/dose IV for 3 doses on days 1, 3, and 5, prior to chemotherapy.

    C. Dexamethasone 12 mg/day IV for 5 days on days 1 to 5 prior to chemotherapy, then 8 mg/day PO for 3 days on days 6 to 8 + palonosetron 0.25 mg/dose IV for 3 doses on days 1, 3, and 5, before chemotherapy.

    D. Granisetron 34.3 mg transdermal patch applied 24 hours before starting chemotherapy and left in place for 7 days (one day after completing emetogenic chemotherapy) + dexamethasone 12 mg/day PO for 5 days on days 1 to 5 prior to chemotherapy, then 8 mg/day PO for 3 days on days 6 to 8 + aprepitant 125 mg PO on day 1 before chemotherapy, then 80 mg/day PO on days 2 to 5.

    E. Any 5-HT$_3$ receptor antagonist daily before chemotherapy for 5 days + aprepitant 125 mg PO on day 1, then 80 mg/day PO on days 2 and 3 before chemotherapy + dexamethasone 8 mg PO daily for 8 days.

5. A 41-year-old female with ovarian cancer presents to the outpatient clinic for a second cycle of carboplatin AUC = 4 mg/mL·min (dosed to achieve systemic exposure consistent with an estimated area under the plasma concentration vs. time curve [AUC]) and docetaxel 75 mg/m^2, both drugs administered intravenously, sequentially, on the first day of a 21-day cycle. The patient's previous (first) treatment cycle was complicated by facial flushing, nausea, and shortness of breath during docetaxel administration. Docetaxel administration was transiently interrupted until symptoms abated, and then resumed at a slower administration rate without recurrent symptoms. Although the patient achieved complete protection from vomiting during the first 24 hours after treatment, she reported experiencing three vomiting episodes during the two days after she received chemotherapy and nausea that persisted throughout the week after treatment in spite of having received outpatient prescriptions appropriate for prophylaxis against delayed symptoms for a moderately emetogenic risk treatment regimen. However, you learn when she returns to clinic for a second cycle of chemotherapy, she had not had her antiemetic prescriptions filled and did not continue antiemetic prophylaxis as planned during the three days that followed her last treatment. The patient's medical history is significant for a history of severe and persistent nausea and vomiting during the first and second trimesters of pregnancy and episodes of motion sickness as a function of where she is seated when traveling by automobile and when she participated in boating excursions during family vacations. Would you modify the patient's antiemetic regimen to prevent or manage persistent symptoms after chemotherapy, and, if so, in what way?

A. Do nothing to modify the previous strategy for antiemetic prophylaxis, but discuss with the patient how compliance with plans for antiemetic prophylaxis while she is an outpatient is an essential part of treatment for her neoplastic disease by preventing debilitating and serious complications associated with uncontrolled emetic symptoms, and doing so improves the likelihood she will be able to complete treatment without compromising her ability to tolerate chemotherapy with respect to doses and scheduling.

B. Consider escalating the aggressiveness of antiemetic prophylaxis to a regimen appropriate for highly emetogenic treatment.

C. Consider adding an anxiolytic before starting chemotherapy and as needed during treatment to prevent the patient from developing anticipatory symptoms.

D. Use the antiemetic regimen previously employed, but add an anticholinergic agent to mitigate symptoms related to motion sickness.

E. Add a dopaminergic (D_2)-receptor antagonist during antineoplastic treatment and for 3 days afterward to "saturate" neuroreceptors unaffected by previously used antiemetics.

6. A 55-year-old female with high-grade astrocytoma returns to your facility to begin her third of seven planned weeks of external beam radiation therapy (RT; 2-Gy fractions, daily for 5 d/wk). Concurrently, she receives temozolomide 140 mg (75 mg/m^2) orally daily, continually, and ondansetron 16 mg orally, daily, for antiemetic prophylaxis. The patient had received antiemetic primary prophylaxis with dexamethasone 4 mg orally, daily, during her first week of treatment in combination with ondansetron 8 mg/day orally, which continued after the 5-day course of dexamethasone was completed, but after experiencing nausea during her second week of temozolomide + RT, her ondansetron dose was increased to 16 mg daily. She presents now with a complaint of persistent nausea not relieved by ondansetron. Which among the following pharmacological interventions would you offer?

   A. Give prochlorperazine 10 mg PO every 6 hours as needed, in addition to ondansetron.

   B. Replace ondansetron with granisetron 2 mg PO daily.

   C. Give olanzapine 10 mg daily PO in addition to ondansetron.

   D. Replace ondansetron with granisetron 2 mg PO daily, and add olanzapine 5 mg PO daily.

   E. Resume giving dexamethasone 4 mg PO daily throughout the remaining duration of RT + temozolomide (approximately 5 weeks) in addition to daily ondansetron.

7. A 58-year-old male with advanced pancreatic ductal adenocarcinoma is to receive adjuvant chemotherapy after pancreatoduodenectomy (Whipple procedure). He presents for combination chemotherapy with oxaliplatin 85 mg/m^2 IV over 2 hours followed by irinotecan 180 mg/m^2 IV over 30 min + leucovorin calcium 400 mg/m^2 IV followed by fluorouracil 400 mg/m^2 by IV injection or short-duration infusion, followed by fluorouracil 2400 mg/m^2 by continuous IV infusion over 46 hours.

The patient's history is significant for the following:

1. Obesity. The patient has lost almost 15 kg in body weight since his diagnosis and surgery, but current body weight and body mass index are 265.5 kg and 38.1 kg/m^2, respectively.

2. A recent DVT treated with warfarin; however, warfarin was discontinued and replaced with enoxaparin 5 days before starting chemotherapy to avoid interaction with fluorouracil.

3. A history of alcohol abuse for approximately 11 years prior to diagnosis of malignant disease.

Following ASCO, MASCC/ESMO, and NCCN guidelines, what antiemetic primary prophylaxis would you provide for this patient?

A. Palonosetron 0.25 mg IV + Rolapitant 180 mg PO + Dexamethasone 8 mg PO on day 1, then Dexamethasone 8 mg/day PO on days 2 to 4

B. Granisetron 10 mg subcutaneously + Dexamethasone 8 mg PO on day 1 + Olanzapine 10 mg PO daily for 4 days starting on day 1

C. Netupitant 300 mg + palonosetron 0.5 mg PO + Dexamethasone 12 mg PO on day 1, then Dexamethasone 8 mg/day PO on days 2 to 4

D. Granisetron 0.1 mg/kg IV + Fosaprepitant 150 mg IV + Dexamethasone 12 mg PO on day 1 + Dexamethasone 8 mg PO once on day 2, then Dexamethasone 8 mg PO twice daily on days 3 and 4

E. Granisetron 2 mg PO + Rolapitant 180 mg PO + Dexamethasone 20 mg PO on day 1, followed by Dexamethasone 8 mg PO twice daily on days 2 and 3

8. With respect to the patient previously described, are there factors that weigh in favor or against his potential response to antiemetic prophylaxis?

A. As a result of age-related senescence, persons approaching their seventh decade of life and older individuals are at greater risk for incomplete emetic control than younger adults.

B. Overweight and obese patients may respond less well to antiemetics given at fixed doses rather than doses calculated as a function of weight.

C. The patient's history of ethanol use favors better antiemetic control than a person without a similar history.

D. Males are less likely than females to achieve complete control of emetic symptoms.

E. Choices B and D

9. A 44-year-old female with an obvious neck mass returns to your clinic for medical care. The patient's disease was diagnosed 7 months prior to her current visit by fine-needle aspiration as consistent with medullary thyroid cancer, but the patient refused surgery at that time and was lost to follow-up. Her voice is hoarse and she complains of some discomfort when swallowing. Workup reveals disease extension beyond the thyroid involving the esophagus to the left of midline and left recurrent laryngeal nerve, but the patient's airway is patent. Again, the patient adamantly states she wishes to avoid surgery, but will accept medical treatment if it does not involve intravenous medications.

She accepts starting treatment with vandetanib 300 mg/day orally, continually, and loperamide as needed for treatment of loose stools and diarrhea, which commonly occur during vandetanib use.

Serum chemistries are found within normal limits prior to starting treatment. A baseline ECG evaluation is unremarkable, and her QT interval (Fridericia corrected) is 432 ms.

What if any antiemetic primary prophylaxis will you prescribe for the patient?

A. Ondansetron dispersible tablets 8 mg PO daily, PRN

B. Metoclopramide 20 mg/day PO 60 minutes before vandetanib + Metoclopramide 10 mg PO every 6 hours PRN

C. Prochlorperazine 10 mg/day PO 60 minutes before vandetanib + Prochlorperazine 10 mg PO every 6 hours PRN

D. Lorazepam 1 mg sublingually every 6 hours PRN

E. Dronabinol 5 mg PO every 8 hours PRN

10. A 74-year-old male diagnosed with stage IIIB small cell lung cancer (T3N2M0) is to receive combination chemotherapy with etoposide 120 mg/m^2 per day for 3 consecutive days (days 1, 2, and 3) and cisplatin 60 mg/m^2 IV over 60 minutes (day 1) every 3 weeks for a total of at least

4 cycles concurrently with thoracic external beam radiation therapy (1.5-Gy fractions, twice daily for 30 fractions weeks 1, 2, and 3).

The patient is to receive antiemetic primary prophylaxis each day chemotherapy and radiation therapy are to be administered, consisting of

Cycle 1 (concurrent chemotherapy and radiation):

Netupitant 300 mg + Palonosetron 0.5 mg PO; Dexamethasone 12 mg PO on day 1; followed by Dexamethasone 8 mg/day PO on days 2, 3, and 4

Prochlorperazine 10 mg PO one hour before each radiation fraction starting on day 5 (day 5, days 8 to 12, and days 15 to 19)

Cycles 2, 3, and 4 (chemotherapy alone):

Netupitant 300 mg + Palonosetron 0.5 mg PO; Dexamethasone 12 mg PO on day 1; followed by Dexamethasone 8 mg/day PO on days 2, 3, and 4

Prochlorperazine 10 mg IV over 30 minutes as needed for breakthrough symptoms

Unfortunately an error in medication administration occurred on the first day of treatment resulting in omission of the planned dose of cisplatin. In remediation for the error, cisplatin is to be given on the second day during the first chemotherapy cycle.

Would you modify the antiemetic regimen for cycle 1, and, if so, in what way?

A. Continue as originally planned without modifying antiemetic prophylaxis planned for the first treatment cycle.

B. Repeat the dose of netupitant 300 mg + palonosetron 0.5 mg PO on day 2.

C. Give Dexamethasone 12 mg instead of an 8-mg dose on day 2.

D. Add to the regimen for cycle 1 olanzapine 10 mg/day PO for 4 days starting on day 2.

E. Give a single dose of a first-generation 5-HT$_3$-receptor antagonist on day 2 before resuming chemotherapy.

ANSWERS TO REVIEW QUESTIONS

1. ANSWER OPTION D: Granisetron 2 mg PO + dexamethasone 12 mg PO + fosaprepitant 150 mg IV prior to chemotherapy, followed by dexamethasone 8 mg/day PO for one dose on day 2, then dexamethasone 8 mg twice daily on days 3 and 4.

DISCUSSION

Combination chemotherapy that includes doxorubicin (an anthracycline) and cyclophosphamide (an "AC" regimen) is categorized by current ASCO, MASCC/ESMO, and NCCN guidelines as presenting high emetic risk. Although docetaxel is also emetogenic, albeit categorized among drugs associated with low emetic risk, guideline-driven recommendations advise prophylaxis appropriate for the most emetogenic component of treatment; therefore, antiemetic prophylaxis appropriate for treatment with high emetic risk is indicated, which includes combination of 5-HT$_3$- and NK$_1$-receptor antagonists with dexamethasone appropriate for preventing emetic symptoms during the acute and delayed phases.

> **Option A** limits glucocorticoid use to only the first day of treatment, which deviates from all three guidelines' recommendations for delayed phase prophylaxis. In addition, concurrent use of aprepitant (or fosaprepitant) with dexamethasone increases the steroid's bioavailability; therefore, a 20 mg dose of dexamethasone in combination with fosaprepitant substantially exceeds the 12 mg dose recommended by MASCC/ESMO, ASCO, and NCCN guidelines.

> **Option B** complies with the components of acute phase prophylaxis. Again, however, a 20 mg of dexamethasone in combination with aprepitant on day 1 exceeds the 12 mg dose recommended by all three guidelines. In addition, dexamethasone was omitted on the days after chemotherapy, which deviates from all three guidelines' recommendations for delayed phase prophylaxis.

> Acute phase prophylaxis described in **Option C** closely resembles all three guidelines' recommendations for acute phase prophylaxis, but a 115 mg dose of fosaprepitant prior to chemotherapy given on a single day followed by aprepitant orally for two additional days is no longer supported by FDA-approved labeling for fosaprepitant or in the guidelines' recommendations for use of fosaprepitant and aprepitant. The addition of dexamethasone on days 2 and 3 (omitting day 4) is similar to ASCO, MASCC/ESMO, and NCCN guidance.

> **Option D** most closely complies with all three professional guidelines by including fosaprepitant on an administration schedule appropriate for the dose administered; granisetron at a dose appropriate for the formulation identified and administration limited to a single dose prior to chemotherapy; and dexamethasone given at a dose appropriate for use with fosaprepitant, and on a schedule and duration of use consistent with ASCO and NCCN guidelines.

> **Option E** eliminates entirely the glucocorticoid component of prophylaxis recommended by all three guidelines for the day of treatment and subsequently, and describes a dose of ondansetron that

exceeds the FDA warnings against intravenously administered single doses >16 mg to prevent serious adverse effects on cardiac electrophysiology.

2. ANSWER OPTION E CHOICES B AND D

DISCUSSION

Dexamethasone and other steroids given systemically for antiemetic prophylaxis often destabilize blood glucose control in diabetic patients, more so in patients whose blood glucose is not well controlled before receiving steroid medications. Increased lability in blood glucose control does not, however, preclude high-potency glucocorticoid use in an antiemetic regimen, but requires more intensive blood glucose monitoring and adjusting and supplementing antidiabetic medications during steroid use, and, subsequently, carefully withdrawing any antidiabetic drugs added or used in place of a patient's home (prechemotherapy) medications to control blood glucose after steroids are discontinued and until blood glucose again stabilizes to within goals for glycemic control. Therefore, an absolute prohibition such as that described in **Option A** is unnecessary as long as healthcare providers and patients recognize the need for more intensive blood glucose monitoring and altering antidiabetic treatment to maintain glycemic control during steroid use.

Option B is correct. Paroxetine is a substrate and potent inhibitor of the cytochrome P450 (CYP) CYP2D6 enzyme, the primary catalyst for phase I metabolism of palonosetron and hydrodolasetron, dolasetron's active metabolite. The HT$_3$-receptor antagonist, rolapitant, should also be avoided for as long as the patient is using paroxetine. Although not a substrate for metabolism by CYP2D6, rolapitant moderately inhibits CYP2D6, and may potentially decrease the rate at which paroxetine is metabolized and eliminated. The rate at which substrates for CYP2D6 are metabolized is often described as "capacity limited" by virtue of two or more substrates in competition, or an amount of one or more substrates that overwhelm enzyme availability. Therefore, the half-life of one or more drugs competing for metabolism catalyzed by CYP2D6 may be substantially increased and, consequently, pharmacodynamic effects associated with pharmacologically active substrates may be exaggerated and persist for unpredictably lengthy periods due to protracted elimination. Ondansetron also is a substrate for CYP2D6, but like palonosetron, it is a substrate for phase I metabolism through alternative catalysts, including CYP3A4, a high-capacity enzyme.

It is unsafe and, therefore, not possible to temporarily discontinue paroxetine during antineoplastic treatment as a means to avoid interaction with other CYP2D6 substrates. Rapid dose decreases and abrupt discontinuation of paroxetine have been associated with a withdrawal syndrome characterized by a variety of severe somatic, psychiatric, and neurological adverse effects.

With respect to **Option C,** there is presently no evidence supporting dose or schedule modification of empirically dosed antiemetics based on extremes of body weight. Among high potency glucocorticoids and 5-HT$_3$- and NK$_1$-receptor antagonists, the safest and most effective antiemetics in clinical use, recommendations for weight-based dosing appear in FDA-approved product labeling only for ondansetron and granisetron, and, with respect to intravenously administered ondansetron, labeling includes warnings against exceeding 16 mg for single doses.

Option D also is correct. Paroxetine use has been associated with aberrations in cardiac electrophysiology including prolongation of ventricular repolarization and, in combination with other CYP2D6 substrate drugs with similar deleterious effects on cardiac conduction, has been implicated in causing torsades de pointes. Both dolasetron and ondansetron have been associated with cardiac QT interval prolongation, which is the basis for contraindications and warnings that appear in current labeling for both products. The potential for serious abnormal arrhythmias is increased by electrolyte abnormalities including hypokalemia and hypomagnesemia and by paroxetine's potential for altering the elimination of 5-HT$_3$-receptor antagonist substrates for metabolism catalyzed by CYP2D6. The patient's healthcare providers should prudently replace magnesium and confirm achieving serum magnesium concentrations within a range of normal values before giving ondansetron intravenously or dolasetron in antiemetic prophylaxis.

An additional consideration about whether one may safely use any 5-HT$_3$-receptor antagonist concomitantly with paroxetine is the potential for developing serotonin syndrome. Current product labeling for all 5-HT$_3$-receptor antagonists includes a warning about a potential for developing signs and symptoms of serotonin syndrome during concomitant use with serotonergic drugs, including selective serotonin reuptake inhibitors. Although the warning stipulates the majority of reports of serotonin syndrome related to 5-HT$_3$-receptor antagonist use occurred in a postanesthesia care unit or an infusion center, it notes serotonin syndrome has occurred as a result of ondansetron alone in overdose, and, in some cases, serotonin syndrome has resulted in fatality.

Option E is the best response, because it acknowledges the validity of both Options B and D.

3. ANSWER OPTION B: Female sex

DISCUSSION

Option A is an attractive choice because gastroparesis and altered gastrointestinal motility associated with diabetes are risk factors for emetic symptoms independent of the emetogenicity of treatment, but the selection is based on inference rather than evidence for altered motility provided by the case history.

Option B, female sex is a well documented risk factor for poor emetic control.

With respect to **Option C**, anxiety preceding antineoplastic treatments often accompanies incipient and frank anticipatory emetic symptoms. Anecdotally, anxiety before and during antineoplastic treatments appears to exacerbate emetic symptoms, but other behavioral disorders including clinical depression, have not been associated with emetic outcomes.

With respect to **Options D, E, and F**, predilection for motion or travel sickness and severe and persistent emetic symptoms during pregnancy, respectively, are recognized risk factors for poor emetic control during antineoplastic treatment, but the case history does not identify either condition. Likewise, constipation, is included among pathological factors associated with altered gastrointestinal motility or obstruction that, when coincident with emetogenic treatment, predispose toward poor emetic control. In addition, constipation is a common side effect associated with paroxetine use, but again, the patient's case history reveals nothing suggesting compromised or altered gastrointestinal motility. Constipation is also an adverse "class effect" associated with $5\text{-}HT_3$-receptor antagonist use. Additional dialog between the patient and her healthcare providers is warranted to establish whether she has experienced difficulty with bowel movements rather than assuming an additional risk factor exists, and to advise the patient about potential effects of antineoplastic and supportive care treatments on bowel function and develop a plan for monitoring and intervening if bowel function changes.

4. ANSWER OPTION D: Granisetron 34.3 mg transdermal patch applied 24 hours before starting chemotherapy and left in place for 7 days (one day after completing emetogenic chemotherapy) + dexamethasone 12 mg/day PO for 5 days on days 1 to 5 prior to chemotherapy, then 8 mg/day PO for 3 days on days 6 to 8 + aprepitant 125 mg PO on day 1 before chemotherapy, then 80 mg/day PO on days 2 to 5.

DISCUSSION

Cisplatin alone or in combination with other emetogenic drugs is associated with high emetic risk. Therefore, in addition to providing antiemetic prophylaxis appropriate for the component of combination chemotherapy with the greatest emetic risk, our strategy from the second through the fifth day of treatment should include medications appropriate to provide protection against both acute- and delayed-phase symptoms. Antiemetic prophylaxis for multiple-day emetogenic treatments has been less well studied than prophylaxis for treatments given on a single day, and professional guidelines are less explicit about how some antiemetics should be used to optimally protect against emetic symptoms associated with multiple-day treatments, particularly drugs formulated for extended-release and those with long half-lives (e.g., granisetron extended-release injection for subcutaneous use, and palonosetron and NK_1-receptor antagonists, respectively). Consequently, some extrapolation and assumptions are required from what is known about the effectiveness of prophylaxis for single-day treatments leavened with knowledge about the pharmacokinetic and pharmaceutical characteristics of available antiemetic products and, if known, patient-specific pharmacogenomic characteristics that may affect drug metabolism. Clinicians also must ascertain whether [1] the emetogenic risk of treatment is the same or varies among treatment days and [2] the physiological changes that underlie acute- and delayed-phase symptoms are operative concurrently, which may require antiemetic prophylaxis appropriate for either one or both phases on each treatment day. When treatment includes drugs with high and moderate emetogenic risks on different days, also consider whether antiemetic prophylaxis against delayed phase symptoms is indicated after emetogenic treatment is completed and the duration for which prophylaxis should continue. Although the present case scenario is realistic, it is simplified by a regimen without daily variation in emetic risk and a patient without concomitant medications or conditions that could complicate antiemetic selection and use.

The drug components identified in **Option A** give protection against both acute- and delayed-phase symptoms during the days on which antineoplastic treatment is given, but the regimen omits prophylaxis against delayed-phase symptoms likely to occur during the days following treatment. In addition, a 20 mg dose of dexamethasone is excessive when given with aprepitant.

Option B deviates from ASCO, MASCC/ESMO, and NCCN guidelines by omitting a high-potency glucocorticoid. Repeated administration of fosaprepitant at a 150 mg dose on an intermittent schedule also is not supported by FDA-approved product labeling or the three professional guidelines.

Option C meets ASCO, MASCC/ESMO, and NCCN guidelines' recommendations for use of a 5-HT_3-receptor antagonist, but repeated administration every second day for a total three doses is an empiric innovation. Although, palonosetron has been studied and found safe at greater doses and administration schedules than what is indicated in product labeling and after repeated doses, the regimen identified in Option C deviates from product labeling and the three professional guidelines. The regimen includes a high-potency glucocorticoid on the days of emetogenic treatment and for three days after completing chemotherapy as recommended by the NCCN guidelines for multiple-day emetogenic treatments, but at a dexamethasone dose on days 1 to 5 less than what is recommended in the absence of aprepitant, fosaprepitant, or netupitant. The regimen also deviates from all three guidelines by completely omitting an NK_1-receptor antagonist in prophylaxis for highly emetogenic treatment.

Option D includes continuous transdermal administration of granisetron from a topically applied patch, a delivery system appropriate for multiple-day emetogenic treatment. A granisetron transdermal system delivers 3.1 mg/day percutaneously during continuous application for up to 7 days. In addition, the regimen includes a high-potency glucocorticoid during emetogenic treatment and for 3 days afterward at doses and administration schedules consistent with ASCO and NCCN recommendations, and for a duration of use approximating both ASCO and NCCN recommendations. Although MASCC/ESMO and NCCN guidelines report on studies in which aprepitant was safely given for five or seven consecutive days, with comparatively better outcomes among patients whose regimens included aprepitant than comparator antiemetic regimens, both guidelines fall short of endorsing aprepitant use at doses and schedules beyond FDA-approved labeling. The NCCN Guidelines take a bolder stance than the other two guidelines by commenting, "...aprepitant 80 mg may be safely administered beyond day 3 of initiating chemotherapy."

Option E recommends any 5-HT$_3$-receptor antagonist daily before chemotherapy, which is not appropriate for sustained and extended-release formulations of granisetron, and arguably not for palonosetron owing to its long half-life. Dexamethasone is included on the days when emetogenic treatment is given, a schedule consistent with all three professional guidelines' recommendations, and for 3 days after chemotherapy is completed which follows ASCO and NCCN recommendations, but the doses stipulated for days 1 to 5 deviate from all three guidelines. As noted for Option D (above), the regimen is consistent with product labeling instructions for NK$_1$-receptor antagonist use, but falls short of what may be needed for multi-day highly emetogenic chemotherapy with respect to the duration of aprepitant use.

5. ANSWER OPTION B: Consider escalating the aggressiveness of antiemetic prophylaxis to a regimen appropriate for highly emetogenic treatment.

DISCUSSION

The three professional antiemetic guidelines are discordant on categorizing emetic risk for carboplatin. The ASCO and MASCC/ESMO guidelines assign moderate risk without qualification. In contrast, the NCCN Guidelines identify emetic risk for carboplatin as a function of systemic exposure (AUC) and attributes high emetic risk to carboplatin doses calculated to achieve an AUC ≥ 4 mg/mL/min.

Although the guidelines do not identify patient sub-groups or characterize risk factors that may predispose toward emetic risk in categorizing individual antineoplastic drugs' emetogenic potential, clinicians should recognize in the present case factors that place the patient at increased risk for poor emetic control during and after chemotherapy, such as female sex, and, from her history, motion sickness and pregnancy complicated by severe persistent emetic symptoms. As a result of poor emetic control during her first treatment cycle, the patient has acquired an additional risk factor that predisposes for poor emetic control during subsequent emetogenic treatments and for developing a conditioned emetic response; that is, anticipatory symptoms. Arguably, initial prophylaxis did not receive a fair trial because the patient did not complete the antiemetic regimen planned for her first treatment cycle, but the aggregate factors both historical and acquired during her previous chemotherapy that predispose toward poor emetic control and carboplatin's mutable emetogenic risk between moderate and high suggest pursuing a more aggressive approach to achieve the goal of antiemetic prophylaxis: complete emetic control with each cycle or course of treatment.

> **Option A** describes rechallenge with the antiemetic regimen previously attempted reinforced by reinstruction and encouraging the patient to comply with plans for self-administered medication and monitoring. A reasonable approach in a patient without risk factors for poor emetic control who will reliably comply with instructions for self-medication, and who will receive treatment for which emetic risk is not contested, but the mitigating risk factors noted above are arguments for antiemetic prophylaxis escalated from the previously planned regimen.

> **Option B** does not dismiss the ASCO and MASCC/ESMO guidelines' categorization of carboplatin's emetic risk, but is informed by the NCCN guidelines that acknowledges some medications labeled moderately emetogenic are highly emetogenic in some patients, and "Based on the patient's experiences, the chemotherapy regimen... may actually be more emetogenic than generally classified..."

> **Option C** is an attractive adjunctive intervention, and may serve to quell what anxiety contributes toward developing and exacerbating emetic symptoms, but evidence for improvement on the effectiveness of antiemetic prophylaxis with a high-potency glucocorticoid combined with 5-HT_3- and NK_1-receptor antagonists is lacking.

> **Options D and E** are empiric approaches to "cover all the bases." Acknowledging neurotransmitters are the principle mediators in initiating and propagating emetic symptoms, anticholinergic and dopaminergic (D_2)-receptor antagonists potentially may add preventative or therapeutic benefit. However, the more prudent course before attempting empiric replacement and supplementation would be to optimize emetic control with high-potency glucocorticoids, and 5-HT_3- and NK_1-receptor antagonists, which, by comparison with anticholinergic and antidopaminergic agents, are more effective and have better therapeutic indices.

6. ANSWER: OPTIONS A OR B

DISCUSSION

The patient is receiving cranial radiation therapy (RT), which is categorized among radiation fields that convey a low emetic risk, and concurrent chemotherapy with temozolomide at a dosage that imparts moderate emetic risk when combined with RT. Although the patient's emetic symptoms were initially controlled with a combination of ondansetron and dexamethasone, the latter drug was discontinued after 5 days of daily use, and the patient developed nausea that was not controlled by ondansetron alone either at the dose initially given or after dose escalation. Although our response for suboptimal and breakthrough emetic symptoms is empiric, published guidelines recommend following a rational approach by either adding an antiemetic that will mechanistically complement ondansetron or by replacing the current intervention with one or more alternative agents.

Option A is consistent with guidelines' recommendations to add agents from a different pharmacological class, which may be enough to mitigate the patient's nausea.

Options B and D include replacing ondansetron with granisetron. Although evidence supporting a difference in outcome after replacing one 5-HT$_3$-receptor antagonist with another is scant, it remains that the intervention sometimes meets with success.

Option C indicates concomitant use of olanzapine and ondansetron. Olanzapine has demonstrated effectiveness in prophylaxis and treatment for acute- and delayed-phase emetic symptoms associated with highly emetogenic chemotherapy, and has been shown to be particularly effective in mitigating nausea. However, there is some cause for concern for adding olanzapine by virtue of the patient's disease and concomitant use of temozolomide, both of which have been implicated as causing or contributing to seizure phenomena. Notably, olanzapine product labeling includes a cautionary warning about use in patients with a history of seizure or with drugs that may decrease the threshold for seizures. Although olanzapine 10 mg/day has been found effective in a prospective, randomized, double-blind, clinical trial, anecdotal reports have suggested antiemetic benefit at different olanzapine doses and schedules, including 5 mg/day for a period of consecutive days.

Healthcare providers should also recognize that ondansetron shares with other 5-HT$_3$-receptor antagonists a potential for perturbing cardiac conduction, which is represented in product labeling as a warning about prolonging the QT/QTc interval. In contrast, product labeling for olanzapine identifies a mean increase in heart rate in comparison with placebo but "...no significant differences between olanzapine and placebo in the proportions of patients experiencing potentially important changes in ECG parameters, including QT, QTc (Fridericia corrected), and PR intervals." However, the CredibleMeds[a] website categorizes olanzapine among drugs that have a conditional risk for causing torsades de pointes: in a setting of hypokalemia or hypomagnesemia concurrent with olanzapine use, or concomitant use of olanzapine with other medications that prolong the QT interval or causes torsades de pointes.

Although the risk of arrhythmias, QT interval prolongation, and torsades de pointe associated with ondansetron is related to the dose/dosage administered and most often associated with intravenous rather than oral administration, the risk of combining ondansetron with another drug with a potential for altering cardiac conduction is worrisome, particularly when other therapeutic options are available.

Option D includes the same change in 5-HT$_3$-receptor antagonist included in Option B and adds olanzapine. Granisetron shares with other 5-HT$_3$-receptor antagonists a potential liability for perturbing cardiac conduction, and although the likelihood of cardiac adverse effects is less with granisetron than dolasetron or ondansetron, product labeling advises granisetron "...should be used with caution in patients with preexisting arrhythmias or cardiac conduction disorders... Patients with cardiac disease, on cardio-toxic chemotherapy, with concomitant electrolyte abnormalities and/or on concomitant medications that prolong the QT interval are particularly at risk."

If not for concerns about risk of altered cardiac conduction and seizure phenomena, the adverse effect profile for granisetron and olanzapine at the doses and administration routes and schedules identified is such that a potential for therapeutic benefit may exceed the risk from concomitant use. Arguably, if the intervention is implemented and proves successful, it will not be possible to know whether a change from granisetron to ondansetron or the addition of olanzapine was sufficient to gain emetic control, or if the combination of both drugs was necessary.

Option E identifies resuming treatment with dexamethasone, which may reestablish control of nausea, but the prospect of a five-week course of treatment at pharmacological doses and the potential for adverse effects related to that course of treatment should inform a decision to seek an alternative associated with less potential metabolic complications and morbidity.

7. ANSWER OPTION E: Granisetron 2 mg PO + Rolapitant 180 mg PO + Dexamethasone 20 mg PO on day 1, followed by Dexamethasone 8 mg PO twice daily on days 2 and 3.

DISCUSSION

Fluorouracil is categorized among drugs with low emetogenic potential by all three professional organizations' guidelines. In contrast, oxaliplatin and irinotecan are categorized as presenting moderate emetic risk by MASCC/ESMO and ASCO guidelines; however, NCCN guidelines acknowledge that both drugs may present greater than moderate risk (i.e., highly emetogenic in some patients). Therefore, it is prudent to initially offer primary prophylaxis appropriate for high emetic risk regimens.

Option A describes palonosetron and rolapitant use consistent with product labeling and NCCN guidelines, but dexamethasone is underdosed both acutely and during the delayed phase.

In **Option B**, a NK_1-receptor antagonist is omitted, and while it may be argued that olanzapine may be used in lieu of a NK_1-receptor antagonist, doing so is not supported by guidelines' recommendations. In addition, the dexamethasone dose stipulated is less than what is recommended for use in a regimen without a NK_1-receptor antagonist (rolapitant excepted), and dexamethasone is not included in prophylaxis after the first day.

Although **Option C** recapitulates ASCO, MASCC/ESMO, and NCCN guidelines' recommendations for antiemetic prophylaxis for chemotherapy with high emetic risk, concomitant use of netupitant, a moderate inhibitor of CYP3A4, with irinotecan is discouraged.

Irinotecan and SN-38, its highly active metabolite, undergo metabolism partially catalyzed by CYP3A4. Concurrent use of medications that inhibit CYP3A subfamily enzymes may increase systemic exposure to irinotecan and SN-38, and consequently, adverse effects associated with irinotecan use.

Option D identifies a granisetron dosage 10-fold greater than what is recommended in FDA-approved product labeling and the three organizations' guidelines for antiemetic prophylaxis. The recommendations for fosaprepitant and dexamethasone use are consistent with ASCO, MASCC/ESMO, and NCCN guidelines.

Option E recapitulates ASCO, MASCC/ESMO, and NCCN guidelines' recommendations, but replaces the NK_1- and $5-HT_3$-receptor antagonist components of prophylaxis specified in Option C with rolapitant and granisetron, respectively. Both rolapitant and granisetron are substrates for metabolism catalyzed by CYP3A4, but do not inhibit the enzyme (CYP3A subfamily enzymes are high-capacity enzymes, generally capable of accommodating multiple substrates that do not inhibit enzyme functionality), and may be safely given concomitantly with irinotecan and other CYP3A subfamily enzyme substrates without clinically important perturbation in competing substrates' metabolism and elimination.

It is worth noting that granisetron shares with other $5-HT_3$-receptor antagonists a potential for adversely affecting cardiac electrophysiology, but the potential varies among agents and is directly related to doses administered and routes of administration that facilitate rapidly attaining high concentrations in blood. The doses, dosages, and dose-rates of delivery approved by the U.S. FDA for marketed granisetron products present a very low potential for altering cardiac conduction. However, the potential for perturbing cardiac electrophysiology may be increased by concurrent use with other drugs with the same liability. Therefore, clinicians are urged to be wary and to employ conservative monitoring for cardiac-related adverse events when administering $5-HT_3$-receptor antagonists with antineoplastics such as oxaliplatin, vandetanib, arsenic trioxide, and other drugs for which QT/QTc prolongation and other adverse effects on cardiac function are identified in product labeling and medical publications.

8. ANSWER OPTION C: The patient's history of ethanol use favors better antiemetic control than a person without a similar history.

DISCUSSION

Option A suggests nonspecific deficits in adult individuals' response to antiemetic medications or increased susceptibility to emetic symptoms as a function of age. Rather, children and young adults are at greater risk for suboptimal emetic control than older adults.

Option B implies a difference in control of emetic symptoms perhaps related to pharmacokinetic differences in drug distribution between lean and overweight or obese persons resulting in subtherapeutic antiemetic drug concentrations in persons whose BMI ≥25 kg/m^2. The assumption is not supported by product labeling for drugs indicated for antiemetic use or by antiemetic use guidelines.

Option C is correct. Nondrinkers are at greater risk for poor emetic control than patients with a history of daily ethanol consumption (>100 g) for several years.

Option D is incorrect. Female sex is a risk factor for poor emetic control, particularly in women who experienced severe or persistent emetic symptoms during pregnancy.

Option E is incorrect.

9. ANSWER OPTION C: Prochlorperazine 10 mg/day PO 60 minutes before vandetanib + Prochlorperazine 10 mg PO every 6 hours PRN

DISCUSSION

Option A is consistent with MASCC/ESMO and NCCN guidelines for antiemetic primary prophylaxis against oral chemotherapy agents with minimal to low emetic risk, and the ondansetron formulation selected will facilitate swallowing whole tablets in a patient who experiences discomfort and has difficulty in swallowing. However, vandetanib has a substantive adverse effect on cardiac conduction such that product labeling is prefaced by a boxed warning advising prescribers that vandetanib:

"…can prolong the QT interval. Torsades de pointes and sudden death have occurred in patients receiving [vandetanib]. Do not use [vandetanib] in patients with hypocalcemia, hypokalemia, hypomagnesemia, or long QT syndrome. Correct hypocalcemia, hypokalemia and/or hypomagnesemia prior to [vandetanib] administration. Monitor electrolytes periodically. Avoid drugs known to prolong the QT interval. Only prescribers and pharmacies certified with the restricted distribution program are able to prescribe and dispense [vandetanib]."

As noted previously, ondansetron labeling identifies ECG changes including QT interval prolongation and torsades de pointes (TdP); and includes recommendations for ECG monitoring in patients with hypokalemia or hypomagnesemia, congestive heart failure, bradyarrhythmias, or patients who use other medications for which QT prolongation is associated with use.

Concomitant vandetanib and ondansetron use seem ill advised when practical alternatives exist.

Option B is also consistent with MASCC/ESMO and NCCN guidelines for antiemetic prophylaxis against oral chemotherapy with minimal to low emetic risk, but the CredibleMeds website[a] identifies for metoclopramide conditions in which it also may cause torsades de pointes, including hypokalemia, hypomagnesemia, or use with another medication that has a liability for causing TdP. Again, for an ambulatory patient who will self medicate remote from medical surveillance and assistance, we should consider less risky alternatives.

Option C is a rational alternative supported by both MASCC/ESMO and NCCN guidelines. If the patient finds swallowing a tablet or capsule problematic, the drug is also available in liquid form

(5-mg/mL solution) and as a suppository for rectal insertion (25 mg/suppository).

With respect to **Option D**, lorazepam is often useful in mitigating psychological effects such as anxiety and agitation in patients who experience trepidation about their disease or its treatment; in preventing the development of anticipatory symptoms, and for the anxiolytic properties benzodiazepines provide in treating anticipatory symptoms; and in mitigating extrapyramidal symptoms such as akathisia, which may occur with dopaminergic-receptor antagonist use; but lorazepam or another benzodiazepine is likely not the first choice for antiemetic prophylaxis or treatment against emetic symptoms associated with drugs known to present an emetic risk.

Option E presents dronabinol for antiemetic primary prophylaxis, an option that is not supported by any of the three guidelines.

10. ANSWER & DISCUSSION: Although contrived, the scenario is plausible. Probably every healthcare provider has or will eventually encounter a situation that is not addressed by guidelines endorsed or mandated by discipline-specific or managed care organizations, or codified standards and policies operative in their practice setting.

For the options identified above, we may extrapolate from empirical evidence in favor of Option A.

With respect to **Option A**; that is, not to alter planned antiemetic prophylaxis, pharmacokinetic measurements in human subjects have established for netupitant an elimination half-life that ranges from approximately 51 to 109 hours with a mean value of approximately 90 hours, and for palonosetron a mean elimination half-life of approximately 40 hours. Consequently, it is reasonable to expect both palonosetron and netupitant to be present systemically and occupying their respective receptor sites only one day after netupitant and palonosetron were given. In addition, netupitant has been shown to exert an inhibitory effect on CYP3A4 catalytic function for days after administration; thereby, increasing the apparent bioavailability of substrates for the enzyme (e.g., dexamethasone). Although an increase in the dexamethasone dose for day 2 from 8 mg to 12 mg likely would do not harm, whether such an incremental dose change would improve emetic control is imponderable. Thus, one may rationalize there is no need increase the dose of dexamethasone initially planned for day 2 as suggested by **Option C**.

Given the pharmacokinetic behavior of both netupitant and palonosetron with respect to their respective elimination half-lives, and, considering only a potential for competitive binding at NK$_1$ and 5-HT$_3$ receptors, respectively, **Option B** and **Option E** appear redundant and unnecessary.

Option D adds olanzapine to the antiemetic regimen without evidence that any additional intervention is necessary, and, considering labeled warnings about the potential for cardiovascular morbidity and death in elderly patients ($\geq$65 y) with dementia-related psychosis attributed to olanzapine use, it may be prudent to forego olanzapine use completely, or at least until antiemetic alternatives without a similar liability have been exhausted.

a. CredibleMeds Worldwide focuses on the detection and prevention of adverse drug interactions, including maintaining a website with lists of drugs that are associated with prolonged QT interval and torsades de pointes and an international registry for patient reports of drug-induced arrhythmias. The site is continuously available to all visitors, but requires user registration (free). At: https://www.crediblemeds.org/ [Accessed: 2 April 2017]

REFERENCES:

1. Basch E, Prestrud AA, Hesketh PJ, et al. Antiemetics: American Society of Clinical Oncology clinical practice guideline update. *J Clin Oncol.* 2011;29:4189–4198.

2. Hesketh PJ, Bohlke K, Lyman GH, et al. Antiemetics: American Society of Clinical Oncology Focused Guideline Update. *J Clin Oncol.* 2016;34:381–386.

3. Roila F, Molassiotis A, Herrstedt J, et al. 2016 MASCC and ESMO guideline update for the prevention of chemotherapy- and radiotherapy-induced nausea and vomiting and of nausea and vomiting in advanced cancer patients. *Ann Oncol.* 2016;27(Suppl 5):v119-v33.

4. Antiemesis, V.1.2017—February 22, 2017. National Comprehensive Cancer Network, Inc., 2017. (Accessed March 9, 2017, at http://www.nccn.org.)

Nutrition 39

Marnie Grant Dobbin

REVIEW QUESTIONS

1. A patient with cancer presents with cachexia and more than 7% weight loss in the past month. He reports that his food intake has been constant even while his weight continues to decrease. He has no gastrointestinal symptoms or fever. The most likely reason for his weight loss is

   A. The patient has an inaccurate perception of his recent intake.

   B. Energy expenditure and nitrogen losses are increased in those with cancer.

   C. Lipolysis has occurred as a result of a preferential use of fat for energy which spares lean body mass.

   D. There is increased turnover of free fatty acids, glucose, and protein.

2. A moderately malnourished patient with stomach cancer is admitted for a gastrectomy to be followed by chemotherapy (leucovorin + 5FU + oxaliplatin). Resting energy expenditure is 1,800 kcal. The patient has been drinking oral nutrition products formulated for postgastrectomy patients, but 1 week after surgery the patient is still unable to tolerate more than 300 kcal a day by mouth. Which is the most appropriate nutrition intervention?

   A. PN should be initiated

   B. A trial of EN via jejunostomy

    C. Track intake; encourage continued use of postgastrectomy oral nutrition product

    D. B and C

3. A woman with end-stage breast cancer and bony metastases has begun treatment for hypercalcemia of malignancy. Her usual diet includes foods high in calcium. Which of the following is NOT indicated?

    A. A low calcium diet to limit exogenous sources of calcium

    B. Discontinuation of drugs that contain vitamin D, calcium, or vitamin A

    C. Rehydration to correct calciuresis-related dehydration

    D. Diuresis to manage or prevent fluid overload

4. What are the most likely reasons for a patient's serum albumin and prealbumin levels to decrease from near normal levels at the time of admission to below reference range 1 week after admission?

    A. Inadequate protein intake

    B. An acute-phase protein response as seen during a fever

    C. Intravascular dilution

    D. Both B and C

5. A 50-year-old male with acute myelogenous leukemia is admitted for an allogeneic hematopoietic stem cell transplant (date of transplant is in 3 days). He has grade III mucositis and diarrhea associated with the busulfan and fludarabine conditioning regimen. These symptoms are expected to continue for > 1 week. He has no edema. Fluid balance is net even. He has central access.

    Height 180 cm, Admission Weight (2 weeks ago): 105 kg = BMI 32.4 kg/m2 (Obesity 1 category)

    Current Weight 99 kg = BMI: 30.6 kg/m2 (Obesity 1 category)

    Labs of nutrition significance are unremarkable except that patient has required potassium replacement (80 mEq/day) to maintain serum potassium within reference range. His albumin level is 4.0 g/dL (within ref range), platelets are 50 k/mcL (below reference range).

Calculated requirements: 2200 kcals (14 kcals/kg actual weight for critically ill obese patients), 119 grams protein/day (1.2 grams protein/kg actual weight)

His mean oral intake in the past 2 weeks has been 900 kcals and 20 grams of protein/day.

What is the appropriate nutrition intervention?

A. As patient is in the obesity 1 BMI category and has an albumin value within reference range, no intervention is indicated at this time. Continue to encourage patient to use nutritionally fortified beverages as recommended by RD.

B. Initiate enteral nutrition.

C. Initiate parenteral nutrition.

D. Initiate peripheral parenteral nutrition.

ANSWERS TO REVIEW QUESTIONS

1. ANSWER: D. The multifactorial causes of weight loss in patients with cancer include cellular and metabolic derangements that lead to depletion of fat and muscle stores. Historically, it was thought that patients with cancer had increased energy expenditure, but measured resting energy expenditure in those with cancer is widely variable and an association with extent of tumor and energy expenditure has not been found. Unlike simple starvation, where glucose turnover is slowed and lean body mass is preserved, there is a maladaptation to starvation in cancer with increased glucose turnover, increase in wasteful metabolic cycles, increased protein turnover, increased muscle protein degradation, and depletion of adipose stores due to increased lipolysis.

2. ANSWER: D. As summarized in the ASPEN Guidelines, "Nutrition support therapy is appropriate in patients receiving active anticancer treatment who are malnourished and who are anticipated to be unable to ingest and/or absorb adequate nutrients for a prolonged period of time (7 to 14 days)." EN is preferred for patients who are unable to maintain adequate nutritional intake by mouth as it maintains the functional integrity of the gastrointestinal tract. EN via jejunostomy feeding tubes can be successful in patients postgastrectomy. PN would only be appropriate if the patient failed an EN trial with appropriate tube placement. Tracking oral intake will allow the tube feeding volume to be adjusted according to oral intake, so that adequate nutrition can be provided, with eventual weaning off of EN.

3. ANSWER: A. Hypercalcemia of malignancy does not respond to a low calcium diet. NCI's PDQ cancer information summary on hypercalcemia indicates that "even though the gut has a role in normal calcium homeostasis, absorption is usually diminished in individuals with hypercalcemia, making dietary calcium restriction unnecessary."

4. ANSWER: D. A patient with low albumin and prealbumin levels may or may not be malnourished. Albumin and prealbumin lack specificity and sensitivity as indicators of nutritional status. They can be reduced by nonnutritional factors such as hypervolemia and inflammation. Earlier reports associating these proteins with nutritional status did not account for the variable of inflammation. These serum hepatic transport proteins are considered negative acute-phase proteins because liver synthesis of these proteins decreases in response to chronic or acute inflammation. C-reactive protein, a positive acute-phase protein, can be measured to help clarify whether active inflammation is present. If C-reactive protein is elevated and albumin or prealbumin are reduced, then inflammation is likely. In order to diagnose a malnutrition syndrome, further information suggesting loss of body cell mass or compromised nutritional intake would be needed. In addition, the half-life of albumin is 18 to 21 days and so a 1-week period is too soon to detect changes in albumin synthesis alone.

5. ANSWER: C. Pt meets criteria to support a diagnosis of malnutrition in adults[1]. He has had a 6% weight loss in less than 1 month, his intake is 41% of his estimated needs for a period of more than five days. B is incorrect as his gastrointestinal tract is not appropriate for enteral nutrition due to grade III mucositis and diarrhea, and also due to low platelets. D is incorrect as peripheral parenteral nutrition is rarely used, and is only appropriate if electrolyte and energy needs are low and in circumstances such as short term need and lack of central access.

REFERENCES:

1. Schlein KM, Coulter SP, Best practices for determining resting energy expenditure in critically ill adults. *Nutr Clin Pract.* 2014;Feb;29(1):44–55.
2. White JV, Guenter P, Jensen G et al. Consensus statement: Academy of Nutrition and Dietetics and American Society for Parenteral and Enteral Nutrition: characteristics recommended for the identification and documentation of adult malnutrition (undernutrition). *JPEN.* 2012 May;36(3):275–283.

Pain and Palliative Care 40

Christina Tafe, Jean-Paul Pinzon, and Ann Berger

REVIEW QUESTIONS

1. A 63-year-old woman, who has a past history of invasive lobular carcinoma of the right breast, mastectomy, and chemotherapy, is brought to the emergency department by her husband, who reports that she has had pain in the middle to lower back for the past three weeks. The pain has become progressively worse in severity, and the patient says that it worsens when she lies down. Since this morning, she has had difficulty walking because of back pain and weak legs. She reports intact bowel and bladder function.

   She has tenderness over the area of the thoracic vertebrae and reduced strength in the lower limb flexors. Magnetic resonance imaging confirms extensive disease consistent with epidural spinal cord compression at the thoracic spine with focal metastases at the T11 and T12 levels.

   In the emergency department, the patient receives a corticosteroid bolus. She is also evaluated by radiation oncology and is scheduled for immediate radiation therapy.

   Which of the following is the strongest prognostic factor for this patient regaining function?

   A. Severity of back pain

   B. Duration of back pain

   C. Current functional status

   D. Level of spinal metastases

   E. Invasive nature of the breast cancer

2. Mrs. Smith, a 59-year-old woman, recently diagnosed with metastatic nonsmall cell lung cancer is receiving standard anticancer therapy in your outpatient oncology practice. Another patient you are seeing, Mr. Jones, a 63-year-old male with the same, recent diagnosis of metastatic nonsmall cell lung cancer is also receiving standard of care therapy, and in addition, is also seeing palliative care specialists for symptom management and psychological support concurrently. What can you definitively say about the prognosis of these patients?

    A. The odds of Mrs. Smith's survival are greater because she is female

    B. The odds of Mr. Jones's survival are lower with palliative care

    C. The odds of Mr. Jones's survival are greater with palliative care

    D. The odds of Mrs. Smith's and Mr. Jones' survival are equivalent

3. A 48-year-old woman with metastatic pancreatic cancer has been having increasing pain and progressive disease despite being on her second clinical trial. She is no longer eligible for treatment protocol. She has been losing weight and spending most of her time in bed, requiring considerable assistance. The patient wants to know how much time she has left. Which of the following would be the best response?

    A. "I really can't tell how much time you have left"

    B. "On average patients with your condition live for about six to nine months"

    C. "It is always hard to predict, but most likely only a few weeks to a few months"

    D. "Only God knows how long someone has to live"

4. A 76-year-old woman with widely metastatic lung cancer was admitted to the hospital after a mechanical fall at home. During her hospitalization, she was found to have a fracture of the right femoral neck and underwent surgical fixation. Before admission, she had been living with her elderly spouse in their own home, with their adult children visiting them daily. She was still seeing her oncologist who was no longer offering anticancer therapy, but has been suggesting she enter hospice care. Her children ask you if the Medicare hospice benefit can help pay

for caregivers. The Medicare hospice benefit will pay for which of the following?

    A. Room and board at a nursing facility for postoperative physical therapy

    B. Long-term care in an inpatient hospice facility

    C. Continuous home nursing care

    D. Respite care at a nursing facility

5. You have been invited to sit on your cancer center's Quality Committee. The Committee is concerned about what some feel to be the excessive use of "aggressive care" at the cancer center, and wish to review the data collected over the past year, which includes patient and family member reported outcomes. Some of the Committee members have seen the preliminary data and suggested implementation of the following strategies to improve the quality of care. Which of the following strategies should be pursued?

    A. Decrease use of chemotherapy at the end of life

    B. Increase capacity of the emergency department

    C. Increase availability of hospital beds for patients who are imminently dying

    D. Monitor for aggressive care "triggers" to palliative care referral

6. A 22-year-old man who has Ewing's sarcoma with diffuse disease to his abdomen, vertebrae, and lungs has severe pain and limited mobility. The disease has compressed his spinal cord, producing paraplegia. He is an inpatient and recently received a palliative care consultation to address his goals, support his decision making, and optimize control of his pain. His primary goal is to preserve his comfort and quality of life.

After one week, the patient's pain has improved, but he remains paraplegic, with paralysis of his legs and no improvement in his bowel or bladder incontinence. He requests assistance with dying from the palliative care team. Which of the following should you do to best respond to this patient's request?

    A. Recommend more aggressively addressing his pain, fatigue, and depression

    B. Recommend spiritual care

C. Have the patient complete a contract for safety and pursue psychiatry consultation

D. Discuss the request with the patient, attempting to identify reasons underlying it

---

7. Mr. Jones is a 54-year-old man who was admitted to the ICU with respiratory distress and was intubated. A chest CT scan revealed a large necrotic mass filling the right hemithorax, obliterating the right and narrowing the left main stem bronchi. Needle biopsy confirmed a diagnosis of non-small cell lung cancer. There is no role for chemotherapy or radiation unless Mr. Jones could be weaned off the ventilator, which was considered doubtful in the setting of his airway obstruction. Mr. Jones is unable to participate in medical decision-making. Social work was able to identify his cousin Mary as the next-of-kin, who is invited to speak with the care team to discuss prognosis and treatment options, including the possibility of withdrawal of life-sustaining treatments. Mary is adamant that all life-sustaining measures be continued despite a previous discussion that Mr. Jones's disease severity will prevent him from ever leaving the ICU, let alone the hospital. Mary expresses hope that, despite the physician's prediction, a miracle will occur that will allow Mr. Jones to leave the hospital. The next best step is to

    A. Schedule another family meeting in the hope of emphasizing Mr. Jones' poor prognosis and low likelihood of meaningful recovery

    B. Tell Mary that hope for a miracle is unreasonable, but that she could still hope that Mr. Jones can be made comfortable

    C. Ask Mary about her spiritual beliefs and how it influences her decision

    D. Involve the ethics committee

---

8. The palliative care team is consulted regarding a 15-year-old girl who has trisomy 21 and has been found to have acute lymphocytic leukemia (ALL). The patient's sibling is a healthy 10-year-old girl who has been misbehaving and performing poorly at school. Her parents report that the 10-year-old girl often awakes during the night. This behavior began shortly after the diagnosis of her sister's leukemia.

After meeting with the patient and family, the palliative care team should do which of the following first?

    A. Advise the parents to address marital tension through counseling

    B. Reassure the family that siblings of cancer patients can have negative emotions affecting behavior

    C. Advise the family to have the sibling undergo counseling in order to achieve increased independence, responsibility, and empathy

    D. Avoid making any recommendations for the sibling so as not to divert psychosocial support from the patient

9. A 75-year-old man who has bone metastases due to prostate cancer was admitted as part of a Phase 1 clinical trial. He has declined dramatically during this hospitalization. His family is considering transition to hospice care. Two nights ago, the patient became unresponsive and developed harsh, gurgling sounds. His son is worried that the gurgling is distressing to his mother. Which of the following should you recommend first?

    A. Transdermal scopolamine

    B. Nebulized saline

    C. Repositioning

    D. Oral suctioning

10. You meet with your 65-year-old breast cancer patient, who is in remission, for follow-up in your outpatient oncology clinic. She tells you she is now widowed, her husband of 35 years passed away suddenly 2 months ago. She tells you she could not eat for the first week after his death. She has support from family and friends, but she still finds herself crying at least 3 to 4 times per day. She tells you she hears her husband's voice now and then, and sometimes thinks she catches a glimpse of him when she turns her head quickly. She finds comfort in looking at old photo albums of her husband. She finds strength in her religious faith and is still able to go to church every week, which was always very important to her and her husband.

    Which of the following would be the most accurate description of her condition?

    A. Post-traumatic stress disorder

    B. Major depressive disorder

C. Grief

D. Complicated grief disorder

---

11. Mrs. White is a 48-year-old with metastatic pancreatic cancer, who is on a clinical trial. Unfortunately she has shown evidence of progressive disease with new lesions in her liver. She has had worsening abdominal pain and is being followed by the palliative care team. She has three children ranging in age from 5 to 14. The children know mom has been ill lately but nothing else. She is thinking about talking with the children and letting them know about her diagnosis, but she is concerned that telling them now will be too traumatic for them. Which of the following would be the best next step?

   A. It is best to wait until the disease is obvious to the children.

   B. Telling the children of the disease may make them less anxious.

   C. Telling the children now will make them too anxious.

   D. She should tell the older child, but the younger child is not at an appropriate developmental age that he will benefit from hearing his mother has cancer.

---

12. A 48-year-old woman whose breast cancer was successfully treated with chemotherapy comes to oncology clinic for management of increasing pain. The patient reports worsening lower-extremity pain that she describes as "burning" and "shooting." The pain is worse at night than during daytime. She has been taking escalating doses of hydromorphone, which has not been effective in controlling her pain, but just makes her feel more sleepy. Which of the following should you prescribe now to help reduce this patient's pain?

   A. Dexamethasone

   B. Topiramate

   C. Gabapentin

   D. Lorazepam

---

13. A 55-year-old woman with early-stage hormone receptor positive breast cancer on adjuvant endocrine therapy arrives to your office for routine visit. She is postmenopausal. She complains of pain on both of her wrists

and hands that started about two months ago. She was evaluated by a rheumatologist and tests for tendinitis, bursitis, and osteoarthritis were negative. She has been taking oxycodone immediate release 5 mg tablets for relief of unrelated low back pain for several years, usually about once or twice per week.

Which of the following is the most likely etiology of the patient's joint pain?

A. Carpal tunnel syndrome

B. Aromatase inhibitor-induced arthralgias

C. Autoimmune disease

D. Opioid hyperalgesia

14. A 70-year-old male with end-stage metastatic lung cancer with painful bone metastases comes to your clinic. Prognosis is poor.

Patient is willing to undergo more treatment but really just wants control of the pain. Mobility is severely limited due to pain and weakness, uses a wheelchair. He lives in the next town. You refer patient to the radiation oncology for consideration of external beam therapy.

The radiation oncologist feels strongly about giving radiation therapy for palliation.

What would be the recommended treatment for your patient?

A. Forego radiation treatment and start morphine drip

B. 30 Gy in 10 fractions

C. 20 Gy in 5 fractions

D. Single 8 Gy fraction

15. A 58-year-old male with a history of metastatic renal cell carcinoma is admitted to the oncology service for worsening pain. His pain previously had been well controlled with twice daily use of hydrocodone 5 mg/acetaminophen 500 mg tablets. His primary focal pain complaint includes left hip pain confirmed by radiography to be osseous metastatic disease. The patient rates his pain as 8/10 on a visual analog scale (VAS) and assessment confirms a clearly uncomfortable gentleman of stated age. Which of the following would be an appropriate initial parenteral analgesic to better control his pain?

A. Propoxyphene

B. Meperidine

C. Hydromorphone

D. Oxycodone

E. Ibuprofen

16. The patient in the previous question now has improved pain control after choosing an appropriate analgesic. The patient is utilizing a total of 100 mg of oral morphine equivalents and has improved pain and functionality with a pain rating of 3/10 on a VAS. Which of the following would be an appropriate long-acting opioid to initiate at this time?

A. Methadone tablets 30 mg PO TID

B. Oxycodone extended release tablets 80 mg PO TID

C. Morphine sulfate extended release tablets 100 mg PO TID

D. Oxycodone immediate release tablets 30 mg PO q4h

E. Fentanyl transdermal patch 25 mcg q72h

17. The same patient in the previous questions continues to have good pain relief (VAS 3/10) after receiving appropriate long and short-acting opioid analgesics. He continues to utilize short-acting analgesics twice daily. In total this utilization equivocates to 30 mg of oral morphine equivalents. He is now ready for discharge home, which of the following would be an appropriate regimen for breakthrough pain that the patient could receive at home?

A. Hydromorphone 8 mg tablets BID prn pain

B. Morphine sulfate immediate release 30 mg tablets BID prn pain

C. Oxycodone immediate release tablets 30 mg BID prn pain

D. Hydromorphone 4 mg tablets BID prn pain

E. Fentanyl transdermal patch 25 mcg q72h

18. A 65-year-old man who has metastatic lung cancer and painful bone metastases reports severe pruritus that started when he began to take morphine for his pain. Pain in his chest wall and legs has been successfully treated with naproxen (500 mg twice daily), sustained-release morphine (60 mg every 12 hours), and short-acting morphine (15 mg orally every 4 hours as needed for breakthrough pain), which he uses two or three

times daily, depending on his level of activity. Because of severe ongoing pruritus, he wants to change his pain medications.

Which of the following should be the management strategy for this patient's chronic cancer-related pain?

   A. Rotate to oxycodone, 60 mg every 12 hours, and oxycodone, 15 mg every 2 hours as needed

   B. Rotate to oxycodone, 30 mg every 12 hours, and oxycodone, 5 to 10 mg every 2 hours as needed

   C. Continue the morphine, hoping to see tolerance develop

   D. Lower the dosage of sustained-release morphine to 30 mg every 12 hours

19. You are a mentor to Dr. Jones, an oncology fellow in his first year of training. Today, Dr. Jones approaches you and states that he is exhausted and getting very little sleep. He is coming off a difficult month-long rotation on the wards, during which time he cared for three long-term patients at the end of their lives. These experiences were stressful and made him feel sad, yet at the same time he tells you he now feels more detached than ever from his patients. You have also noticed that Dr. Jones seems increasingly distant with not only his patients but also his colleagues. What would you recommend to him?

   A. Bright light therapy

   B. St. John's Wort

   C. An SSRI

   D. Mindfulness meditation

20. A 65-year-old male with nonsmall cell lung CA is admitted to the ICU with worsening dyspnea. He is found to have a large right-sided pleural effusion requiring thoracentesis and placement of chest tube for drainage. Despite some moderate relief, patient continues to experience some dyspnea, which keeps him awake at night and provokes some anxiety. Serum hemoglobin and hematocrit are within normal range. He is opioid naïve. Which of the following would be the appropriate next step?

   A. Nebulized morphine

   B. Parenteral morphine

C. Supplemental oxygen via nasal cannula

D. Lorazepam

---

21. A 55-year-old man who has worsening nonsmall cell lung cancer has started a new second-line chemotherapy. Forty-eight hours after finishing his most recent chemotherapy session, he comes to the emergency department for intravenous hydration. Physical examination is significant for active bowels sounds and a soft, nontender abdomen without rigidity or guarding. The patient continues to vomit periodically and cannot retain any oral intake despite 3 L of fluid. Which of the following drugs has proven efficacy for treating nausea and vomiting in patients such as this?

A. ABH gel (Ativan, Benadryl, and Haldol)

B. Lorazepam

C. Dexamethasone

D. Octreotide

---

22. A 62-year-old male with a history of Cushing's disease secondary to pituitary macroadenoma, status-post transsphenoidal surgical resection and treated for gross residual disease with adjuvant radiation therapy 5400 cGy in thirty fractions, comes to oncology clinic for complaint of fatigue of one year's duration. He found himself with increased sleep duration, up to 10 to 11 hours per night. He had generalized fatigue with no focal weakness. The fatigue affected him in such a way that he had to cut back work from full time to part time. He consistently felt exhausted after a full night of sleep. His fatigue persisted long after his radiation therapy was completed. He was seen by endocrinology and urology. He had extensive lab workup including serum cortisol, ACTH stimulation test, thyroid function tests, testosterone level, complete blood count and metabolic panel all of which produced normal results. One year follow-up MRI of the pituitary showed overall reduction in the size of the intrasellar and suprasellar mass, with no evidence of recurrent disease. He did not meet screening criteria for clinical depression. What would be an appropriate next step to address the patient's fatigue?

A. duloxetine

B. methylphenidate

C. modafinil

D. red blood cell transfusion

23. A 25-year-old male with osteosarcoma has had chronic pain for several years and was previously well managed on an opioid regimen consisting of extended release morphine. Last month he underwent surgery on his left femur for localized disease progression and has recovered well, but his pain has escalated requiring increases in his opioid regimen. As a result, he has had worsening constipation. He has tried using multiple agents simultaneously with some improvement. He feels he needs to continue this regimen although he admits it can be burdensome and expensive. He asks you to help minimize the number of agents he is taking.

    Which of the following agents your patient is taking for opioid-induced constipation should be discontinued?

    A. Polyethylene glycol

    B. Docusate sodium

    C. Sorbitol

    D. Senna

24. A 74-year-old retired police officer with his metastatic prostate cancer comes to your clinic for a periodic health evaluation accompanied by his daughter. He lives alone at home, but his daughter visits him daily and helps with meal preparation. The patient recently lost his beloved wife to dementia. She died 8 months ago, 3 days after their fiftieth wedding anniversary.

    In clinic, his daughter reports that he has been feeling weaker, has had no appetite, and has not been eating or drinking much. He usually spends all day in bed and has stopped doing the things he used to enjoy, such as playing golf and visiting with friends. He also has had difficulty sleeping at night and has been drinking several glasses of hard liquor every night to help him sleep. On further questioning, the patient says, "My life is worthless. Now that my wife is gone, I have no reason to live. I want to hurry up and die." Which of the following should you do now?

    A. Ask the patient if he has had thoughts about suicide

    B. Start the patient on citalopram

    C. Start the patient on methylphenidate

    D. Refer the patient to a psychiatry clinic

25. **A** 67-year-old female with metastatic colorectal cancer and an estimated survival of less than 3 months presents to the hospital with symptoms of increasing abdominal pain, intractable nausea and vomiting. Imaging studies reveal incomplete small bowel obstruction. Her serum albumin is 1.7 g/dL. Functional status is poor. She is being seen by general surgery and operative approaches are being considered. The hospital is in a rural area and there are few GI specialists available. Which of the following would be the best treatment approach for this patient?

    A. Resection and primary anastomosis

    B. Metoclopramide, scopolamine, and octreotide

    C. Endoscopic stent placement

    D. Start patient on morphine drip

26. A 70-year-old woman with widespread breast cancer has had hallucinations and mild agitation for the past week. She appears confused and disoriented, but is not violent and is not hurting herself or anyone else. She is becoming more troubled by the voices she is hearing. Which of the following would be the most appropriate initial treatment for her delirium?

    A. Lorazepam 2 mg PO q1h PRN

    B. Olanzapine 10 mg PO q4h PRN

    C. Midazolam 1 mg IV q1h PRN

    D. Haloperidol 0.5 mg PO q1h PRN

27. Mr. Sanchez is a 70-year-old Spanish-speaking man who presented to the hospital with dyspnea and chest pain, and was found to have a mass obstructing a bronchiole and pleural effusion. He was diagnosed with metastatic lung cancer. You are the oncologist and wish to organize a family meeting to discuss prognosis and goals of care. The meeting will include Mr. Sanchez, his wife, and the hospital social worker. Mr. Sanchez speaks only Spanish. His wife speaks both English and Spanish, and states that she has acted as the interpreter during previous meetings with physicians. You took Spanish in high school and have some basic language skills. The best next step would be

    A. Plan ahead of the meeting to use a live professional interpreter

    B. Find a hospital employee nearby who speaks Spanish to act as an interpreter

C. Mrs. Sanchez should act as the interpreter because she is his wife

D. Conduct the family meeting in Spanish yourself to the best of your ability

28. An 80-year-old woman who has end-stage leukemia decided to enroll in home hospice care after her functional status declined. Her chief caregivers are her adult children, who have been tremendously helpful to her, but have busy lives of their own and are trying to balance their own family and work obligations.

Your patient feels that she is becoming a burden to others. Her increasing debility is very distressing to her. In fact, she hopes for "the end to come sooner." She reveals to you that she has been consciously eating and drinking less and less each day in hopes of hastening her death. She asks whether she can completely stop eating and drinking. She is not depressed and her pain is well-controlled. In order for you to support this patient's decision to stop eating and drinking, which of the following must be present?

A. Decision-making capacity

B. Intractable pain

C. An advance directive

D. Enrollment in hospice care

29. A 67-year-old male diagnosed with human papilloma virus–positive oropharyngeal cancer is undergoing combination radiation therapy and chemotherapy. He currently reports sore throat and difficulty swallowing solid foods for the past 3 months. You recommend a prophylactic feeding tube, which the patient refuses.

Subsequently, after one of his radiation therapy sessions, his wife brings him to the emergency department with dizziness and fatigue. He is found to be severely dehydrated. You see him in the emergency department and once again recommend a feeding tube, to which he responds, "I have seen too many friends and family members suffer and die with feeding tubes. I just want to die gently and with dignity when my time comes."

Which of the following is the best initial response to the patient?

A. "You must consent to artificial nutrition if you want to continue radiation therapy for the cancer."

B. "Artificial nutrition is beneficial in your situation and will probably improve the quality of your life."

C. "You have the right to refuse treatment. I respect your decision."

D. "We need you to sign a Physician Orders for Life-Sustaining Treatment (POLST) form stating that you are refusing tube feedings."

30. You are ward attending on the hematology service this month. You are seeing a 32-year-old female, Ms. Snow, with sickle-cell disease who is regularly admitted to the hospital with frequent pain crises. She has severe, sharp pain in her knees, lower back, and shoulder. She describes the pain as 10/10 in intensity. She was last in the hospital 2 weeks ago with the same complaints. Her scans have not changed since one year ago, ruling out avascular necrosis or osteomyelitis. She receives ketamine for pain when she is hospitalized, but as an outpatient you have her on long-acting oxycodone for pain. She was started on 20 mg twice daily one year ago. Since that time, her opioid requirement has gradually increased. She is currently on 80 mg twice daily.

During interdisciplinary rounds, her nurse tells you that the dose of hydromorphone Ms. Snow now requires is much greater than the dose she required the last time she took care of her 6 months ago. The social worker states that although Ms. Snow has had numerous health difficulties this past year, she has managed to make all her regular outpatient visits, has no history of incarceration, and maintains a healthy relationship with her 12-year-old son.

Which of the following would be the best description of Ms. Snow's current situation?

A. Increased pain

B. Tolerance

C. Opioid use disorder

D. Dependence

ANSWERS TO REVIEW QUESTIONS

1. ANSWER: C. Current functional status

Rationale:

Cord compression in cancer patients is an emergency and warrants immediate administration of corticosteroids, and consultation and evaluation for potential surgery and radiation therapy. The best prognostic factor for post-treatment functional recovery is the pre-treatment functional status. The severity and duration of pain, disease burden (invasive lobular carcinoma in this case), and level of disease are helpful in making the diagnosis; however, they are not primary prognostic factors for post-treatment regaining of function.

REFERENCES:

Kim RY, Spencer SA, Meredith RF, et al. Extradural spinal cord compression: analysis of factors determining functional prognosis—prospective study. *Radiology.* 1990;176:279–282.

Martenson JA Jr, Evans RG, Lie MR, et al. Treatment outcome and complications in patients treated for malignant epidural spinal cord compression (SCC). *J Neurooncol.* 1985;3:77–84.

2. ANSWER: C. The odds of Mr. Jones's survival are greater because he is receiving palliative care

Rationale:

It is a common misconception that receiving palliative care is equivalent to end-of-life care, and that it somehow shortens the longevity of people living with serious illness. In a pivotal study based on a randomized controlled trial published in the *New England Journal of Medicine* in 2010, it was found that early outpatient palliative care in addition to usual oncology care for metastatic nonsmall cell lung cancer not only improved physical symptoms, depression, and sense of well-being, but also showed a survival benefit of two months when compared to the control group. In addition, early outpatient palliative care led to reduced use of high intensity high cost care, such as chemotherapy, emergency department visits, and hospitalization at the end-of-life. While the authors could not identify the exact reason for the survival benefit, the lower rate of hospitalization and chemotherapy at the end of life in the palliative care group may have been important factors.

REFERENCE:

Temel et al. Early palliative care for patients with metastatic non–small-cell lung cancer. *N Engl J Med.* 2010;363:733–742.

3. ANSWER: C. "It is always hard to predict, but most likely only a few weeks to a few months"

Rationale:

Prognostic disclosures are generally best done by giving accurate estimates with ranges, as well as disclosure of uncertainty. In general, performance status has been considered to be the single most powerful prognostic factor in cancer, with rule-of-thumb guidelines for patients with solid tumors and declining PS that KPS 40 to 60 have median survivals in the 1 to 3 month range. Choice A would not be correct because in this case performance status has some predictive value.

Choice B would be an overestimation. In patients with advanced cancer, physicians tend to overestimate when predicting survival. One study showed the proportion of accurate clinical prediction of survival (CPS) to be 35%, while the proportion of patients living shorter than CPS was 45%. While choice D may be reassuring to some, it would be inappropriate to assume all people have a belief in a divine being. This patient is asking for a clear, rational response.

REFERENCES:

Barbot, A. et al. (2008). Assessing 2-month clinical prognosis in hospitalized patients with advanced solid tumors. *J Clin Oncol*. 26(15);2538–2543.

Amano, et al. The accuracy of physicians' clinical predictions of survival in patients with advanced cancer. *JPSM*. 2015;50(2):139–146.

4. *ANSWER: D.* Respite care at a nursing facility

Rationale:

Hospice covering the room and board at a nursing facility while the family decides between long-term care at a facility or caregivers in the home represents respite care, which is one of the four levels of care that hospice provides. Hospice pays for room and board when a patient is receiving respite care at a contracted facility for 5 days or when a patient is receiving general inpatient hospice care for uncontrolled symptoms. However, this patient is not demonstrating uncontrolled symptoms and so would not qualify for general inpatient hospice care.

Hospice care is appropriate when a patient's goals are for nonlife-prolonging treatment, which would exclude inpatient physical therapy at a nursing facility. Physical therapy for this purpose would be consistent with acute rehabilitation under Medicare. Hospice must provide all treatments and interventions related to a patient's terminal diagnosis; however, caregivers and room and board at a facility are not covered under the hospice benefit. Provision of a bedside nurse for at least 8 hours in a 24-hour period in the patient's home, which constitutes continuous home care, or admission to an inpatient hospice facility for acute care, is available when a patient has uncontrolled symptoms necessitating intensive nursing support. However, this patient is not having uncontrolled symptoms and so does not qualify for a higher level of hospice care.

REFERENCE:

The Hospice Manual. Centers for Medicare & Medicaid Services. http://www.gpo.gov/fdsys/pkg/CFR-2011-title42-vol3/pdf/CFR-2011-title42-vol3-part418-subpartD.pdf. Accessed December 13, 2014.

5. ANSWER: D. Monitor for aggressive care "triggers" to palliative care referral

Rationale:

Despite increasing evidence that high-intensity treatments may not be associated with better patient quality of life, outcomes or caregiver bereavement, patients with advanced-stage cancer continue to receive aggressive medical care at the end of life. A recently published prospective study of Medicare claims data from 2003 to 2011 concluded that reports of better end-of-life care by family members of decedents with colorectal or lung cancer were associated with avoidance of ICU admissions within 30 days of death, hospice services >3 days, and death outside the hospital setting. The authors suggest that efforts to monitor physicians practices to utilize aggressive care and refer to palliative care would likely result in more patient-centered care and improved quality of end-of-life care. This study did not find any differences in family-reported quality outcomes based on other variables, such as whether or not chemotherapy was received in the last two weeks of life, or repeated use of emergency visits near death, although these factors have been endorsed by several organizations as indicators of overly aggressive care at the end of life.

REFERENCES:

Wright, et al. Family perspectives on aggressive cancer care near the end of life. *JAMA* 2016;315(3):284–292.

Wright et al. Associations between end of life discussions, patient mental health, medical care near death and caregiver bereavement adjustment. *JAMA.* 2008;300(14):1665–1673.

Teno et al. Family perspectives on end of life care at the last place of care. *JAMA.* 2004;291(1):88–93.

6. ANSWER: D. Discuss the request with the patient, attempting to identify reasons underlying it

Rationale:

The patient's request for assistance with dying can be challenging, and investigation of such a request is an important issue for the palliative care team. The most appropriate choice is to further explore this patient's wishes. His pain is currently not an issue, as stated. The patient might benefit from spiritual care and discussion with a psychiatrist, but the primary action should be exploring his request for assistance with dying. Patients who experience loss of autonomy or the sense of self may request this type of assistance.

REFERENCE:

Hendry M, et al. Why do we want the right to die? A systematic review of the international literature on the views of patients, carers and the public on assisted dying. *Palliative Med.* 2013;27(1):13–26.

7. ANSWER: C. Ask Mary about her spiritual beliefs and how it influences her decision

Rationale:

Most individuals would like physicians to ask about their spiritual and religious beliefs. In addition, patients who report that their spiritual needs are supported by the medical team are more likely to receive hospice care than those who report their spiritual needs were unsupported. Although it would be reasonable to again discuss prognosis, the cousin's belief in miracles can reflect spiritual beliefs, which may take precedence over a physician's opinion of prognosis despite adequate communication of prognosis. One study of surrogates of incapacitated critically ill patients at high risk for death found that only 2% based their views of prognosis solely on the physician's prognostic estimate. Rather, these surrogates used a combination of sources including knowledge of the patient's intrinsic qualities and will to live; their observations of the patient; their beliefs in the power of their support and presence, and optimism, intuition, and faith. Survey data have shown that most respondents believed that divine intervention from God could save a person even if the physician told them futility had been reached.

Without knowing more about the cousin's spiritual and religious beliefs and having a good understanding of what a "miracles means for her," reframing of her hope would be premature and could be perceived as condescending. Involving the ethics committee without taking the previous steps would not likely be effective.

REFERENCES:

Widera EW, Rosenfeld KE, Fromme EK, Sulmasy DP, Arnold RM. Approaching patients and family members who hope for a miracle. *J Pain Symptom Manage*. 2011 Jul;42(1):119–125.

Boyd EA, Lo B, Evans LR, et al."It's not just what the doctor tells me:" factors that influence surrogate decision-makers' perceptions of prognosis. *Crit Care Med*. 2010;38:1270e1275.

Jacobs LM, Burns K, Bennett Jacobs B. Trauma death: views of the public and trauma professionals on death and dying from injuries. *Arch Surg*. 2008;143:730e735.

Balboni TA, Paulk ME, Balboni MJ, et al. Provision of spiritual care to patients with advanced cancer: associations with medical care and quality of life near death. *J Clin Oncol*. 2010;28:445e452.

8. ANSWER: B. Reassure the family that siblings of cancer patients can have negative emotions affecting behavior

Rationale:

Although marital tension and distress increase after the diagnosis of illness in a child, there is not a notable increase in divorce rates among parents of children with cancer. Sibling response to cancer is complex and multidimensional. Negative outcomes among siblings, such as feeling ignored and isolated due to loss of attention, are often experienced after the cancer diagnosis. Negative outcomes often diminish over time. Siblings can also experience positive outcomes of increased responsibility, independence, empathy, and compassion. It is routine for pediatric palliative care teams to focus on all members of the family, including minor siblings.

In this case, the immediate next step is to reassure the family about the sibling's behaviors and explain the underlying reasons for the behavior. The step after reassuring the family about the sibling's behaviors would be to counsel the parents about constructive strategies to support the patient and the sibling and help them cope with this difficult situation. Many pediatric palliative care programs have mental health counselors as integral members of the team, and they are ideally suited to help and counsel the parents and the siblings of seriously ill children.

REFERENCES:

Melissa A. Alderfer, Kristin A, et al. Psychosocial adjustment of siblings of children with cancer: a systematic review. *Psycho-Oncology*. 2010;19:789–805.

Abby R, Rosenberg K, Baker S. Systematic review of psychosocial morbidities among bereaved parents of children with cancer. *Pediatr Blood Cancer*. 2012;58:503–512.nt

9. ANSWER: C. Repositioning

Rationale:

At the end of life, respiratory secretions occur commonly. These secretions have been colloquially termed "the death rattle" and are described as a gurgling sound produced during inspiration and expiration. They are thought to be due to excessive airway secretions, and it is unclear whether they are uncomfortable for the patient. Families and friends in attendance appear to be more distressed and therefore ask for treatment of the symptom. Repositioning can decrease the secretions without adverse effects. Several antimuscarinic agents have been used, but they have not been shown to be superior to placebo and can result in distressing symptoms such as urinary retention and dry mouth. Nebulized saline will not decrease the secretions. Suctioning can cause more physical discomfort.

REFERENCES:

Kehl KA, Kowalkowski JA. A systematic review of the prevalence of signs of impending death and symptoms in the last 2 weeks of life. *Am J Hosp Palliat Care*. 2013;30:601–616.

Wee B, Hillier R. Interventions for noisy breathing in patients near to death. *Cochrane Database Syst Rev*. 2008 Jan 23;(1):CD005177. doi: 10.1002/14651858.CD005177.pub2.

Hwang IC, Ahn HY, Park SM, et al. Clinical changes in terminally ill cancer patients and death within 48 h: When should we refer patients to a separate room? *Support Care Cancer*. 2013;21:835–840.

Morita, T, Ichiki T, Tsunoda J, et al. A prospective study on the dying process in terminally ill cancer patients. *Am J Hosp Palliat Care*. 1998;15:217–222.

Hui D, Dos Santos R, Chisholm G, et al. Clinical signs of impending death in cancer patients. The Oncologist. 2014;19:1–7.

10. ANSWER: C. Grief

Rationale:

Normal grief is the emotional process of reacting to the death of a loved one. It occurs in most people following a loss. It is time-limited, begins soon after a loss, and largely resolves within the first year or two. It is not uncommon for the bereaved to have dreams, illusions, and even hallucinations of the deceased. Complicated grief (CG) occurs in about 10% to 20% of the bereaved. This is a persistent or prolonged period of intense loss. Symptoms must cause marked dysfunction in social, occupational, or other important domains. In the most recent revision of the Diagnostic and Statistical Manual of Mental Disorders (DSM V), CG was relabeled as persistent complex bereavement disorder. Insecure attachment styles, weak parental bonding in childhood, childhood abuse and neglect, female gender, low perceived social support, supportive marital relationships, and low preparation for the loss are all felt to be risk factors for CG. CG shares characteristics with major depressive disorder (suicidal ideation, preoccupation with worthlessness) and post-traumatic stress disorder (re-experiencing intrusive thoughts of the deceased, avoidance of reminders of the deceased and emotional numbness). However these are separate entities differentiated by precipitating events, risk factors, course of illness and response to intervention. In this case, the patient is experiencing sorrow but is also able to engage in activities that were meaningful to her, such as going to church, therefore A, B, and D are incorrect.

REFERENCES:

Markowitz AJ, Rabow MW. Caring for bereaved patients: "All the doctors just suddenly go." *JAMA.* 2002;287(7):882.

Shear K, Frank E, Houck PR, Reynolds CF, 3rd. Treatment of complicated grief: a randomized controlled trial. *JAMA.* 2005 Jun 1;293(21):2601–2608.

Prigerson HG, Horowitz MJ, Jacobs SC, et al. Prolonged grief disorder: Psychometric validation of criteria proposed for DSM-V and ICD-11. *PLoS Med.* Aug 2009;6(8).

Zisook S, Simon NM, Reynolds CF, 3rd, et al. Bereavement, complicated grief, and DSM, part 2: complicated grief. *J Clin Psychiatry.* Aug 2010;71(8):1097–1098.

11. *ANSWER: B.* Telling the children of the disease may make them less anxious

Rationale:

There is a widespread misconception that disclosing news about a dying family member to children is damaging and detrimental to their emotional well-being and development. A high quality longitudinal study of bereaved children showed that separation anxiety symptoms begin prior to death of a family member. Interventions when a family death is impending are important to prevent complicated grief. Clear and honest communication with children is always recommended

REFERENCES:

Rauch PK, Muriel AC. Raising an emotionally healthy child when a parent is sick. New York, NY: McGraw-Hill; 2005.

Rosenheim, E., Reicher, R. (1985). Informing children about a parent's terminal illness. *J Child Psychol Psychiatry.* Allied Disc. 26:995–998.

Siegel, K., Raveis, V., Karus, D. (1996). Pattern of communication with children when a parent has cancer. In L. Baider & L. Cooper (Eds) *Cancer and the family*, pp 109–128. John Wiley and Sons: New York.

Kaplow JB. Saunders J. Angold A. Costello EJ. Psychiatric symptoms in bereaved versus nonbereaved youth and young adults: a longitudinal epidemiological study. *J Am Acad Child Adolesc Psychiatry.* Nov. 2010;49(11):1145–1154.

12. *ANSWER: C.* Gabapentin

Rationale:

It is important during a pain assessment to identify key words, which characterize the nature of the pain. In this case, the descriptors "burning" and "shooting" indicate neuropathic pain. This type of pain is defined as nonsomatic pain due to abnormal nerve signaling, which may be due to mechanisms such as peripheral nerve injury or central sensitization. Classic examples include postherpetic neuralgia and diabetic peripheral neuropathy. Typically opioids are not helpful. Antidepressant and anticonvulsant therapies have been studied and shown to be effective for neuropathic pain.

There is strong evidence that gabapentin is useful in the management of neuropathic cancer pain. Dexamethasone would not be appropriate, as there is no evidence of inflammation. Lorazepam would be the wrong choice, as there is no evidence of muscle cramping and the patient is already confused. Topiramate can be used for neuropathic pain but is widely thought to be second-line therapy for neuropathic pain relief.

REFERENCES:

Wiffen PJ, McQuay HJ, Edwards JE, Moore RA. Gabapentin for acute and chronic pain. *Cochrane Database Syst Rev.* 2005;(3)CD005452.

Caraceni A, Zecca E, Bonezzi C, et al. Gabapentin for neuropathic cancer pain: a randomized controlled trial from the Gabapentin Cancer Pain Study Group. *J Clin Oncol.* 2004;22:2909–2917.

Serpell MG; Neuropathic Pain Study Group. Gabapentin in neuropathic pain syndromes: a randomised, double-blind, placebo-controlled trial. *Pain.* 2002;99:557–566.

13. ANSWER: B. Aromatase inhibitor-induced arthralgias

Rationale:

In postmenopausal women, aromatase inhibitor therapy is increasingly common because it is associated with fewer long-term serious toxicities compared to tamoxifen. However, aromatase inhibitors cause arthralgias in 40% to 50% of patients, which can influence adherence to therapy and can lead to treatment discontinuation in a minority of cases. BMI has been shown to be a positive predictor for AI-associated musculoskeletal symptoms. The mechanism underlying the development of this toxicity remains unclear. The patient has no known etiology for carpal tunnel syndrome, which makes this diagnosis unlikely. There is no evidence of autoimmune disease. She is on minimal amounts of opioids making hyperalgesia unlikely.

REFERENCE:

Henry NL, Giles JT, Ang D, et al: Prospective characterization of musculoskeletal symptoms in early stage breast cancer patients treated with aromatase inhibitors. *Breast Cancer Res Treat.* 111:365–372, 2008.

14. ANSWER: D. Single 8 Gy fraction

Rationale:

Studies suggest equivalent pain relief following 30 Gy in 10 fractions, 20 Gy in 5 fractions, or a single 8 Gy fraction. A single treatment is more convenient but may be associated with a slightly higher rate of retreatment to the same site. Strong consideration should be given to a single 8 Gy fraction for patients with a limited prognosis or with transportation difficulties.

REFERENCES:

Lutz S, et al; American Society for Radiation Oncology (ASTRO). Palliative radiotherapy for bone metastases: an ASTRO evidence-based guideline. *Int J Radiat Oncol Biol Phys.* 2011 Mar 15;79(5):965–976.

Chow E, Zheng L, Salvo N, Dennis K, Tsao M, Lutz S. Update on the systematic review of palliative radiotherapy trials for bone metastases. *Clin Oncol (R Coll Radiol).* 2012 Mar;24(2):112–124.

15. ANSWER: C. Hydromorphone

Rationale:

The patient currently is in a "pain crisis" warranting utilization of stronger analgesics. Based on DOME (daily oral morphine equivalents), 1 mg of intravenous hydromorphone is approximately four times as strong as the hydrocodone the patient had previously taken. Additionally, propoxyphene, oxycodone, and ibuprofen are not available parenterally. Meperidine has metabolites that can be epileptogenic.

REFERENCE:

Ann M. Berger, John L. Shuster, Jr., and Jamie H. Von Roenn. *Principles and Practice of Palliative Care and Supportive Oncology*, 4th ed. Lippincott Williams & Wilkins, 2013.

16. ANSWER: E. Fentanyl transdermal patch 25mcg q72h

Rationale:

When initiating a long-acting opioid after achieving control of acute pain, the long-acting opioid should be initiated at roughly 50% of the DOME. Among the choices offered, choice E the fentanyl transdermal patch provides 50 mg or roughly 50% of the required analgesia. All the other choices provide much stronger doses of opioids, which could possibly result in adverse effects.

REFERENCE:

Ann M. Berger, John L. Shuster, Jr., and Jamie H. Von Roenn. *Principles and Practice of Palliative Care and Supportive Oncology*, 4th ed., Lippincott Williams & Wilkins, 2013.

17. ANSWER: D. Hydromorphone 4 mg tablets BID prn pain

Rationale:

Among the choices listed, choice D is the only one that provides the 30 mg of DOME; all the other choices provide much stronger doses of opioids, which could possibly result in adverse effects.

REFERENCE:

Ann M. Berger, John L. Shuster, Jr., and Jamie H. Von Roenn. *Principles and Practice of Palliative Care and Supportive Oncology*, 4th ed.,Lippincott Williams & Wilkins, 2013.

18. ANSWER: B. Rotate to oxycodone, 30 mg every 12 hours, and oxycodone, 5 to 10 mg every 2 hours as needed.

Rationale:

The patient's baseline long-acting morphine daily dose was 120 mg, with a minimum short-acting morphine dose of 30 mg daily, which yields a total daily dose of 150 mg. The morphine-to-oxycodone ratio is generally accepted to be 1.5:1; so this patient's morphine-equivalent daily dose of oxycodone would be 100 mg. With the use of a cross-tolerance conversion of 25% to 50%, the daily dose of oxycodone would be 60 mg. Thus, the every-12-hour dose of long-acting oxycodone would be 30 mg.

Rotation to oxycodone, 60 mg every 12 hours, and oxycodone, 15 mg every 2 hours as needed, does not take into account the concept of cross-tolerance or the accepted oxycodone-to-morphine equianalgesic conversion, thus putting the patient at risk for both possible opioid toxicity from another agent and the emergence of additional oxycodone opioid adverse effects due to incomplete cross-tolerance. Tolerance to opioid-induced pruritus should develop in approximately 7 to 10 days, although in rare cases no tolerance develops and refractory symptoms persist despite treatments. Lowering the dosage of sustained-release morphine to 30 mg every 12 hours is incorrect because pruritus is not necessarily a dose-response phenomenon.

REFERENCES:

Nuckols TK, Anderson L, Popescu I, et al. Opioid prescribing: a systematic review and critical appraisal of guidelines for chronic pain. *Ann Intern Med.* 2014;160:38–47.

Fine PG, Portenoy RK. Ad Hoc Expert Panel on Evidence Review and Guidelines for Opioid Rotation. Establishing "best practices" for opioid rotation: conclusions of an expert panel. *J Pain Symptom Manage.* 2009;38:418–425.

Pergolizzi J, Boger RH, Budd K, et al. Opioids and the management of chronic severe pain in the elderly: consensus statement of an International Expert Panel with focus on the six clinically most often used World Health Organization Step III opioids (buprenorphine, fentanyl, hydromorphone, methadone, morphine, and oxycodone). *Pain Pract.* 2008 Jul-Aug;8(4):287–313.

19. ANSWER: D. Mindfulness meditation

Rationale:

Up to 60% of practicing physicians report symptoms of burnout, defined as emotional exhaustion, depersonalization (treating patients as objects), and low sense of accomplishment. Physician burnout has been linked to poorer quality of care, including patient dissatisfaction, increased medical errors, and lawsuits and decreased ability to express empathy. Substance abuse, automobile accidents, stress-related health problems, and marital and family discord are among the personal consequences reported. Burnout can occur early in the medical educational process. Nearly half of all third-year medical students report burnout and there are strong associations between medical student burnout and suicidal ideation.

One proposed approach to addressing loss of meaning and lack of control in practice life is developing greater mindfulness—the quality of being fully present and attentive in the moment during everyday activities. Mindfulness meditation is a secular contemplative practice focusing on cultivating an individual's attention and awareness skills. Participation in a mindful communication program was associated with short-term and sustained improvements in well-being and attitudes associated with patient-centered care.

REFERENCE:

Krasner, et al. Association of an educational program in mindful communication with burnout, empathy, and attitudes among primary care physicians. Krasner, et al. *JAMA*. 2009;302(12):1284-1293. doi:10.1001/jama.2009.1384.

20. *ANSWER: B.* Parenteral morphine

Rationale:

The use of systemic opioids has been well established in numerous studies and meta-analyses as the standard of care for symptomatic relief of dyspnea. A well-designed randomized, controlled trial of oxygen vs ambient air, delivered by nasal cannula, in patients with advanced illness and dyspnea showed no benefit of oxygen over ambient air delivered by nasal cannula. Nebulized morphine has not been shown to be of greater benefit than systemic opioids. While benzodiazepines can be helpful in refractory dyspnea, they would not be the next best step in this case.

REFERENCES:

Bruera E, Sweeny C, and Ripamonti C. Dyspnea in patients with advanced cancer. In: Berger A, Portenoy R and Weissman DE, eds. *Principles and practice of palliative care and supportive oncology.* 2nd ed. New York, NY: Lippincott-Raven; 2002.

Chan KS et al. Palliative medicine in malignant respiratory diseases. In: Doyle D, Hanks G, Cherney N, and Calman N, eds. *Oxford Textbook of Palliative Medicine*, 3rd ed. New York, NY: Oxford University Press; 2005.

Viola R et al. The management of dyspnea in cancer patients: a systematic review. *Supp Care Cancer.* 2008;16:329–337.

Bruera E, et al. Nebulized versus subcutaneous morphine for patients with cancer dyspnea: a preliminary study. J Pain Symptom Manage. 2005 Jun;29(6):613–618.

21. *ANSWER: C.* Dexamethasone

Rationale:

Corticosteroids have proven efficacy in the treatment of delayed chemotherapy-induced nausea. Their mechanism of action is not totally clear, although some effect on prostaglandins has been proposed.

Application of ABH gel (lorazepam, diphenhydramine, haloperidol) to the patient's wrist as needed for nausea is common practice, but the data have been based on patient recall. Prospective studies examining ABH gel use have shown no more effectiveness in controlling nausea or vomiting than placebo. There are no data indicating effectiveness for lorazepam in delayed chemotherapy-induced nausea. The only settings where it is expected that lorazepam may help treat chemotherapy-induced nausea are in patients who demonstrate anticipatory nausea when they think about chemotherapy, or on the day of treatment prior to any chemotherapy administration. Octreotide is used to decrease gastrointestinal secretions and may have some efficacy regarding vomiting in patients with mechanical bowel obstruction or severe chemotherapy-induced diarrhea. Its mechanism of action does not have an impact on any receptors or physiologic mediators that factor into delayed nausea from chemotherapy.

REFERENCES:

Fletcher DS, Coyne PJ, Dodson PW, et al. A randomized trial of the effectiveness of topical "ABH Gel" (Ativan(R), Benadryl(R), Haldol(R)) versus placebo in cancer patients with nausea. *J Pain Symptom Manage.* 2014 Nov;48(5):797–803. doi: 10.1016/j.jpainsymman.2014.02.010. Epub 2014 May 2.

Smith TJ, Ritter JK, Poklis JL, et al. ABH gel is not absorbed from the skin of normal volunteers. *J Pain Symptom Manage.* 2012;43(5):961–966.

Weschules DJ. Tolerability of the compound ABHR in hospice patients. *J Palliat Med.* 2005;8(6):1135–1143.

22. *ANSWER: B.* methylphenidate

Rationale:

Methylphenidate has been shown to effectively improve symptoms of fatigue in cancer patients. A positive response is usually seen within a few days of initiation of the medication. The patient did not meet screening criteria for depression. There have been anecdotal reports of duloxetine as improving energy, however, in this case it would not be the preferred treatment. Modafinil may be an option, but it is more expensive, and has not been proven to be more effective for cancer-related fatigue than other psychostimulants. Transfusion would be of no benefit for fatigue in absence of anemia.

REFERENCES:

Morrow GR, Shelke AR, Roscoe JA. Management of cancer-related fatigue. *Cancer Investigation.* 2005; 23:229–239.

Qu D, Zhang Zm Yu X, et al. Psychotropic drugs for the management of cancer-related fatigue: a systematic review and meta-analysis. *Eur J Cancer Care.* 2015

23. *ANSWER: B.* Docusate sodium

Rationale:

Constipation is a common occurrence in hospitalized patients, particularly for patients who are on opioids for pain. Although the use of certain laxatives, particularly docusate-based softeners, is widespread and commonplace, there is little quality evidence supporting the efficacy of docusate in constipation prevention or treatment. A randomized, placebo-controlled trial of docusate use in hospice patients showed it was no better than placebo in the management of constipation. There are indirect costs of docusate, which include pharmacy inventory management and distribution; nursing administration time; polypharmacy and pill burden; and downstream investigations (e.g., clostridium difficile testing) in the case of laxative-induced diarrhea. For these reasons, the use of docusate should be avoided in favor of more effective agents.

REFERENCES:

Lee, MD, MPH, et al. Research Letter: "Less Is More: Pattern of Inpatient Laxative Use: Waste Not, Want Not." *JAMA Internal Medicine*, published online June 20, 2016.

Rapid Response Reports CADTH. Dioctyl sulfosuccinate or docusate (calcium or sodium) for the prevention or management of constipation: A review of the clinical effectiveness. Ottawa, ON: Canadian Agency for Drugs and Technologies in Health; 2014.

Tarumi Y, Wilson MP, Szafran O, and Spooner GR. Randomized, double-blind, placebo-controlled trial of oral docusate in the management of constipation in hospice patients. *J Pain Symptom Manage.* 2013;45(1):2–13.

24. ANSWER: A. Ask the patient if he has had thoughts about suicide

Rationale:

The patient in this question presents a clinical picture of depression, as he exhibits anhedonia, a sense of worthlessness, and a desire for an early death. He is at very high risk for suicide, being an elderly male who lives alone and has a major physical illness, has lost a vital relationship, and has a history of alcohol usage. He also has been socially isolating himself by staying in bed all day and stopping his typical social activities. The best immediate next step in the care of this patient is to assess him for suicidality. Gentle exploration about any thoughts of suicide will provide the patient with an outlet to discuss these sensitive issues and divulge any plans he may have or ideas he is contemplating related to suicide.

While both methylphenidate and citalopram can help palliate his depression, neither drug is the best immediate next step. Referral to a psychiatry clinic is appropriate. However, given the patient's high risk of suicide, he needs immediate assessment and management, which may include hospitalization for management of suicidality in some situations.

REFERENCES:

Block SD. Assessing and managing depression in the terminally ill patient: ACP-ASIM end-of-life care consensus panel. American College of Physicians - American Society of Internal Medicine. *Ann Intern Med.* 2000;132:209–218.

Department of Veterans Affairs. Suicide Risk Assessment Guide: Reference Manual. Internet reference:www.mentalhealth.va.gov/docs/suicide_risk_assessment_reference_guide.pdf   Accessed December 13, 2014.

25. ANSWER: B. Metoclopramide, scopolamine and octreotide

Rationale:

There is good evidence to support the use of antiemetics, antisecretory agents and somatostatin analogues in the setting of malignant bowel obstruction (MBO). In this case, the patient has incomplete obstruction; however, in the case of complete obstruction, metoclopramide should be avoided. Specific parameters have been repeatedly identified in cohorts less likely to benefit from surgical intervention. These include complete small bowel obstruction (SBO) as opposed to partial SBO or large bowel obstruction, nongynecological cancer, ascites, low serum albumin, and white cell count outside normal range. In addition to this, age >65, malnutrition and a general decrease in functional status have been described as negative prognostic features. The feasibility of stent placement depends on the presence of experts and available technologies. While using opioids for cancer-related pain is reasonable, this would be inadequate treatment of MBO in which symptoms of nausea and vomiting need to be addressed.

REFERENCES:

H.J.M. Ferguson et al. *Ann Med and Surg.* 2015;4:264–270.

L. Helyer, A.M. Easson, Surgical approaches to malignant bowel obstruction. *J Support. Oncol.* 2008;6:105–113.

J.C. Henry, S. Pouly, R. Sullivan, et al., A scoring system for the prognosis and treatment of malignant bowel obstruction. *Surgery* 152(2012) 747–756.

Laval et al, Review Article, Recommendations for bowel obstruction with peritoneal carcinomatosis. *J Pain Symptom Manage.* 2014 July;48(1).

26. *ANSWER: D.* Haloperidol 0.5 mg PO q1h PRN

Rationale:

Haloperidol is the first-line for the treatment of delirium. Benzodiazepines can be used for sedation in cases of severe hyperactive delirium, but may worsen symptoms, especially in the elderly. While olanzapine is effective for delirium, it is no more effective than haloperidol and is more expensive.

REFERENCES:

Breitbart W, Alici Y. Evidence-based treatment of delirium in patients with cancer. *J Clin Oncol.* 2012;30:1206–1214.

Breitbart W, Bruera E, Chochinov H, Lynch M. Neuropsychiatric syndromes and psychological symptoms in patients with advanced cancer. *J Pain Symptom Manage.* 1995;10:131–141.

27. *ANSWER: A.* Plan ahead of the meeting to use a live professional interpreter

Rationale:

Medical interpreters have expertise in interpretation as opposed to ad hoc interpreters (i.e., family members, hospital staff). Errors in interpretation occur less commonly with professional interpreters and patient satisfaction is higher. Live interpreters are preferable to telephone interpreters because nonverbal communication, such as body language and emotional cues, can be vital to goals of care discussions and can be easily missed by a telephone interpreter. Family members may not accurately translate what is said by the physician. This may be due to a lack of familiarity with medical terminology in either language, discomfort with what is being discussed in the family meeting, or overwhelming emotions or personal beliefs. Physicians who can speak a second language should use an interpreter unless they have native fluency in that second language and know medical terminology in that second language.

REFERENCES:

Schenker Y, et al. "Her Husband Doesn't Speak Much English": Conducting a Family Meeting with an Interpreter. *J Palliat Med*. 2011 Nov 22.

Butow PN, Goldstein D, Bell ML, et al. Interpretation in consultations with immigrant patients with cancer: how accurate is it? *J Clin Oncol*. 2011;29(20):2801–2807.

28. ANSWER: A. Decision-making capacity

Rationale:

Patients who have a terminal illness may express the wish to die and ask their physician how to hasten their death. A thorough assessment of the reasons leading to this request should occur first, including evaluation and management of depression, to determine whether there is unaddressed or untreated physical or emotional distress. For patients whose suffering remains intolerable despite palliative efforts, there are legally and ethically accepted methods of hastening one's death. Stopping eating and drinking is ethically viewed as withdrawal of a life-sustaining treatment. Patients who are able to make their own decisions may choose to stop oral nutrition and hydration. The act of voluntarily stopping eating and drinking is an expression of control and autonomy in the patient who has decision-making capacity.

The patient does not need to have intractable physical symptoms to voluntarily stop eating and drinking, as this is not a physician-directed intervention. The patient retains decision-making capacity, and so the physician does not need to follow or refer to previously documented wishes, such as an advance directive stating that she does not want life-prolonging measures. It is not a requirement that the patient should already be receiving hospice care in order to make this decision.

REFERENCES:

Ivanovic N, Buche D, Fringer A. Voluntary stopping of eating and drinking at the end of life - a 'systematic search and review' giving insight into an option of hastening death in capacitated adults at the end of life. BMC *Palliat Care*. 2014;13:1.

Quill TE, Lo B, Brock DW. Palliative options of last resort: a comparison of voluntarily stopping eating and drinking, terminal sedation, physician-assisted suicide, and voluntary active euthanasia. *JAMA*. 1997;278:2099–2104.

29. ANSWER: B. "Artificial nutrition is beneficial in your situation and will probably improve the quality of your life."

Rationale:

In most patients who have advanced cancer, artificial nutrition is not indicated because it does not increase longevity or improve functional status. However, these principles do not apply in patients with intact performance status who are suddenly unable to orally take food or hydration, especially in patients with head and neck cancer who are undergoing radiation therapy, as is the case with this patient. The patient is currently severely dehydrated as a result of his inability to take any food or fluids; thus, it is likely that the radiation oncologists will be hesitant to continue radiation therapy if he does not receive supplemental nutrition and hydration. However, stating that "You must consent to artificial nutrition if you want to continue radiation therapy for the cancer" is antagonistic and will probably erode the doctor-patient relationship. It would be more effective to gently encourage the patient to consent to a feeding tube by stating that his specific cancer is one of the few for which feeding tubes are indicated and beneficial. While respect for patient autonomy is one the guiding ethical principles of medical care, this necessitates informed decision-making for the patient. The physician's role is to provide expert guidance and counsel to patients based on best evidence. While it is appropriate for all patients who have a serious illness to complete a Physician Orders for Life-Sustaining Treatment (POLST) form, this option is incorrect as the initial response to this patient.

REFERENCES:

Casarett D, Kapo J, Caplan A. Appropriate use of artificial nutrition and hydration: fundamental principles and recommendations. *N Engl J Med.* 2005;353:2607–2712.

Physician Orders for Life-Sustaining Treatment (POLST). POLST for Healthcare Providers. http://capolst.org/polst-for-healthcare-providers/. Accessed December 13, 2014.

30. ANSWER: B. Tolerance

Rationale:

Tolerance is the physiologic phenomenon that can occur when opioids are used for pain in the long-term setting. It is the need to increase a drug to achieve the same effect. There is no evidence to indicate increased pain in this case. Physical dependence is the development of a withdrawal syndrome when a drug is suddenly discontinued or an antagonist is administered. While it is likely opioid withdrawal can occur if the oxycodone is withheld, it is not enough to describe the current situation and is clinically irrelevant in this case.

Opioid use disorder (OUD) includes signs and symptoms that reflect compulsive, prolonged self-administration of opioid substances that are used for no legitimate medical purpose or, if another medical condition is present that requires opioid treatment, that are used in doses greatly in excess of the amount needed for that medical condition. Individuals with OUD tend to develop such regular patterns of compulsive drug use that daily activities are planned around obtaining and administering opioids. Opioids are usually purchased on the illegal market but may also be obtained from physicians by falsifying or exaggerating general medical problems or by receiving simultaneous prescriptions from several physicians. Most individuals with OUD have significant levels of tolerance and will experience withdrawal on abrupt discontinuation of opioid substances. Opioid use disorder can be associated with a history of drug-related crimes (e.g., possession or distribution of drugs, forgery, burglary, robbery, larceny, receiving stolen goods). While this case demonstrates opioid tolerance, there is no evidence that Ms. Snow is engaging in aberrant or harmful behaviors.

REFERENCES:

Sees KL, Clark HW. Opioid use in the treatment of chronic pain: assessment of addiction. *J Pain Symptom Manage*. 1993;8:257–264.

Eisendrath SJ. Psychiatric aspects of chronic pain. *Neurology*. 1995;45:S26-S34.

Passik SD, Kirsh KL, Portenoy RK. Understanding aberrant drug-taking behavior: addiction redefined for palliative care and pain management settings. *Principles and Practice of Supportive Oncology Updates*. 1999;2:1–12.

Diagnostic and Statistical Manual of Mental Disorders, 5th edn. (Copyright 2013). American Psychiatric Association.

Central Venous Access Device 41

Peter A. Zmijewski and Hannah W. Hazard-Jenkins

REVIEW QUESTIONS

1. What is the inner most layer of the vein that is damaged with repeat trauma from peripheral venipuncture?

    A. Tunica intima

    B. Tunica adventitia

    C. Tunica media

    D. All of the above

    E. None of the above

2. Which of the following is NOT a contraindication for long-term central venous access device?

    A. Ongoing bloodstream infection

    B. Prior central venous access device

    C. Thrombosis of the vessel

    D. Uncontrolled coagulopathy

    E. None of the above

3. Which of the following central venous access devices is completely internalized (no part of the device is exposed)?

    A. PICC

    B. Hickman

C. Infusaport

D. TCC

E. PIV

---

4. Which of the following should be taken into consideration when deciding which central venous access device to use?

    A. Osmolality of the infusate

    B. Patient preference

    C. Duration of treatment

    D. Location of treatment

    E. All of the answers are correct

---

5. Which of the below central venous access devices is the most likely to cause major complications such as pneumothorax and hemothorax?

    A. Midline catheter

    B. PICC

    C. PIV

    D. Right internal jugular TCC

    E. Left subclavian vein infusaport

ANSWERS TO REVIEW QUESTIONS

1. ANSWER: A. Tunica intima

Rationale:

The tunica intima is the inner most layer of the vein and comprises a thin layer of endothelial cells that allow for nutrient and oxygen exchange. The tunica media is the middle layer and the vein has a thin layer of muscular cells and a scan amount of connective tissue. The tunica adventitia is the outermost layer and is the thickest and predominantly connective tissue.

2. ANSWER: B. Prior central venous access device

Rationale:

Ongoing blood stream infection is contraindicated due to the extremely high risk of seeding the implanted device and perpetuating the infection. An occluded vessel means the catheter would not be able to be placed in the appropriate location. Ongoing coagulopathy places the patient at high risk for bleeding complications such as hematoma and hemothorax. Catheters may be placed if there were prior catheters but it may be worthwhile to Doppler the venous system to see if the vein is still patent.

3. ANSWER: C. Infusaport

Rationale:

The infusaport is the only device that is completely under the skin; the TCC, PICC, Hickman, and peripheral IV all have components of the system externalized.

4. ANSWER: E. All of the Answers are correct

Rationale:

All are important considerations when choosing a line. If a patient is getting a high osmolar liquid, externalized lines are better so as to ensure the therapy is not infused into the subcutaneous tissues. If a patient is receiving therapy in and out of the hospital, peripheral IVs will not last.

5. ANSWER: E. Left subclavian vein infusaport

Rationale:

All catheters mentioned except for the infusaport are placed peripherally and do not involve venipuncture to the large central veins that can cause a risk of hemothorax/pneumothorax.

Procedures in Medical Oncology **42**

Kerry Ryan and George Carter

REVIEW QUESTIONS

1. A 34-year-old male presents to your oncology office with a newly diagnosed stage Burkitt's Cell Lymphoma. He is complaining of headaches and his wife states he has unstable gait and fallen several times at home. What should your next step be?

    A. Perform an emergent lumbar puncture to rule out leptomeningeal disease.

    B. Prescribe the patient pain medication for his headache.

    C. Perform a MRI or CT of his brain before preceding to a lumbar puncture.

2. A 56-year-old male with stage IV Diffuse Large B Cell Lymphoma presents for his staging workup following 6 cycles of R-CHOP. You are planning on doing a bone marrow on him today to complete his re-staging. Four months ago he has had a deep venous thrombosis and is now on enoxaparin 100 mg/kg subcutaneously twice daily. He took his morning dose, two hours ago. Do you proceed with the bone marrow today?

    A. Yes

    B. No

3. A 64-year-old female presents with metastatic ovarian cancer and is short of breath. She is found to have a large right sided pleural effusion and you decide to perform a thoracentesis. The ultrasound machine has broken. What intercostal spaces should you perform a thoracentesis through?

    A. Ninth or tenth intercostal space

    B. Seventh or eighth intercostal space

    C. Sixth or seventh intercostal space

    D. Fifth or fourth intercostal space

4. A 31-year-old with newly diagnosed acute lymphoblastic leukemia undergoes a lumbar puncture to evaluate for CNS involvement. It is an uncomplicated procedure; however, the next day she is complaining of a severe headache and cannot get out of bed without her headache worsening. She is given oxycodone and told to remain recombinant. After 48 hours she is still complaining of a severe headache. What should be considered next?

    A. Intravenous hydration

    B. Nonsteroidal medication

    C. Abdominal binder

    D. Epidural blood patch

5. A 65-year-old female with ovarian cancer presents with abdominal pain and distention. Imaging of her abdomen demonstrates dilated loops of bowel and a large amount of ascites. What is the most appropriate procedure to perform next?

    A. Paracentesis without ultrasound

    B. Paracentesis with ultrasound

    C. Insertion of a urinary catheter

    D. Insertion of a nasogastric tube

ANSWERS TO REVIEW QUESTIONS

1. ANSWER: C. A contraindication to performing a lumbar puncture is the presence of unequal pressures between the supratentorial and infratentorial compartments. This is usually deduced from the following characteristics on imaging of the brain: midline shift; loss of suprachiascmatic and basilar cisterns; posterior fossa mass; loss of superior cerebellar cistern; or loss of the quadrigeminal plate cistern. When a patient presents with neurologic symptoms, imaging of the brain is necessary prior to performing lumbar puncture.

2. ANSWER: B. No, anticoagulation should be held prior to a bone marrow biopsy, if safe to do so. This is not an emergent need for this bone marrow to be performed, so a delay of one or two days would not be harmful. Also, since the patient is three months past the deep venous thrombosis, the risk of holding the medication for a short period of time is relatively low. The patient should hold his enoxaparin 24 hours prior to the bone marrow. If the patient was on coumadin they should be transitioned over to a low-molecular heparin, and this should be held 24 hours prior to the bone marrow.

3. ANSWER: B. In the absence of ultrasound guidance, a thoracentesis should be performed through the seventh or eighth intercostal space.

4. ANSWER: D. This patient is suffering from a postlumbar puncture headache and has not found benefit from initial conservative therapy. Hydration and abdominal binders have not shown benefit in treating postlumbar puncture headaches. Epidural blood patches should be considered next.

5. ANSWER: D. A nasogastric tube should be placed first in patients with bowel obstruction prior to performing a paracentesis.

Basic Principles of Radiation Oncology 43

Chirag Shah, Nikhil P. Joshi, and Bindu Manyam

REVIEW QUESTIONS

1. Radiation therapy can be delivered in multiple different forms. At this time, the most common form of therapeutic radiation is delivered with a linear accelerator which utilizes

   A. High energy protons

   B. Low energy neutrons

   C. High energy photons

   D. Alpha particles

2. High energy photons interact with matter to cause biologic damage. Its most common interactions with matter can best be described as

   A. Indirectly ionizing, indirect action

   B. Directly ionizing, direct action

   C. Indirectly ionizing, direct action

   D. Directly ionizing, indirect action

3. Heavy charged particles interact with matter to manifest biologic damage. Its most common interactions with matter can best be described as

   A. Indirectly ionizing, indirect action

   B. Directly ionizing, direct action

   C. Indirectly ionizing, direct action

   D. Directly ionizing, indirect action

4. Clinical radiation oncology commonly utilizes fractionation, where multiple small doses of radiation are given daily. One fundamental principle of fractionation is repair, which is important because of what factor?

   A. It allows for cells to move to more sensitive phases of the cell cycle.

   B. It allow for DNA damage to be fixed.

   C. It allows for tumor growth.

   D. It allows for normal tissue cells to address sublethal damage.

5. Repopulation represents a challenge for clinicians during fractionated radiotherapy. Which of the following represents a strategy to limit the impact of repopulation?

   A. Extend duration of treatment

   B. Shorten duration of treatment

   C. Split treatment course

   D. Reduce total dose

6. Patients receiving radiation therapy typically undergo a workflow to ensure safe and effective treatment. Which of the following is not part of the standard treatment workflow?

   A. Simulation

   B. Quality assurance

   C. Treatment planning

   D. Volume study

7. Linear accelerators can deliver treatment with either photons or electrons. When using photons which of the following components must be in place which is not present when using electrons?

   A. Scattering foils

   B. Light field

   C. Target

   D. Jaws

8. Radiation therapy can cause side effects. Which of the following would be an unexpected toxicity with breast radiation?

    A. Fatigue

    B. Skin redness

    C. Chest wall pain

    D. Diarrhea

9. Stereotactic radiosurgery/Stereotactic body radiation therapy represents techniques where high doses are delivered in a single or a few treatments. Which of the following treatment sites is not commonly treated with SBRT at this time?

    A. Lung cancer

    B. Breast cancer

    C. Spine metastases

    D. Brain metastases

10. Brachytherapy is routinely used to treat many cancers. Which of the following is not a site typically treated with brachytherapy?

    A. Gynecologic cancers

    B. Prostate cancer

    C. Breast cancer

    D. CNS malignancies

ANSWERS TO REVIEW QUESTIONS

1. ANSWER: C

Rationale:

Radiation therapy delivered by a linear accelerator comes in the form of high-energy photons, which are created when electrons strike a target, creating photons.

REFERENCE:

McDermott PN, Orton CG. X-ray production II: basic physics and properties of resulting x-rays. In: McDermott PN, Orton CG, ed. *The Physics of & Technology of Radiation Therapy*. 1st ed. Madison, WI: Medical Physics Publishing; 2010:5:1-5:29.

2. ANSWER: A

Rationale:

High-energy photons primarily work by indirect ionization, generating secondary particles (electrons). DNA damage is then caused primarily by indirect action where the secondary electrons produce free radicals that interact and damage DNA.

REFERENCE:

Hall EJ, Giaccia AJ. Physics and chemistry of radiation absorption. In: Hall EJ, Giaccia AJ, ed. *Radiobiology for the Radiologist*, 6th ed. Philadelphia, PA: Lippincott Williams & Wilkins; 2006:5–15.

3. ANSWER: B

Rationale:

Unlike photons, heavy charged particles are directly ionizing, in that they do not commonly produce secondary particles to produce DNA damage. They are also primarily direct acting in that they do not commonly generate free radicals to cause DNA damage.

REFERENCE:

McDermott PN, Orton CG. X-ray production II: basic physics and properties of resulting x-rays. In: McDermott PN, Orton CG, ed. *The Physics of & Technology of Radiation Therapy*. 1st ed. Madison, WI: Medical Physics Publishing; 2010:5:1-5:29.

4. ANSWER: D

Rationale:

Repair is essential for fractionation and allows for normal tissue to repair sublethal damage, reducing toxicity. Tumor cells are able to repair sublethal damage as well but due so less efficiently enhancing the therapeutic ratio associated with fractionation.

REFERENCE:

Hall EJ, Giaccia AJ. Time, dose, and fractionation in radiotherapy. In: Hall EJ, Giaccia AJ, ed. *Radiobiology for the Radiologist*, 6th ed. Philadelphia, PA: Lippincott Williams & Wilkins; 2006:378–397.

5. ANSWER: B

Rationale:

Repopulation, while allowing normal tissue to recover, is a major challenge for clinicians as malignancies can also repopulate reducing tumor control. The most common strategy to limit this, is to shorten the duration of treatment.

REFERENCE:

Hall EJ, Giaccia AJ. Time, dose, and fractionation in radiotherapy. In: Hall EJ, Giaccia AJ, ed. *Radiobiology for the Radiologist*, 6th ed. Philadelphia, PA: Lippincott Williams & Wilkins; 2006:378–97.

6. ANSWER: D

Rationale:

Radiation therapy centers typically have a standardized workflow to ensure quality and safety. This begins with a consultation which is followed by a simulation. Subsequently, cases are planned in the treatment planning system and then reviewed. Treatment plans undergo quality assurance checks as well to ensure safety.

REFERENCE:

McDermott PN, Orton CG. External beam radiation therapy units. In: McDermott PN, Orton CG, ed. *The Physics of & Technology of Radiation Therapy*. 1st ed. Madison, WI: Medical Physics Publishing; 2010:9:1-9:45.

7. ANSWER: C

Rationale:

Photons are generated in the linear accelerator when electrons interact with the target. Scattering foils are used only in electron mode while a flattening filter is used in photon mode. The light field is present for both types of treatment. Jaws remain in place for both types of treatment.

REFERENCE:

McDermott PN, Orton CG. External beam radiation therapy units. In: McDermott PN, Orton CG, ed. *The Physics of & Technology of Radiation Therapy*. 1st ed. Madison, WI: Medical Physics Publishing; 2010:9:1-9:45.

8. ANSWER: D

Rationale:

Radiation therapy typically causes side-effects based on the site of treatment with common toxicities associated with breast radiation being fatigue and skin erythema. Diarrhea could be expected for GI or GU radiation therapy cases.

REFERENCE:

Hall EJ, Giaccia AJ. Dose-response relationships for model normal tissues. In: Hall EJ, Giaccia AJ, ed. *Radiobiology for the Radiologist*, 6th ed. Philadelphia, PA: Lippincott Williams & Wilkins; 2006:303–326.

9. ANSWER: B

Rationale:

Increasing data supports the use of SBRT in early-stage non-small cell lung cancers while data is available supporting the use of SRS for brain and spine metastases with excellent rates of local control noted. Breast cancer is primarily treated with whole breast irradiation or in some cases brachytherapy but SBRT is not commonly used at this time.

REFERENCES:

McGarry RC, Papiez L, Williams M, et al. Stereotactic body radiation therapy of early-stage nonsmall-cell lung carcinoma: phase I study. *Int J Radiat Oncol Biol Phys.* 2005;63:1010–1015.

Timmerman R, Paulus R, Galvin J, et al. Stereotactic body radiation therapy for inoperable early stage lung cancer. *JAMA* 2010;303:1070–1076.

RTOG 0631: A Phase II/III Study of Image-Guided Radiosurgery/SBRT for Localized Spine Metastasis. Available at: https://www.rtog.org/ClinicalTrials/ProtocolTable/StudyDetails.aspx?study=0631. Accessed August 20, 2016.

Kotecha R, Vogel S, Suh JH, et al. A cure is possible: a study of 10-year survivors of brain metastases.

Vicini F, Shah C, Tendulkar R, et al. Accelerated partial breast irradiation: An update on published Level I evidence. *Brachytherapy.* 2016;15:607–615.

10. ANSWER: D

Rationale:

Brachytherapy is a standard of care treatment approach in the management of prostate cancers as monotherapy for low-risk prostate cancer and as part of boost treatment for high-risk cases. Brachytherapy can be used in breast cancer to deliver APBI. It also remains an essential component in the treatment of gynecologic cancers particularly endometrial and cervical malignancies.

REFERENCES:

Stone NN, Stock RG. 15-year cause specific and all-cause survival following brachytherapy for prostate cancer: negative impact of long-term hormonal therapy. *J Urol.* 2014;192:754–759.

Martinez AA, Shah C, Mohammed N, et al. Ten-year outcomes for prostate cancer patients with Gleason 8 through 10 treated with external beam radiation and high-dose-rate brachytherapy boost in the PSA era. *J Radiat Oncol.* 2016;5:87–93.

Morris JW, Tyldesley S, Pai HH, et al. ASCENDE-RT: A multicenter randomized trial of dose-escalated external beam radiation therapy (EBRT-B) versus low-dose-rate brachytherapy (LDR-B) for men with unfavorable-risk localized prostate cancer. *J Clin Oncol.* 2015;33:s7:3.

Vicini F, Shah C, Tendulkar R, et al. Accelerated partial breast irradiation: An update on published Level I evidence. *Brachytherapy.* 2016;15:607–615.

Harkenrider MM, Block AM, Alektiar KM. American Brachytherapy Task Group Report: Adjuvant vaginal brachytherapy for early-stage endometrial cancer. A comprehensive review. *Brachytherapy.* 2016 May 3 [Epub ahead of print].

Viswanthan AN, Thomadsen B. American Brachytherapy Society consensus guidelines for locally advanced carcinoma of the cervix. Part 1: general principles. Brachytherapy 2012;11:33–46.

Clinical Genetics 44

Holly Jane Pederson and Brandie Heald

REVIEW QUESTIONS

1. A 28-year-old woman presents with a lump and is diagnosed with a triple-negative breast cancer. There is no family history of breast cancer. Her father who is of Ashkenazi Jewish descent was an only child and is healthy. What genetic testing do you recommend?

   A. None—there is not family history of cancer

   B. *BRCA1/2* sequencing including BART

   C. *TP53* testing

   D. Multisite 3 testing

   E. Multisite 3 testing with reflex to gene panel testing.

2. She is found to harbor one of the three founder mutations seen in the Ashkenazi population, 185delAG, in *BRCA1*. This finding may have important treatment implications in that

   A. *BRCA* associated cancers may have better response to dose-dense anthracycline taxane chemotherapy regimens.

   B. *BRCA* associated cancers may have a better response to platinum agents than sporadic cancers.

   C. *BRCA* associated cancers may have a better response to therapies such as poly-(ADP) ribose polymerase inhibitors.

   D. B and C

   E. All of the above

3. A 40-year-old woman is recently diagnosed with breast cancer. She reports a prior history of colorectal hamartomatous polyps, and on physical examination you note that she is macrocephalic. Which gene or gene(s) are on the top of your differential?

   A. *BMPR1A* and *SMAD4*

   B. *BRCA1* and *BRCA2*

   C. *PTEN*

   D. *STK11*

4. A 45-year-old male comes to you for a second opinion. He was diagnosed with colon cancer a month ago after presenting with fatigue, dyspnea on exertion, and right upper quadrant abdominal pain. Colonoscopy revealed a large nonobstructing tumor at the hepatic flexure and biopsy showed a poorly differentiated, mucinous-producing colon adenocarcinoma. Staging studies showed local extension into the liver capsule but no intrahepatic lesions or widespread metastatic disease was seen. His family history is significant for a mother diagnosed with uterine carcinoma at the age of 47, a maternal aunt with ovarian cancer diagnosed in her 50s, and her daughter who was recently found to have a brain tumor. His maternal grandfather died when the patient was very young from what he thinks was either stomach or pancreatic cancer. What gene mutation does this patient likely harbor?

   A. Germline mutation of *APC*

   B. Somatic mutation of the *CDH1* gene and subsequent loss of E-cadherin

   C. Germline mutation of *MSH2*

   D. Germline mutation of *STK11*

5. A gastroenterologist refers a 50-year-old patient to you who underwent a baseline colonoscopy and was found to have a transverse colon cancer in the setting of a couple hundred adenomas. The patient has four siblings in their 40s and an 11 year old son and 13 year old daughter. Which of the following is the least appropriate recommendation?

   A. The patient's children should have a colonoscopy at this time.

   B. The patient should have an upper endoscopy.

C. The patient should have examination of his thyroid.

D. The patient should have *APC* and *MUTYH* testing.

6. You are asked to see a 45-year-old woman who is recently found to carry a BRCA1 mutation. She is aware of the association between BRCA1 and pancreatic cancer and wonders if she should have screening. There is no family history of pancreatic cancer and she is a nonsmoker. Choose the FALSE statement below:

   A. Reassure her that pancreatic cancer is rare and only 3% of cases are linked to known genetic cancer susceptibility syndromes or inherited disease.

   B. She should embark on pancreatic cancer screening with MRCP (magnetic resonance cholangiopancreatolography) alternating with EUS (endoscopic ultrasonography).

   C. Patients with Peutz-Jegher's syndrome, regardless of family history, should be considered for screening.

   D. BRCA2, PALB2, or P16 mutation carriers with one or more affected first-degree relatives should be screened for pancreatic cancer.

7. You are asked to advise a 45-year-old woman who was recently diagnosed with invasive lobular carcinoma and was found to carry a CDH1 mutation. There is no family history of diffuse gastric cancer, and she is having difficulty with the decision around prophylactic gastrectomy. You share with her the following to assist with these decisions and advice for her 20-year-old son:

   A. Screening for diffuse gastric cancer (GC) with intensive annual endoscopy and gastric biopsies has a high sensitivity and specificity for gastric cancer detection.

   B. Her estimated lifetime risk for the development of gastric cancer is 10%.

   C. Her son does not need to test for the genetic mutation as gastric cancers occur late and he is not at risk for breast cancer.

   D. Patients with hereditary diffuse gastric cancer are often asymptomatic in the early stages and tend to present late with symptoms such as weight loss, abdominal pain, nausea, dysphagia and early satiety.

8. A 26-year-old woman is diagnosed with ER+/PR+/HER2+ invasive ductal carcinoma of the breast and is found to carry a germline TP53 mutation, conferring the diagnosis of Li Fraumeni syndrome (LFS). Neither of her parents carry the mutation and she is concerned about her 5-year-old son. She would also like to have another child. Choose the INCORRECT statement below:

   A. LFS is a rare autosomal dominant syndrome characterized by increased risk for soft tissue sarcomas, osteosarcoma, premeno-pausal breast cancer, central nervous system tumors, adrenocorti-cal carcinoma, and leukemia.

   B. Cancers do not affect the pediatric population—therefore, children need not be tested until the age of 18.

   C. Pre-implantation genetic diagnosis is an option for her for future pregnancies to avoid passing down the mutation to future offspring.

   D. The de novo mutation rate for LFS is between 7% to 20%, explaining the negative tests in her parents.

9. Which of the following syndrome(s) is/are appropriate to offer predictive genetic testing to minors (age <18)?

   A. MUTYH-associated polyposis

   B. Familial adenomatous polyposis, Peutz-Jeghers syndrome, juvenile polyposis syndrome

   C. Hereditary breast ovarian cancer syndrome and Lynch syndrome

   D. Any hereditary cancer syndrome

10. You have a 30-year-old female patient who has tested positive for a germline *CDH1* mutation. At the age of 24 she underwent a prophylactic gastrectomy. Which organ is at the next highest risk for developing a malignancy?

   A. Breasts

   B. Thyroid

   C. Pancreas

   D. Colon

ANSWERS TO REVIEW QUESTIONS

1. ANSWER: E. Any woman with triple-negative breast cancer under the age of 60 should have genetic testing so choice A is incorrect. The three Ashkenazi founder mutations represent the majority of germline mutations in BRCA1 and BRCA2 in the Ashkenzi Jewish population. This patient also meets NCCN criteria for testing for Li Fraumeni syndrome, so the strategy that makes the most sense in her testing is to test first for the Jewish founder mutations, and to reflex to a gene panel test if no mutation is initially identified.

REFERENCES:

Robson M, Dabney MK, Rosenthal G, et al. Prevalence of recurring BRCA mutations among Ashkenazi Jewish women with breast cancer. *Genet Test.* 1997;1:47-51.

Genetic/Familial High-Risk Assessment: Breast and Ovarian. NCCN, 2016. (Accessed October 9, 2016,

Couch FJ, Hart SN, Sharma P, et al. Inherited mutations in 17 breast cancer susceptibility genes among a large triple-negative breast cancer cohort unselected for family history of breast cancer. *J Clin Oncol.* 2015;33:304–311.

Fackenthal JD, Olopade OI. Breast cancer risk associated with BRCA1 and BRCA2 in diverse populations. *Nat Rev Cancer.* 2007;7:937–948.

2. ANSWER: D. Among neoadjuvant regimens, sequential anthracycline-taxane chemotherapy represents a commonly used standard of care, but there is no evidence that BRCA-associated cancers are associated with improved response to this regimen. BRCA-associated cancers do have a greater response to therapies such as poly-(ADP) ribose polymerase inhibitors and platinum agents than sporadic cancers.

REFERENCES:

Byrski T, Huzarski T, Dent R, et al. Pathologic complete response to neoadjuvant cisplatin in BRCA1-positive breast cancer patients. *Breast Cancer Res Treat.* 2014;147:401–405.

Tutt A, Robson M, Garber JE, et al. Oral poly(ADP-ribose) polymerase inhibitor olaparib in patients with BRCA1 or BRCA2 mutations and advanced breast cancer: a proof-of-concept trial. *Lancet.* 2010;376:235–244.

von Minckwitz G, Schneeweiss A, Loibl S, et al. Neoadjuvant carboplatin in patients with triple-negative and HER2-positive early breast cancer (GeparSixto; GBG 66): a randomised phase 2 trial. *Lancet Oncol.* 2014;15:747–756.

3. ANSWER: C. Breast cancer and gastrointestinal tract hamartomatous polyps are among the most common features in women with PTEN-hamartoma tumor syndrome caused by pathogenic variants in PTEN. The majority of patients with this syndrome will have macrocephaly.

REFERENCES:

Genetic/Familial High-Risk Assessment: Breast and Ovarian. NCCN, 2016. (Accessed October 9, 2016,

Heald B, Mester J, Rybicki L, Orloff MS, Burke CA, Eng C. Frequent gastrointestinal polyps and colorectal adenocarcinomas in a prospective series of PTEN mutation carriers. *Gastroenterology*. 2010;139:1927–1933.

Tan MH, Eng C. RE: Cowden syndrome and PTEN hamartoma tumor syndrome: systematic review and revised diagnostic criteria. *J Natl Cancer Inst*. 2014;106:dju130.

4. *ANSWER: C.* This patient has the classic presentation of colon cancer in a family history consistent with Lynch syndrome. Colon cancer associated with Lynch syndrome is typically found in the right colon and, despite the aggressive histologic features, does not metastasize as often as sporadic cases. Lynch syndrome is caused by germline mutations of the MMR genes, including *MSH2*.

REFERENCES:

Giardiello FM, Allen JI, Axilbund JE, et al. Guidelines on genetic evaluation and management of Lynch syndrome: a consensus statement by the US Multi-Society Task Force on colorectal cancer. *Gastroenterology*. 2014;147:502–526.

Evaluation of Genomic Applications in P, Prevention Working G. Recommendations from the EGAPP Working Group: genetic testing strategies in newly diagnosed individuals with colorectal cancer aimed at reducing morbidity and mortality from Lynch syndrome in relatives. *Genet Med*. 2009;11:35–41.

5. *ANSWER: A.* This patient's presentation of a couple hundred colonic adenomas could be due to the diagnosis of familial adenomatous polyposis (FAP, caused by pathogenic *APC* variants) or *MUTYH*-associated polyposis (MAP, caused by pathogenic *MUTYH* variants). Both of these syndromes are associated with upper gastrointestinal tract cancers and increased risk of thyroid carcinoma. However, APC variants are inherited in an autosomal dominant manner, in which case the patient's children would have a 50% chance of inheriting the variant and also having FAP, while MAP follows an autosomal recessive pattern of inheritance, in which case the patient's siblings have a 25% chance of having the syndrome and his children would have a very low risk. Therefore, it is not worth exposing his children to the risk of colonoscopy until genetic testing can help to clarify the diagnosis.

REFERENCES:

NCCN. Genetic/Familial High-Risk Assessment: Colorectal Version 2.2016. 2016.

Sieber OM, Lipton L, Crabtree M, et al. Multiple colorectal adenomas, classic adenomatous polyposis, and germ-line mutations in MYH. *N Engl J Med*. 2003;348:791–799.

Lubbe SJ, Di Bernardo MC, Chandler IP, Houlston RS. Clinical implications of the colorectal cancer risk associated with MUTYH mutation. *J Clin Oncol*. 2009;27:3975–3980.

Sampson JR, Dolwani S, Jones S, et al. Autosomal recessive colorectal adenomatous polyposis due to inherited mutations of MYH. *Lancet*. 2003;362:39–41.

Jenkins MA, Croitoru ME, Monga N, et al. Risk of colorectal cancer in monoallelic and biallelic carriers of MYH mutations: a population-based case-family study. *Cancer Epidemiol Biomarkers Prev*. 2006;15:312–314.

6. *ANSWER: B.* Patients who carry BRCA1 mutations do have a 1-2.8 relative risk for the development of pancreatic cancer, but unless they have a first-degree relative with pancreatic cancer, screening is not recommended. Patients with Peutz-Jegher's syndrome (who generally carry germline STK11 gene mutations) have a very high (132-fold) risk of pancreatic cancer and should undergo screening.

REFERENCES:

- Canto Marcia Irene et al. International Cancer of the Pancreas Screening (CAPS) Consortium summit on the management of patients with increased risk for familial pancreatic cancer. *Gut.* 2013;62:339–347.
- Overbeek Kasper A. et al. Surveillance for neoplasia in the pancreas. *Best Pract Res Clin Gastroenterol.* 2016;30:971–986.

7. ANSWER: D. The lifetime cumulative risk for diffuse GC reaches >80% by age 80 years. The median age at diagnosis is 38 years, with the range varying greatly from 14 to 82 years. Surveillance remains challenging and gastrectomy is recommended between the ages of 18 and 40. Her son would be considered for prophylactic gastrectomy even at his age, and may also choose to consider reproductive assistance to avoid passing the mutation to his offspring.

REFERENCES:

- Tan Ryan and Ngeow Joanne. Hereditary diffuse gastric cancer: What the clinician should know. *World J Gastrointest Oncol.* 2015 September 15;7(9):153–160.
- NCCN Genetic /Familial High Risk Assessment: Breast and Ovarian. *JNCCN.2017;15:9–20*

8. ANSWER: D. Adrenocortical carcinomas occur in the first 5 years of life. CNS tumors are biphasic with the first peak in childhood and the second peak at 20 to 40 years of age. Soft tissue sarcomas occur in the first 5 years, and osteosarcomas and leukemias are common in the pediatric population. Her young child should have testing.

REFERENCE:

- Valdez Jessica et al. Li-Fraumeni syndrome: a paradigm for the understanding of hereditary cancer predisposition. *Br. J. Haematol.* 2017;176(4): 539–552.

9. ANSWER: B. Familial adenomatous polyposis syndrome, Peutz-Jeghers syndrome, and juvenile polyposis syndrome are all conditions that, on average, onset in the teenage years with polyp development. Therefore, a change in medical management would be indicated in the teenage years if the child was found to carry a mutation. It is generally not endorsed by the American Society of Human Genetics or the American College of Medical Genetics to test minors for adult onset hereditary cancer syndrome such as hereditary breast ovarian cancer syndrome, Lynch syndrome, or MUTYH-associated polyposis. There is limited to no medical benefit to test a minor and the potential psychosocial harms to the minor outweigh the benefits (Wilfond BS. Points to consider: ethical, legal, and psychosocial implications of genetic testing in children and adolescents.

REFERENCE:

- American Society of Human Genetics Board of Directors, American College of Medical Genetics Board of Directors. *Am J Hum Genet.* 1995;57:1233–1241.

10. *ANSWER: A.* Women with germline CDH1 mutations have up to a 42% risk of developing breast cancer.

REFERENCE:

(Hansford S, Kaurah P, Li-Chang H, et al. Hereditary Diffuse Gastric Cancer Syndrome: CDH1 Mutations and Beyond. *JAMA oncology* 2015;1:23-32).

Basic Principles of Immuno-Oncology 45

Jason M. Redman, Julius Strauss, and Ravi A. Madan

REVIEW QUESTIONS

1. A 67-year-old gentlemen with prostate cancer returns to your clinic for follow-up. Eight years ago, he underwent definitive radical prostatectomy for moderate risk prostate cancer. All margins and resected lymph nodes were negative. Four years ago he developed biochemically recurrent disease which was observed without treatment until 2 years ago when he developed low-volume metastatic disease seen on CT scans. At that time he was started on androgen deprivation therapy with a marked decrease in his PSA. Follow-up scans since then have shown no further growth in his metastatic disease. However, at his last visit and visit again today you notice that his PSA is again increasing. The gentlemen is asymptomatic. A check of his testosterone level shows that it is <20 ng/ml. You are concerned that he has developed metastatic castration resistant disease and decide to discuss sipuleucel-T with the patient as a possible therapeutic option. When speaking with your patient which statement about sipuleucel-T below would be correct?

    A. Data suggests that patients with higher baseline PSA values benefit more from sipuleucel-T than patients with lower baseline PSA values.

    B. Sipuleucel-T has been shown to provide a PFS benefit but no OS benefit in a phase III clinical trial of men with minimally symptomatic mCRPC.

    C. Sipuleucel-T has been shown to provide an OS benefit but no PFS benefit in a phase III clinical trial of men with minimally symptomatic mCRPC.

    D. PSA values decline by more than 50% in the majority of patients receiving sipuleucel-T

2. A 74-year-old female with metastatic NSCLC returns to your clinic for follow-up. She was a heavy smoker for many years and previous genetic testing has revealed no actionable EGFR, ALK, or ROS1 mutations. She was recently started on nivolumab after having disease progression on cisplatin and alimta. She returns today for her first restaging scan on nivolumab. Her disease looks to be improving with treatment and you estimate about a 20% reduction in her disease. Unfortunately, the patient has noticed a maculopapular rash worsening over the past week, which now covers 20% of her body surface area, is pruritic, and has been limiting her ability to perform routine chores around the house. The rash does not appear urticarial in nature and she denies any other new medications, foods, or lifestyle changes. She has no other symptoms. Assuming this is an immune-mediated rash from nivolumab, what would be the most appropriate next step?

   A. Discontinue nivolumab and start patient on prednisone 1mg/kg or an equivalent steroid dose until disease improves to grade 0 to 1 followed by a steroid taper over at least a month.

   B. Prescribe topical steroids and dose reduce nivolumab from 3mg/kg to 1.5 mg/kg every 2 weeks.

   C. Prescribe topical steroids and continue with treatment without dose reduction.

   D. Prescribe topical steroids and hold the next dose until the rash improves to grade 0-1.

3. A 56-year-old man with metastatic renal cell cancer to the lung comes to your clinic for follow-up. He had previously had progressive disease on sunitinib and was recently started on nivolumab. He returns today for his first restaging scan on nivolumab. His scan shows what appears to be overall stable disease; however, there are ground glass infiltrates throughout his bilateral lung fields. More concerning the patient appears to be tachypnic on exam and using accessory muscles of respiration. He reports worsening dyspnea over the past week and a half with an associated dry cough without any other symptoms of fever or leg swelling. His O_2 sat in the office is 87% but improved to 95% on O_2 2L/min via nasal cannula. You make the decision to admit him to work up the dyspnea. He undergoes a bronchoscopy which is negative for any infectious agents. You are concerned that the patient may have pneumonitis due to nivolumab and

elect to start him on systemic steroids with a plan to taper the steroids over at least a month following improvement in his symptoms to grade 0 to 1. In addition to starting systemic steroids what other action is most appropriate to consider?

A. Start prophylaxis against encapsulated bacteria

B. Start prophylactic antifungals

C. Start prophylactic antibiotics against PCP

D. Start prophylaxis against VZV

4. A 63-year-old female with locally advanced melanoma returns to your clinic for follow-up. She had noticed an enlarging irregularly shaped hyperpigmented lesion on her left shin over the past three months. Exam by her dermatologist was suspicious for melanoma without any clinically palpable lymph nodes. She underwent an excisional biopsy, which confirmed the diagnosis of melanoma and showed a thickness of 1.75 mm. She went on to complete wide local excision of the lesion as well as a sentinel lymph node biopsy. Pathology showed good margins around the lesion (>2cm), but unfortunately sentinel lymph node biopsy was positive. A PET scan showed no evidence of metastases. Two weeks ago she completed lymphadenectomy, which returned with one positive node bearing 0.5 mm of tumor involvement. She now comes to you to discuss adjuvant therapy for her stage III melanoma, which has been completely resected. When speaking with her, which of the below statements about adjuvant therapy would be correct?

A. Both interferon alpha 2b and ipilimumab are FDA-approved options for her as adjuvant therapy

B. Nivolumab is an FDA-approved option for her as adjuvant therapy

C. Interferon alpha 2b is the only FDA-approved option for her as adjuvant therapy

D. Aldesleukin (IL-2) is the only FDA-approved option for her as adjuvant therapy

5. A 55-year-old male with metastatic colorectal cancer is referred to your clinic to be evaluated for a clinical trial. He has previously been treated with and progressed through FOLFOX, FOLFIRI with bevacizumab, trifluridine and tipiracil, and regorafenib. He has not received anti-EGFR

therapy as previous testing has shown a KRAS mutation in codon 12. Prior testing of mismatch repair protein expression showed positive expression of MLH1, MSH6, and PMS2 and negative expression of MSH2. Just prior to seeing you he had Foundation One gene testing done, which showed mutations in P53, KRAS, and PIK3CA. Which of the following results suggests that this patient may respond to immune checkpoint inhibitors?

   A. Presence of KRAS mutation in codon 12

   B. Positive MLH1 expression

   C. Negative MSH2 expression

   D. Presence of PIK3CA mutation

6. A 72-year-old female with metastatic nonsquamous NSCLC returns to your office for follow-up. She previously received cisplatin/pemetrexed with stable disease and has been on pemetrexed maintenance the past few months. On review of her scans today you notice progressive disease. You discuss the scans with her as well as potential second-line therapies. She is particularly interested in possible immune checkpoint therapies as a next step. In discussing these therapies with her which of the following statements are true?

   A. Atezolizumab is FDA-approved for second-line treatment of metastatic NSCLC if there is positive PD-L1 expression on tumor biopsy.

   B. Nivolumab is FDA-approved for second-line treatment of metastatic NSCLC if there is positive PD-L1 expression on tumor biopsy.

   C. Pembrolizumab is FDA-approved for second-line treatment of metastatic NSCLC if there is positive PD-L1 expression on tumor biopsy.

   D. Avelumab is FDA-approved for second-line treatment of metastatic NSCLC if there is positive PD-L1 expression on tumor biopsy.

7. A 42-year-old female with metastatic melanoma to her lungs returns to your clinic for follow-up. Genetic testing has shown her disease to be BRAF V600 wild type. She was recently started on nivolumab, which she has tolerated well aside from a grade 1 rash. On review of CT scan today

you notice that the three lesions in her lung are about 30% to 40% bigger than when she started treatment some weeks ago. She is feeling well and denies pain, cough, or shortness of breath. You are not sure whether these finding represent pseudoprogression or true progression. In your discussion with your patient, which of the following statements about pseudoprogression would be most accurate?

A. Pseduoprogression occurs in the majority of patients being treated with immune checkpoint inhibitors.

B. Pseudoprogression occurs commonly (20% to 50%) among patients being treated with immune checkpoint inhibitors.

C. Pseudoprogression occurs in 10% to 20% of patients being treated with immune checkpoint inhibitors.

D. Pseudoprogression occurs rarely (<10%) among patients being treated with immune checkpoint inhibitors.

8. A 69-year-old man with metastatic head and neck cancer to the lungs returns to your clinic for follow-up. He has a long history of smoking and his tumor stained negative for P16. He recently progressed on cetuximab, 5-FU, platinum combination therapy. Since then he had been on pembrolizumab 200 mg every 3 weeks. Initial restaging scans after 9 weeks on pembrolizumab showed stable disease. During your discussion with the patient he asks you if it is still possible for him to get see a response to treatment and if he can and does get a response, how long is that response expected to last. Which of the following statements would most accurately answer his questions?

A. The median response time to pembrolizumab is 2 months but patients may respond more than a year after starting treatment. The median duration of response is greater than a year.

B. The median response time to pembrolizumab is 2 months but patients may respond more than a year after starting treatment. The median duration of response is 8 months.

C. Nearly all patients who will have responses to pembrolizumab will have had responses by 2 months. The median duration of response is greater than a year.

D. Nearly all patients who will have responses to pembrolizumab will have had responses by 2 months. The median duration of response is 8 months.

9. A 35-year-old man comes to your clinic for follow-up of his classical Hodgkin's lymphoma. He was originally diagnosed with stage IIIB disease, which was treated with ABVD x 6 cycles resulting in a complete remission. Unfortunately, two years later he was found to have disease recurrence. He received induction chemotherapy with DHAP and underwent an autologous HSCT resulting in another complete remission. Unfortunately, 6 months later he is again diagnosed with disease recurrence. He tells you that he has heard that nivolumab was recently FDA-approved for Hodgkin's lymphoma and asks if it would be appropriate to consider that for him at this point. Which of the following responses is most accurate?

   A. Nivolumab is FDA approved for treatment of Hodgkin's that has relapsed after a single multiagent chemotherapy regimen.

   B. Nivolumab is FDA approved for Hodgkin's lymphoma that has relapsed after autologous HSCT.

   C. Nivolumab is FDA approved for Hodgkin's lymphoma that has relapsed after autologous HSCT and post-transplant brentuximab vedotin.

   D. Nivolumab is FDA approved for Hodgkin's lymphoma that has relapsed either after autologous or allogeneic HSCT.

10. A 70-year-old female with a history of urothelial carcinoma of the bladder returns to your clinic for follow-up. Nine months ago she underwent neo-adjuvant treatment with dose dense MVAC followed radical cystectomy for muscle invasive bladder cancer. Pathology revealed T2bN0 disease. At the time of her surgery there was no evidence of metastatic disease. At her last visit 3 weeks ago she was found to have two new pulmonary nodules largest of which was 2.5 cm in diameter. She recently underwent biopsy of this nodule, which unfortunately was consistent with urothelial carcinoma. She is disappointed with the results of the biopsy but is optimistic about potential immunotherapy as a next step. Which of the following agents is currently FDA approved in this clinical setting?

   A. Ipilimumab

   B. Aldesleukin (IL-2)

   C. Bacillus Calmette-Guérin (BCG)

   D. Atezolizumab

ANSWERS TO REVIEW QUESTIONS

1. ANSWER: C. A phase III trial (IMPACT trial) randomized 512 patients with minimally symptomatic mCRPC to receive sipuleucel-T every 2 weeks for a total of 3 doses, or placebo. Patients receiving sipuleucel-T had a 4.1-month improvement in median OS (25.8 vs. 21.7 months; HR 0.78; 95% CI,0.61 to 0.98; $P = 0.03$). No significant PFS difference was noted and only 2.6% of patients receiving sipuleucel-T were observed to have confirmed PSA declines (>50%). When patients enrolled in the IMPACT trial were separated into quartiles based upon baseline PSA (<22 ng/mL >22 ng/mL to 50.1 ng/mL, >50.1 ng/mL to 134.1 ng/mL, >134.1 ng/mL), those in the lowest PSA quartile benefited the most from sipulecuel-T with a HR of 0.51 (0.31 to 0.85) compared with 0.84 (0.55 to 1.29) for patients in the highest quartile. This translated into a survival benefit of 13 months over the placebo group in the lowest PSA quartile as compared with only 2.8 months for patients in the highest PSA quartile.

REFERENCES:

1. Kantoff PW, Higano CS, Shore ND, et al. Sipuleucel-T immunotherapy for castration-resistant prostate cancer. *N Engl J Med.* 2010;363:411–422.
2. Schellhammer. Lower baseline prostate-specific antigen is associated with a greater OS benefit from sipulecuel-T in the immunotherapy for prostate adenocarcinoma treatment (IMPACT) trial. *Urology.* June 2013.

2. ANSWER: D. This patient is having a moderate grade (grade 2) immune-related adverse drug skin reaction. A grade 1 rash is limited to less than 10% BSA (grade 1). A grade 3 rash covers more than 30% BSA or is associated with local superinfection requiring po antibiotics. Further treatment with nivolumab would likely exacerbate her skin condition and may result in further complications or the need for hospitalization. For moderate (grade 2) immune mediated adverse reactions, the nivolumab package insert and FDA recommended that treatment be held until the side effects have resolved or improved to at least grade 1. Topical steroids would be appropriate here for symptom relief. Systemic oral steroids followed by a steroid taper would likely be excessive here. They are generally reserved for grade 3 to 4 immune-related adverse drug reactions. No recommendation exists to dose reduce nivolumab for adverse drug reactions.

3. ANSWER: C. Prophylactic antibiotics against pneumocystis pneumonia should be administered to patients on long-term immune suppression with steroids. While there are no specific guidelines on what length of steroid treatment warrants PCP prophylaxis, it is reasonable to offer PCP prophylaxis for steroid treatment longer than a month. While these patients may potentially develop fungal infections or zoster if they are on steroids for long enough, the biggest concern would be PCP. There is no role for prophylaxis against encapsulated bacteria. A bronchoscopy to rule out infectious agents as well as lymphangitic spread of disease is an important consideration in cases of presumed pneumonitis.

4. *ANSWER: C.* Both interferon alpha 2b and ipilimumab have FDA approval as adjuvant therapy for melanoma with regional lymph node involvement (stage III) after surgical resection including complete lymphadenectomy. Both agents' approvals are based on phase III trials showing significant improvement in median recurrence free survival versus placebo or observation. However, FDA approval of alpha 2b as adjuvant therapy is limited to patients who have had complete surgical resection, including lymphadenectomy within the past 84 days. While FDA approval of ipilimumab as adjuvant therapy is limited to patients containing regional lymph nodes with more than 1 mm of pathologic tumor involvement. Given our patient was treated with definitive surgery two weeks ago but has only 0.5 mm of pathologic tumor involvement in her regional lymph nodes, the only FDA-approved adjuvant therapy for her would be interferon alpha 2b. Had her lymph node had more than 1mm of tumor involvement, answer A would also have been correct. Neither nivolumab nor aldesleukin are FDA approved as adjuvant therapy for melanoma.

REFERENCES:

1. Eggermont AM, Suciu S, Testori A, et al. Long-term results of the randomized phase III trial EORTC 18991 of adjuvant therapy with pegylated interferon alfa-2b versus observation in resected stage III melanoma. *J Clin Oncol.* 2012 Nov 1;30(31):3810.
2. Eggermont AM, Chiarion-Sileni V, Grob JJ, et al. Adjuvant ipilimumab versus placebo after complete resection of high-risk stage III melanoma (EORTC 18071): a randomised, double-blind, phase 3 trial. *Lancet Oncol.* 2015 May;16(5):522–530.

5. *ANSWER: C.* Mismatch repair (MMR) deficient tumors have been found to have a higher response rate to immune checkpoint inhibition than mismatch repair proficient tumors. IHC testing in a mismatch repair proficient tumor should show positive expression of MLH1, MSH2, MSH6, and PMS2. Negative expression of any of these in a tumor makes the tumor MMR deficient. In a phase II study of pembrolizumab in patients with progressive metastatic carcinoma, 4 of 10 (40%) patients with MMR deficient colorectal cancers had an objective response compared with 0 of 18 (0%) patients with MMR proficient colorectal cancers. In addition, objective responses were observed in 5 of 7 (71%) patients with mismatch repair deficient noncolorectal cancers. MMR deficiency usually results in high microsatellite instability (MSI). Tumors with high MSI status are more likely to respond to immune checkpoint inhibitors than microsatellite stable (MSS) tumors.

REFERENCE:

Le DT, Uram JN, Wang H, et al. PD-1 Blockade in Tumors with Mismatch-Repair Deficiency. *N Engl J Med.* 2015;372:2509–2520.

6. *ANSWER: C.* Atezolizumab, nivolumab and pembrolizumab are all FDA approved for second-line treatment of metastatic NSCLC (squamous and adeno) following previous platinum-based chemotherapy. However, FDA approval of pembrolizumab for metastatic NSCLC is dependent on positive tumor expression of PD-L1 (>1%) using an FDA-approved assay. Nivolumab and atezolizumab are FDA approved for second-line treatment of NSCLC regardless of tumor PD-L1 expression. Currently avelumab is not approved for NSCLC.

7. ANSWER: D. A recent study retrospectively looked at 356 patients with a variety of cancers (i.e., melanoma, lung, breast) receiving immune checkpoint inhibitors and found that only 6% of patients developed pseudo progression by immune related response criteria.

REFERENCE:

Kurra V, Sullivan RJ, Gaino JF, et al. Pseudoprogression in cancer immunotherapy: Rates, time course and patient outcomes. *J Clin Oncol.* 34, 2016 (suppl; abstr 6580).

8. ANSWER: A. In the phase Ib trial that led to FDA approval of pembrolizumab in patients with HNSCC, the median time to response was two months but ranged from two to as many as 17 months. The median duration of response was not reached after a median 12.5 months of follow-up. These timeframes for median time to response and duration of response are consistent in both nivolumab and pembrolizumab and across a variety of tumor types.

REFERENCE:

Mehra R, Seiwert TY, Mahipal A, et al. Efficacy and safety of pembrolizumab in recurrent/metastatic head and neck squamous cell carcinoma (R/M HNSCC): Pooled analyses after long-term follow-up in KEYNOTE-012. *J Clin Oncol.* 34, 2016 (suppl; abstr 6012)

9. ANSWER: C. Nivolumab has received FDA approval for Classical Hodgkin lymphoma that has relapsed or progressed after autologous HSCT and post-transplantation brentuximab vedotin. This approval was based on a small cohort of 23 patients with refractory classical Hodgkin's lymphoma who were treated with pembrolizumab and showed an ORR of 87%, including 17% with a complete response and 70% with a partial response. 78% of the patients had previously received autologous HSCT and 78% of the patients had previously received brentuximab vedotin. Nivolumab should be given with extreme caution after an allogeneic transplant. There have been reported cases of hyperacute GVHD in this setting.

REFERENCE:

Ansell SM, Lesokhin AM, Borrello I, et al. PD-1 blockade with nivolumab in relapsed or refractory Hodgkin's lymphoma. *N Engl J Med.* 2015;372:311–319.

10. ANSWER: D. Atezolizumab, an anti-PD-L1 antibody, has FDA approval for the treatment of patients with locally advanced or metastatic urothelial carcinoma who have progressed following platinum-based chemotherapy or have disease progression within 12 months of neoadjuvant or adjuvant treatment with platinum-based chemotherapy. This approval was based on a phase II study where 316 patients with metastatic urothelial carcinoma who had disease progression on platinum-based chemotherapy were given atezolizumab 1200 mg every 3 weeks. The ORR was 15%, with 91% of responses still ongoing after 24 weeks of follow-up. Currently ipilimumab and aldesleukin are not FDA approved for urothelial carcinoma. BCG is only approved for urothelial carcinoma in situ or as adjuvant therapy for local Ta or T1 nonmuscle invasive urothelial carcinoma after resection with high risk of recurrence.

REFERENCE:

Hoffman-Censits J, Grivas P, Van Der Heijden M, et al. IMvigor 210, a phase II trial of atezolizumab (MPDL3280A) in platinum-treated locally advanced or metastatic urothelial carcinoma (mUC). *J Clin Oncol.* 2016;34(suppl 2S):abstr 355

Anticancer Agents 46

Erin F. Damery and Thomas E. Hughes

REVIEW QUESTIONS

1. **Testing point:** Recognize appropriate counseling points when prescribing lenalidomide for the treatment of multiple myeloma.

   Stem: GA is a 65-year-old post-menopausal female started on lenalidomide and dexamethasone for newly diagnosed multiple myeloma.

   Question: Which of the following is a correct counseling point for the patient regarding her new medication regimen?

   Key and Distractors:

   A. Start taking aspirin 81 to 325 mg daily to prevent venous thrombotic events.

   B. Do not take any proton pump inhibitors or H2 antagonists as they will decrease the absorption of lenalidomide.

   C. Two negative pregnancy tests will be needed prior to her starting therapy.

   D. She can pick up her prescription at her local pharmacy.

2. **Testing point:** Identify pertinent drug interactions with ibrutinib.

   Stem: JJ is a 75-year-old male who has started on ibrutinib for CLL. His medication list includes amlodipine 10 mg daily, metoprolol succinate 50 mg daily, fluticasone nasal spray, pravastatin 20 mg daily, and St. John's Wort for depression.

   Question: What change should be made to the patient's medication list?

Key and Distractors:

Correct answer and distractors, lettered A to D

A. Empirically reduce the dose of amlodipine to 5 mg daily as ibrutinib will inhibit the metabolism of amlodipine.

B. Discontinue St. John's wort and initiate an alternative antidepressant.

C. Add aspirin 325 mg daily for prophylaxis of venous thrombotic events.

D. Reduce the dose of pravastatin due to the risk of muscular toxicity in combination with ibrutinib.

3. **Testing point:** The certified oncologist should be able to identify the correct mutation and drug pairing for lung cancer.

Stem: FR is a 58-year-old male with metastatic NSCLC whose molecular testing returned prior to starting treatment. His tumor is reported as follows: EGFR +, PD-L1 +, ALK -, ROS1 -.

Question: What is an appropriate first-line treatment option for this patient based on his molecular testing?

Key and Distractors:

A. Afatinib

B. Crizotinib

C. Pembrolizumab

D. Ceritinib

4. **Testing point:** Recognition of appropriate interventions for drug-induced pulmonary interstitial lung disease associated with certain agents.

Stem: A 45-year-old patient with pancreatic cancer presents with new onset dyspnea, cough, and fever. He was initiated on erlotinib and gemcitabine 7 months prior to this presentation and his last staging evaluation demonstrated a partial response. A pulmonary CT scan is suggestive for interstitial lung disease. A bronchoscopy is negative for any infectious etiology and biopsies are consistent with interstitial lung disease.

Question: What action should be taken in regards to his erlotinib and gemcitabine therapy?

Key and Distractors:

    A. Discontinue erlotinib and continue gemcitabine.

    B. Discontinue gemcitabine and continue erlotinib.

    C. Discontinue both agents and evaluate for an alternative regimen.

    D. Resume therapy with both agents once symptoms resolve.

5. **Testing point:** Recognition of interventions needed for auto-immune toxicities associated with ipilimumab.

    Stem: A 27-year-old male with stage 3 melanoma is initiated on ipilimumab for adjuvant therapy following resection and lymphadenectomy. He presents 10 months into his adjuvant therapy with severe diarrhea (grade 3) consistent with enterocolitis with a negative workup for infectious disease.

    Question: What action should be taken in regards to his ipilimumab therapy?

Key and Distractors:

    A. Discontinue ipilimumab.

    B. Discontinue ipilimumab and initiate high-dose corticosteroids.

    C. Hold ipilimumab and resume at a 50% dose reduction after resolution of symptoms.

    D. Hold ipilimumab, initiate high-dose coriticosteroids, and then resume ipilimumab therapy at full dose after resolution of symptoms.

6. **Testing point:** Recognize the appropriate premedication or concomitant therapy required for pemetrexed therapy.

    Stem: A 55-year-old female is being evaluated for initiation of pemetrexed and cisplatin for therapy of metastatic nonsmall cell lung cancer.

    Question: What premedication or concomitant therapy should be considered for pemetrexed?

Key and Distractors:

    A. Folic Acid, cyanocobalamin (vitamin B-12), and pyridoxine (vitamin B-6)

    B. Folic Acid, cyanocobalamin (vitamin B-12), and dexamethasone

C. Dexamethasone followed by leucovorin rescue after each pemetrexed dose

D. Cyanocobalamin (vitamin B-12) and leucovorin rescue after each pemetrexed dose

---

7. **Testing point:** Recognition of the toxicity profile of bortezomib as related to the route of administration

   Stem: A patient is going to be initiated on bortezomib therapy for multiple myeloma.

   Question: What toxicity is less likely to occur when bortezomib is administered by subcutaneous injection as compared to intravenous infusion?

Key and Distractors:

A. Myelosuppression

B. Fever, chills, and rigors

C. Orthostatic hypotension

D. Peripheral neuropathy

---

8. **Testing point:** Knowledge of carboplatin dosing methodology.

   Stem: A 35-year-old patient with ovarian cancer is presenting for her first cycle of paclitaxel and carboplatin therapy. The estimated creatinine clearance is calculated at 135 ml/min and the target AUC is 6.

   Question: What should the calculated dose of carboplatin be using the Calvert equation and current FDA guidance?

Key and Distractors:

A. 900 mg

B. 960 mg

C. 810 mg

D. 750 mg

9. **Testing point:** Knowledge of available drug therapies for patients with Chronic Myelogenous Leukemia who have a documented T315I mutation.

   Stem: A 65 year old female with chronic myelogenous leukemia has disease progression after receiving both imatinib and dasatinib. A mutational analysis has revealed that she has a T315I mutation.

   Question: What pharmacologic therapies can be utilized which have shown activity in patients with the T315I mutation?

Key and Distractors:

   A. Nilotinib and Bosutinib

   B. Nilotinib and Ponatinib

   C. Ponatinib and Omacetaxine mepesuccinate

   D. Bosutinib and Omacetaxine mepesuccinate

10. Testing point: Identify the appropriate genotyping or phenotyping for individual antineoplastic agents.

    Stem:

    Question: Genotyping or phenotyping for polymorphisms of the enzyme thiopurine S-methyltransferase (TPMT) can assist in the identification of patients who are homozygous deficient or low or intermediate metabolizers to identify patients who are at greater risk of toxicity of which antimetabolite antineoplastic drugs?

Key and Distractors:

    A. Fludarabine and clofarabine

    B. Fluorouracil and capecitabine

    C. Cytarabine and pentostatin

    D. Mercaptopurine and thioguanine

ANSWERS TO REVIEW QUESTIONS

1. ANSWER: A

Rationale:

It is recommended to start VTE prophylaxis in patients who are taking lenalidomide for the treatment of multiple myeloma. Specifically, patients who have 0 to 1 individual or multiple myeloma risk factors may take aspirin 81 to 325 mg once daily. Patients with at least 2 individual or multiple myeloma risk factors should receive prophylaxis with full-dose warfarin or low-molecular weight heparin (equivalent to enoxaparin 40 mg once daily). Individual risk factors include BMI ≥ 20 kg/m^2, prior VTE, CVAD or pacemaker, chronic renal disease, diabetes, acute infection, immobilization, surgery, use of erythropoietin and blood clotting disorders. Myeloma-related risk factors include multiple myeloma *per se*, and hyperviscosity. Distractors: Lenalidomide has no drug interactions reported with acid suppressing agents. As a postmenopausal female, pregnancy tests will not be required as part of the Revlimid REMS program. Revlimid is dispensed through specialty pharmacies approved by the Revlimid REMS program.

REFERENCES:

Revlimid [package insert]. Summit, NJ: Celgene Corporation; 2017.

National comprehensive Cancer Network. Cancer-Associated Venous Thromboembolic Disease (Version 1.2016). www.nccn.org. Accessed May 15, 2017. Revlimid REMS program website.

2. ANSWER: B

Rationale:

Ibrutinib is a substrate of CYP3A. It is recommended to avoid concomitant use of strong CYP3A inducers such as St. John's Wort, carbamazepine, rifampin and phenytoin while taking ibrutinib. Distractors: A: ibrutinib is not an enzyme inhibitor and should not impact the metabolism of amlodipine; C: ibrutinib is not associated with venous thrombotic events; C: ibrutinib will not impact the metabolism of pravastatin increasing the risk of muscular toxicity.

REFERENCE:

Imbruvica [package insert]. Sunnyvale, CA: Pharmacyclics LLC; 2017.

3. ANSWER: A

Rationale:

Afatinib is approved for first-line use in NSCLC in patients with an EGFR exon 19 deletion or exon 21 substitution. Crizotinib and ceritinib are not indicated since the patient is ALK negative. Patients who are PD-L1 positive and have genetic aberrations should progress on FDA-approved therapies for these mutations prior to treatment with pembrolizumab.

REFERENCES:

Gilotrif [package insert]. Ridgefield, CT: Boehringer Ingelheim Pharmaceuticals, Inc.;2016.

Keytruda [package insert]. Whitehouse Station, NJ: Merck & Co., Inc.; 2017.

4. ANSWER: C

Rationale:

Product labeling for both erlotinib and gemcitabine recommend discontinuation of therapy for new onset or progressive pulmonary symptoms if interstitial lung disease is diagnosed.

REFERENCES:

Tarceva [package insert] San Francisco, CA, Genentech, Inc. 2016

Gemzar [package insert] Indianapolis, IN, Eli Lilly and Company 2017

5. ANSWER: B

Rationale:

Product labeling for ipilimumab recommend permanent discontinuation of therapy and initiation of high-dose corticosteroids for severe enterocolitis.

REFERENCE:

Yervoy [package insert] Princeton, NJ; Bristol-Myers Squibb Company 2017

6. ANSWER: B

Rationale:

Product labeling recommends initiating vitamin supplementation with folic acid and cyanocobalamin prior to initiating pemetrexed and to continue supplementation throughout therapy. Dexamethasone is also recommended to be given the day prior, the day of and the day after pemetrexated therapy to reduce the incidence and severity of cutaneous reactions.

REFERENCE:

Alimta [package insert] Indianapolis, IN, Eli Lilly and Company. 2015

7. ANSWER: D

Rationale:

There is a lower incidence of peripheral neuropathy when bortezomib is administered by subcutaneous injection compared to intravenous infusion. The other toxicities are not commonly seen or have not been shown to be different depending on route of administration.

REFERENCE:

Velcade [package insert] Cambridge, MA, Millenium Pharmaceuticals, Inc. 2017

8. ANSWER: A

Rationale:

The calvert equation would lead to a calculated dose of 900 mg if the creatinine clearance is capped at 125 ml/min which is recommended by the FDA guidance.

Dose (in milligrams) = (Target AUC) x (GFR + 25)

REFERENCES:

Paraplatin [package insert] Princeton, NJ. Bristol-Myers Squibb Inc. 2010
FDA guidance on Carboplatin dosing 2010

9. ANSWER: C

Rationale:

Ponatinib is the only tyrosine kinase inhibitor, which has activity in CML patients with the T315I mutation. Omacetaxine mepesuccinate acts independently of BCR-ABL binding and is approved for CML patients with resistance and/or intolerance to two or more TKI's.

REFERENCES:

Synribo [package insert]. North Wales, PA. Teva Pharmaceuticals 2015.
Iclusig [package insert]. Cambridge, MA. Ariad Pharmaceuticals 2016

10. ANSWER: D

Rationale:

TMPT genotyping or phenotyping would only be helpful for mercaptopurine and thioguanine.

REFERENCES:

Purinethol [package insert]. Sellersville, PA. Gate Pharmaeuticals 2011
Tabloid [package insert]. Research Triangle Park, NC. GlaxoSmithKline 2009